Evidence-Based Research in Ayurveda against COVID-19 in Compliance with Standardized Protocols and Practices

Authored by

Acharya Balkrishna

University of Patanjali and General Secretary at Patanjali Research Foundation Trust
Haridwar
India

Evidence-Based Research in Ayurveda Against COVID-19 in Compliance with Standardized Protocols and Practices

Author: Acharya Balkrishna

ISBN (Online): 978-981-5051-18-6

ISBN (Print): 978-981-5051-19-3

ISBN (Paperback): 978-981-5051-20-9

Bentham Science Publishers Pte. Ltd.
80 Robinson Road #02-00
Singapore 068898
Singapore
Email: subscriptions@benthamscience.net

BENTHAM SCIENCE

Message

Ayurveda is a rich legacy that we as Indians are fortunate to have inherited from our ancestors. However, the lack of proper guidelines has kept this system of medicine less organized and limited its spread for a long time. To streamline such precious knowledge, the Ministry of AYUSH has organized India's traditional systems of medicine under one umbrella with tangible, pragmatic guidelines to align them with other medicinal systems across the globe. Several aspects of this book by Acharya Balkrishna orient Ayurveda in a direction that holds promise to bridge the gap between modern and traditional systems of medicine. This precise effort of bridging the gap is evident from the meticulous scientific affirmation generated by Patanjali Research Institute, in support of Ayurvedic remedy for COVID-19. This excellent compendium of preclinical and clinical data has the potential to serve as a general guide for developing Ayurvedic formulations into modern forms of medications.

Prof. (Dr.) Sunil Kumar Joshi,

Vice-Chancellor,

Uttarakhand Ayurved University,

Haridwar, Uttarakhand, India

CONTENTS

FOREWORD

The COVID-19 pandemic has emerged as a global health emergency of international concern since its first identification, resulting in millions of deaths and economic disruption. The healthcare systems across the globe are at the hilt and being tested for effective management against COVID-19. Employing our ancient traditional system and integrative approach, our nation has dealt with this bolstering virus competently, which is evident from the significantly low mortality rates in India. Param Pujya Acharya Ji, with his sheer dedication, astute guidance, pragmatic approach, and deep knowledge of the ancient Indian traditional system of medicine, has written a new success story by developing an effective medicine against COVID-19.

Patanjali Research Institute, Haridwar, Uttarakhand, is a lineage representative of ancient Indian Vedic and sage traditions. A team of dedicated scientists at Patanjali Research Institute has worked relentlessly to develop Ayurvedic formulations into effective medicine by screening close to 1500 phytochemicals from more than 200 medicinal plants. This was a path-finding journey with experiences shared in this book titled **"Ayurveda against COVID-19"**. We hope that this body of work will serve as a capstone of guidance to develop a new series of Ayurvedic formulations into medicines that would be acceptable to the modern medical and scientific fraternity worldwide.

By sharing our research through this book, we wish to reach a greater and wider readership and, in the process, hope to materialize our humble efforts towards ensuring the well-being of humankind worldwide.

May this excellence of scientific practice in Ayurveda find its due destination!

Swami Ramdev

President and Co-founder
Patanjali Yogpeeth
Haridwar, Uttarakhand
India

PREFACE

The year 2020 has posed a grave challenge for humankind in the form of a new coronavirus, SARS-CoV-2. The outbreaks witnessed by the world back in 2002 and 2012 due to SARS and MERS, respectively, now appear to be insignificant in front of the current pandemic. The virus was officially named coronavirus disease 2019 (COVID-19) by WHO in March 2020, after due diligence of the first case being reported in Wuhan, Province of China. This pandemic has divided the current age into two eras: pre-COVID-19 and post-COVID-19, in every respect, some of which are obvious immediately, like, healthcare and finance, while others, like education and politics, are yet to be revealed. All these changes are primarily adaptive, and yet we are still not well-adapted to this selection pressure. The world as one entity has stood up in solidarity to face this challenge in all spheres of life, healthcare, and medicine being at the forefront. While on field, it is the medical personnel who are relentlessly fighting an apparently never-ending battle against COVID-19. In the laboratories, it is the scientists putting their heart and soul to find a solution to end this battle that is draining humankind both physically and emotionally.

We still do not have a cure for COVID-19 despite the fact that the etiology and pathology of this disease have been thoroughly worked out. Modern medicine is grappling to cope with the current situation with no specific treatment against COVID-19. Our hopes for the re-purposed modern medicines fell flat with unfavorable outcomes of clinical trials conducted involving them. So, after a transient flash of hope for a potential cure for COVID-19, we are apparently, still in the darkness as at the beginning of this year. Alternative medicines are coming up with promising reports but establishing a medicine from an alternative system is difficult with no standard operating protocols to do so in place.

The ancient Indian medicinal system, Ayurveda, is at the core of the working mandate of Patanjali Research Institute (PRI), governed by Patanjali Research Foundation Trust (PRFT), Haridwar, India. PRFT has been following the rapid evolution of COVID-19 very closely right from the day when the first case was reported. Probably, that is the reason, today, PRFT can confidently declare that it has found a way to fight COVID-19, although the solution is only recognized as an immunity booster, preliminary and interim outcomes from surveys, observational clinical studies, and completed and continuing clinical trials speak more favorably towards this solution being a cure rather than a mere prophylactic in the form of an immunity booster. This book is a chronicle of this journey of PRFT from fields (medicinal herbs) to clinics (medicines being used in clinical trials) via research laboratories at Patanjali Research Institute (PRI) for developing solutions for COVID-19. Additionally, this work is also expected to be a capstone to guide how one can develop traditional medicines into forms acceptable by modern medical practitioners worldwide.

PRFT has been actively involved in finding a cure for COVID-19 since WHO expressed its concern last January, even before declaring this to be an outbreak. In fact, computational studies from PRFT after coming into the public domain as pre-prints triggered several groups to take up similar studies that have now resulted in a huge database of phytochemicals with predicted antiviral potentials against SARS-CoV-2. Even before this, revered Swami Ramdev Ji recommended the use of decoctions of herbs (which were later used in these medicines) as a home remedy for protection against COVID-19. These recommendations were based on Ayurvedic medicines prescribed for ailments with corresponding etiologies. So, it is evident that what we have offered humankind in the form of a Coronil kit is the outcome of our deep-rooted traditional scientific knowledge. We believe that this piece of work would be like a beacon to whosoever wishes to develop our ancient Ayurvedic prescriptions into a form acceptable to the practitioners of modern medicine.

CONSENT FOR PUBLICATION

Not applicable.

CONFLICT OF INTEREST

The author declares no conflict of interest, financial or otherwise.

ACKNOWLEDGEMENT

Declared none.

Acharya Balkrishna
The University of Patanjali and
General Secretary at Patanjali Research
Foundation Trust
Haridwar
India

CHAPTER 1

Virtual Screening and Computational Study

Abstract: This chapter discusses the virtual screening of phytochemicals and computational validation of identified ones as potential antiviral agents against the SARS-CoV-2 virus. In addition, we have provided an outline of how to conduct virtual screening and computer validation to identify potential lead compounds for further studies, including their formulation, chemical characterization, validation, and licensing, which have been addressed in the next chapter.

Keywords: ACE 2, Molecular docking, Molecular dynamic simulation, RBD, SARS-CoV-2, Scutellarein, Tinocordiside, Withanone.

1.1. SARS-COV-2 OUTBREAK AND HELPLESSNESS OF MANKIND

On 8th December 2019, a pneumonia case of unknown cause was reported in Wuhan, province of China, and hence, started the COVID-19 nightmare (Lu *et al.*, 2020). By the first week of January 2020, a new strain of coronavirus was identified by the Chinese Centre for Disease Control and Prevention (CCDCP), which was never associated with humans earlier (Kruse, 2020; Zhu *et al.*, 2020). Soon after, on 10th January 2020, the World Health Organization (WHO) acknowledged this report and tentatively referred to the novel coronavirus as 2019-nCoV. Within just three days, the first case of the new disease was reported in Thailand. The disease started spreading like wildfire, and by the end of the month, on 30th January 2020, WHO recognized it as a Public Health Emergency of International Concern and, on 11th March 2020, exactly one month after naming the disease as COVID-19, WHO declared it as a pandemic. With its anniversary just shy of a month, the COVID-19 situation, if anything, has become more rampaging.

The opening remarks of Dr. Tedros Adhanom Ghebreyesus, the current Director-General of WHO, in a media briefing on COVID-19 on 26th October 2020, are far from putting our minds at ease. According to him, the third week of October 2020 witnessed the highest number of COVID-19 cases worldwide. Several countries in the Northern Hemisphere are experiencing a concerning rise in the active COVID-

Acharya Balkrishna

19 cases that require hospitalizations, filling up the intensive care units to the capacity in some places (WHO, 2020). Initial ripples created in the global economic matrix due to preventive shutdown measures against COVID-19 have now multiplied to a colossal magnitude. The pandemic has plunged the global economy into a severe contraction. The World Bank has forecasted a 5.2% shrinkage in the global economy this year, making it the deepest recession since the Second World War (The World Bank, 2020). Another lockdown would, for sure, swallow the world economy in a never-to-be-recovered abyss. The magnitude of this shock keeps mounting with the continued lack of a specific cure for COVID-19.

1.2. MOLECULAR ETIOLOGY OF COVID-19

SARS-CoV-2 is recognized as a member of the sister clade of the prototype human and bat Severe Acute Respiratory Syndrome Coronaviruses (SARS-CoVs) (Gorbalenya *et al.*, 2020). Coronaviruses are zoonotic pathogens that can transmit from animals to humans. They are large positive-stranded RNA viruses, with host specificity among avian and mammalian species and are responsible for ailments of the central nervous system, upper and lower respiratory and gastrointestinal tracts (Huynh *et al.*, 2012; Yu *et al.*, 2015; Salata *et al.*, 2019; Gralinski and Menachery, 2020). There are seven coronaviruses identified so far, out of which, OC43, 229E, HKU1, and NL63 are mild ones, whereas SARS-CoV, MERS-CoV, and SARS-CoV-2 are extremely virulent in humans. SARS-CoV and MERS-CoV appeared in 2002 in China, causing Severe Acute Respiratory Syndrome, and in 2012 in Saudi Arabia, causing Middle East Respiratory Syndrome, respectively (Ksiazek, 2003; Stadler *et al.*, 2003; Zaki *et al.*, 2012; Zeng *et al.*, 2018). The epidemiological and clinical knowledge base of COVID-19, although building up fast, still falls behind the swift evolution found in the virus (Huang *et al.*, 2020s; Hui *et al.*, 2020). Therefore, the whole world is left with the only option of employing stringencies, like social distancing and lockdowns, to face this challenge until a cure or a vaccine against it is developed. The present COVID-19 pandemic has put us in a war-like situation, requiring strategic planning in all areas. Developing treatments, identifying cures, and formulating intervention strategies to fight back the COVID-19 outbreak has become our most important concern. Fortunately, studies, by now, have confirmed the molecular pathway of COVID-19 virulence that involves ACE-2, AT1, and TMPRSS2. Many studies have been reported, and several others are ongoing to find a cure using these target molecules.

Coronaviruses enter the target animal cells by binding to cell-surface-associated receptors. During viral infection, entry of the virus into the host cell is a critical step that can be exploited for antiviral therapy (Bupp and Roth, 2005). So, entry inhibition by targeting viral receptor binding through neutralizing antibodies (NABs) is an obvious option that works well in most cases. There are also certain small molecules (like RFI-641 and VP-14637) that inhibit the entry of several viruses, including respiratory syncytial virus (Razinkov, *et al.*, 2001; Douglas, *et al.*, 2003). SARS-CoV entry into the host cell is mediated by the Receptor-Binding Domain (RBD) of its spike glycoprotein (S-protein). S-protein binds to the host cell receptor Angiotensin-Converting Enzyme-2 (ACE-2) (Prabakaran, *et al.*, 2006; Adedeji, *et al.*, 2013). The coronavirus S-protein is a structural protein conferring the crown-like morphology to the virus particles. It is ~1200 aa long, belongs to Class-I viral fusion proteins, and contributes to the cell receptor binding, tissue tropism, and pathogenesis (Millet and Whittaker, 2015). It contains several conserved domains and motifs, and the trimetric S-protein is processed at the S1/S2 cleavage site by host cell proteases. The protein is cleaved (or primed) at a conserved sequence AYT↓M (located 10 aa downstream of SLLR-ST) into an N-terminal S1-ectodomain that recognizes a cognate cell surface receptor and a C-terminal S2membrane-anchored protein involved in viral entry (Bosch, Bartelink and Rottier, 2008; Matsuyama *et al.*, 2010; Millet and Whittaker, 2015). The SARS-CoV S1-protein contains a conserved RBD, which recognizes the host ACE-2. The interacting interface of RBD of S1 and ACE-2 implicates 14 aa in the S1 of SARS-CoV (Li *et al.*, 2005). Among them, 8 residues are strictly conserved in SARS-CoV-2 S protein, supporting the observations that SARS-CoV-2 uses the SARS-CoV receptor ACE-2 for entry and the serine protease TMPRSS2 for S protein priming (Lan *et al.*, 2020; Wan *et al.*, 2020). The receptor-binding domain (RBD) of viral coat spike (S) protein binds to transmembrane ACE-2. Viral coat fuses with host cell membrane only after the viral coat S protein gets primed, that is, cleaved at S1/S2 and the S2' sites by host cellular serine protease, TMPRSS2 (Hoffmann *et al.*, 2020). The RBD of SARS-CoV-2 S protein differs largely from the SARS-CoV at the C-terminus, but the difference does not affect its capability to engage the ACE-2 receptor (Tian *et al.*, 2020). Therefore, RBD has been an attractive target for researchers to abrogate coronavirus infection. Reports suggested that certain human antibodies recognized RBD on the S1 domain of SARS-CoV and inhibited the viral infection by blocking its attachment to ACE-2 (Anand *et al.*, 2003; Dau and Holodniy, 2009). Consequently, three possible mechanisms, namely, targeting ACE-2 receptor, RBD of S protein, and the interaction between ACE-2 and RBD are proposed, which are schematically depicted in Fig. **(1.1)**, through which SARS-CoV-2 entry/infusion can be abrogated.

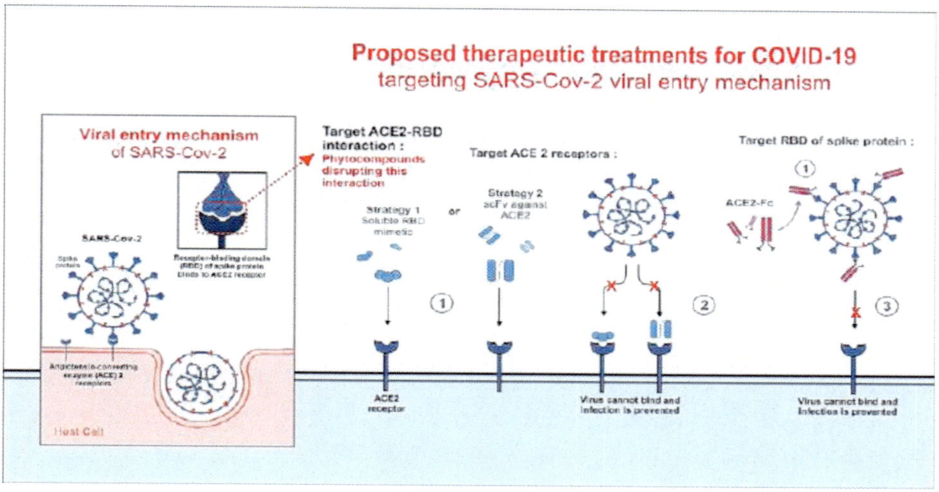

Fig. (1.1). The proposed mechanisms to block the entry of SARS-CoV-2 into host cells. The mechanism behind SARS-CoV-2 entry into the host cell is provided. Three proposed models are depicted where COVID-19 infection can be abrogated by blocking the interaction of RBD of the spike (S) protein and ACE-2. In one of the approaches, ACE-2-RBD interaction can be destabilized by small molecules. In the second approach, ACE-2 can be blocked with RBD mimetics or single-chain antibody fragment (scFv) against ACE-2. In yet another approach, RBD of SARS-CoV-2 S protein can be blocked using the ACE-2 extracellular domain. An Fc domain fused to ACE-2 would facilitate prolonged circulation of the biologic (ACE-2-Fc). The observations made in this study support the strategy to block or weaken the interaction between RBD and ACE-2 by using phytocompounds of natural origin. *[Courtesy:* (Balkrishna, Pokhrel, *et al.*, 2021)*; Under CCBY License].*

1.3. FINDING THE CURE: HOPE *VERSUS* REALITY

ACE 2 is one of the crucial factors of the renin-angiotensin system (RAS), which is a major physiological regulator of body fluid volume, electrolyte balance, and arterial pressure. Renin converts angiotensinogen to angiotensin I (Ang I). Angiotensin-converting enzyme1 (ACE 1) then converts ANG I to ANG II. ANG II manifests its biological actions through angiotensin type 1 (AT1) and type 2 (AT2) receptors. The main role of ACE-2 is the degradation of Ang II, resulting in the formation of angiotensin 1–7 (Ang 1–7), which opposes the actions of Ang II. Thus, ACE-2/angiotensin 1-7 axis is another arm of RAS, which generally shows the opposite effect to the ACE 1/angiotensin II axis. While ANG II can induce strong vasoconstriction, pro-inflammatory effects, and pro-fibrotic effects, Ang 1-7 exhibits antiproliferative, antiapoptotic, and mild vasodilating abilities. These result in several cardiovascular protective effects, including antithrombosis, antimyocardial hypertrophy, antifibrosis, antiarrhythmic, and antiatherogenic, along with preventing heart failure and attenuating vascular dysfunction related to metabolic syndrome. The disruption of the subtle balance between ACE 1 and ACE-2 can lead to the dysregulation of blood pressure. ACE-2 is widely expressed in cardiomyocytes, cardiac fibroblasts, and coronary endothelial cells, which are also a regulator of heart function. Studies have found that overexpression of ACE-2 can prevent or even reverse the heart failure phenotype, whereas loss of ACE-2 can accelerate the progression of heart failure (Guo, *et al.*, 2020). ACE-2 is substantially increased in type 1 and type 2 diabetes patients who are treated with Angiotensin-converting enzyme inhibitors (ACEIs) and angiotensin receptor blockers (ARBs, acting on AT1) (Wan *et al.*, 2020). Similarly, hypertension is also treated with ACEIs and ARBs, which results in an upregulation of ACE-2 (Li, Zhang, and Zhuo, 2017). These findings confirmed the earlier observation that blocking either Ang II synthesis or activity-induced increases in cardiac ACE-2 gene expression (Ferrario, *et al.*, 2005). Higher ACE-2 expression might lead to a higher risk of SARS-CoV-2 infection (Guo *et al.*, 2020). A study by Ali et al., 2013, showed that chronic AT2 receptor activation increased renal ACE-2 activity and attenuated AT1 receptor functions (Ali, Wu, and Hussain, 2013). Abundant expression of ACE-2 in a population of alveolar cells expressing AT2 explained the severe alveolar damage after infection. Moreover, when AT1 and AT2 are activated, they lead to the increased expression of pro-inflammatory mediators, such as interleukin-8/Cytokine-induced Neutrophil Chemoattractant-3 and interleukin-6, triggering an inflammatory process in the lungs and other organs (Cava, Bertoli and Castiglioni, 2020). Some clinicians suspect the driving force in many terminally ill patients' downhill trajectories is a disastrous overreaction of the immune system known as a "cytokine storm"; in this regard, interleukin-1β (IL-1β) and interleukin 6 (IL-6) play a major role. Reduced innate antiviral defenses coupled with exuberant inflammatory cytokine production are the defining and driving feature of COVID-19.

While, initially, COVID- 19 was thought to be affecting the human respiratory system, accumulating evidence shows that this infection can reach beyond the lungs. It can invade and rampage almost all the organs in the body. The "cytokine storm" is believed to be the reason behind this.

The use of ACEIs/ARBs might be a double-edged sword in COVID-19. On the one hand, it might reduce the severity of lung damage caused by the infection, while on the other, it can lead to an increased risk of SARS-CoV-2 infection. Besides, patients with COVID-19 also showed potential cardiac injuries and RAS activation. SARS-CoV-2 infection possibly influences the balance between angiotensin II and angiotensin 1-7, whereas ACEIs/ ARBs can block the RAS and protect the heart and other organs, which are susceptible to injury caused by the RAS activation (Guo *et al.*, 2020). TMPRSS2 mediated cleavage of membrane-bound ACE-2 augmented cellular uptake of SARS-CoV, and this over-expression of TMPRSS2 facilitated cellular uptake of soluble SARS-CoV (Heurich *et al.*, 2014). Therefore, from the above review of literature on ACE-2 and TMPRSS2, we can conclude that upregulation of ACE-2 can increase chances of viral entry, blocking AT1 receptor can upregulate ACE-2, AT2 receptor can affect ACE-2 differently from AT1 receptor, over-expression of TMPRSS2 will facilitate viral uptake by the cells, and IL-6 is over-expressed in response to COVID-19 infection. As evident, serious anticipated drawbacks and unforeseen side-effects co-exist with the investigable available treatment options holding potential against COVID-19 infection.

Early this year (February 2020), a WHO COVID-19 research forum recommended a large randomized clinical trial for four re-purposed antiviral drugs that were hoped to have at least a moderating effect on the rate of mortality. These four drugs were Remdesivir, Hydroxychloroquine, Lopanivir-Ritonavir combination, and Interferon- beta 1a. The registered WHO Solidarity Trial (ISRCTN83971151, NCT04315948) began in March. It involved 11266 patients across 405 hospitals in 30 countries. Two thousand seven hundred fifty patients were given Remdesivir, 954 received Hydroxychloroquine, 1411 Lopinavir, 651 Interferon plus Lopinavir, 1412 only Interferon, and 4088 received no study drug. Eligible patients were 18 years or more of age and hospitalized with a diagnosis of COVID-19, not known to have received any of the study drugs with no contraindication to them either. The primary end-point, *i.e.*, the main aim of the study, was to assess the effects of the study drugs on the mortality of hospitalized patients. As a secondary objective of the study, the effects of the drugs on the initiation of ventilation and hospitalization durations were also monitored. The protocol was approved by the local and WHO ethics committee as compliant with Helsinki Declaration and Good Clinical Practice principles, and national trial regulations. The study was an open-label, randomized one, in which the inpatients were randomized equally between whichever drug was locally available, and the control subjects, healthcare providers, and the patients were aware of the drug being administered. The daily doses used were the ones already recommended for other diseases. This trial was adaptive, which means it allowed the removal of drugs showing no promise. Hydroxychloroquine and Lopanivir were discontinued for futility on June 18th and July 4th, 2020, respectively. None of the four study drugs reduced mortality, initiation of ventilation, or hospitalization duration. This is from an interim report of the WHO Solidarity Trial, unfortunately, showing enough evidence to move away from these four drugs in the treatment of SARS-CoV-2. This report was enough to crush the high hopes that were held for these drugs as promising treatment options for the SARS-CoV-2 infection. With this unfortunate turn of events, we needed to take a fresh look at the challenge at hand. We need to open our minds and be receptive to alternative options existing in traditional medicines systems (WHO Solidarity Trial Consortium, 2020). The reason for disease severity is not what matters anymore now. The hope of identifying a cure soon enough is what everybody is holding on to.

1.4. THE WAY FORWARD: AYURVEDA AGAINST COVID-19

Needless to mention that COVID-19 has sent the world into a medical crisis, one which, if not contained or prevented, might take a serious toll on the economy of India and the world alike. Despite herculean efforts by the government of India, the rapid spread of COVID-19 infection calls for an imminent need for realizing treatment and intervention options to stop the crisis from spiralling out of control.

Undeniably, modern medical science faces a very difficult challenge in the form of SARS-CoV-2. COVID-19 infection affects individuals with weak immunity more severely. Therefore, enhancing immunity is definitely one of the ways doctors across the globe have been using for treating COVID-19 cases. High doses of vitamin C, known to boost immunity, have been administered to COVID-19 patients in China and elsewhere in the world with promising results, reminding us of Benjamin Franklin's words, "An ounce of prevention is worth a pound of cure."

As Hippocrates said, "He will manage the cure best who has foreseen what is to happen from the present state of matters." So, our battle against COVID-19 started even before the World Health Organization (WHO) recognized this highly infectious new influenza-like disease caused by SARS-CoV-2 coronavirus to be a pandemic in March early this year. We engaged in rigorous bioprospecting with the help of *in silico* tools to identify medicinal herbs based on their constituent phytocompounds, which could potentially jeopardize the host-viral interactions, attenuate viral propagation within the host cell and hinder viral packaging. The rationale behind these efforts was in the existing knowledge of Ayurveda, one of the world-renowned forms of Indian traditional medicine that mentions several immunity-boosting therapeutics.

To combat the COVID-19 virus with Ayurveda, we have screened close to 1000 phytochemicals from more than 100 medicinal plants, *in-silico* and still counting. We looked for their binding affinities to COVID-19 essential proteins and host protein interactions. We have discovered that natural phytochemicals in Ashwagandha, Giloy, and Tulsi indeed have the potential to combat COVID-19 and its pathogenicity. The major phytochemicals that we found to be potentially effective against SARS-CoV-2 entry into host cells are withanone and tinocordiside, present in Ashwagandha (*Withania somnifera*) and Giloy (*Tinospora cordifolia*), respectively (Balkrishna, Pokhrel, and Varshney, 2020; Balkrishna, Pokhrel, *et al.*, 2021). Similarly, Scutellarein, present in Tulsi

(*Ocimum sanctum*), was found to be a potent inhibitor of SARS-CoV-2 RNA-dependent RNA polymerase (RDRP) (unpublished data). We recognized the urgent requirement for immunity boosters and recommended Ashwagandha (*W. somnifera*), Giloy (*T. cordifolia*), and Tulsi (*O. sanctum*) as the immunity-boosting herbs, with potential against new coronavirus infection.

1.4.1. Scientific Rationale Behind Pure Extract of Ashwagandha (*W. somnifera)* as Anti- SARS-CoV-2 Agent

W. somnifera or Ashwagandha is a well-known medicinal plant used in traditional medicines for more than 3,000 years. This plant extract and its bioactive compounds are used in the prevention and treatment of many diseases, such as arthritis, impotence, amnesia, anxiety, cancer, neurodegenerative and cardiovascular diseases, and others.

1.4.1.1. Pharmacological Perspective of Using Ashwagandha

Immunomodulatory Activities: Immunomodulatory potential of Ashwagandha was tested in experimental azoxymethane-induced colon cancer in mice. Animals were treated with 400 mg/kg of *W. somnifera* extract once a week for four weeks orally. *W. somnifera* significantly altered the level of leucocytes, lymphocytes, neutrophils, immune complexes, and immunoglobulins (Ig) A, G, and M. Furthermore, the root extract of *W. somnifera* was also tested for immunomodulatory effects in three myelosuppression models in mice: cyclophosphamide, azathioprine or prednisolone. A significant increase in haemoglobin concentration, red blood cell count, white blood cell count, platelet count, and body weight was observed in WS-treated mice compared to untreated control mice. The effect of *W. somnifera* was also studied on the function of mouse macrophages obtained from mice treated with the carcinogen ochratoxin A (OTA), and it significantly decreased the chemotactic activity of the macrophages and associated Interleukin-1 (IL-1) and tumour necrosis factor-alpha (TNF-α) production (Mishra, Singh and Dagenais, 2000). The immunomodulatory effect of *W. somnifera* was also assessed in IgE-mediated anaphylaxis, observed as a reduction of ovalbumin-induced paw oedema in animals treated with its extract at doses of 150 and 300 mg/kg. The results were compared with the standard drug disodium cromoglycate. Cyclophosphamide-induced immunosuppression was counteracted by treatment with *W. somnifera*, revealing a significant increase in hemagglutinating antibody responses and hemolytic antibody responses towards sheep red blood cells (Agarwal *et al.*, 1999).

***Pulmonary Hypertension** (PH):* The effect of *W. somnifera* root powder on monocrotaline (MCT)-induced PH in rats has been studied. Preventive treatment with 50 and 100 mg/kg *W. somnifera* significantly reduced the Right Ventricular Systolic Pressure (RVSP) and all markers of Right Ventricular Hypertrophy (RVH) in MCT-challenged rats. There was an improvement in inflammation, oxidative stress and endothelial dysfunction, and attenuation of proliferative markers and apoptotic resistance in lungs (Kaur *et al.*, 2015).

***Chronic Obstructive Pulmonary Disease** (COPD):* Ashwagandha has been given to patients with COPD due to its rejuvenating and strengthening effects. It has been shown to reduce tiredness, frequency of breathing trouble, and cough attacks (Singh, 2015).

***Pulmonary Fibrosis** (PF):* The potential of one of the many bioactive metabolites in Ashwagandha, Withaferin A, to target pulmonary fibrosis (PF) has been tested in EMT and fibrotic events induced by TGF-β1 in alveolar epithelial cells and human fetal lung fibroblasts. Treatment with Withaferin A reduced the progression of PF by modulating the EMT-related cell markers (Kaur, *et al.*, 2015) both *in vivo* and *in vitro*. Withaferin A ameliorated the expression of inflammatory cytokines as well as attenuated the expression of pro-fibrotic proteins. Expression of angiogenic factors was also inhibited by Withaferin A. Collectively, Withaferin A could probably prove as an efficient and potential therapeutic against PF (Bale *et al.*, 2018).

Toxicological Studies: Toxicological aspects of *W. somnifera* were evaluated to check whether it induced any negative impact on the human body. The liver, spleen, lungs, kidneys, thymus, adrenals, and stomach were examined histopathologically and were all found to be normal after treatment with an estimated dose of 200 mg/kg/day for four weeks in rats (Kulkarni and Dhir, 2008), suggesting a rather safe profile of Ashwagandha extracts.

1.4.1.2. Computational Evidence for W. somnifera as Anti-SARS-CoV-2 Agent

SARS-CoV-2 engages the host cell ACE-2 through its spike (S) protein receptor-binding domain (RBD). We have shown that the natural phytochemical from *W. somnifera*, withanone, has distinct effects on viral RBD and host ACE-2 receptor complex. It was found that withanone docked very well in the binding interface of the ACE 2-RBD complex. It was found to move slightly towards the interface centre on 50 nanoseconds molecular dynamic simulation and abolished interacting salt bridges (Fig. **1.2**) (Balkrishna, Pokhrel, *et al.*, 2021).

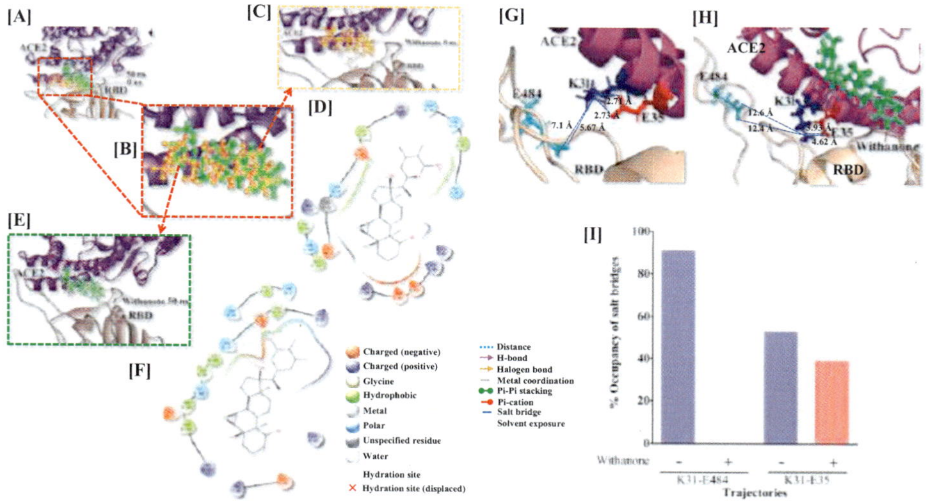

Fig. (1.2). Withanone docks at the interface of ACE 2-RBD complex and shifts slightly towards the centre of the interface, modulating several molecular interactions in the process. **[A]** Initial and final position of Withanone in the ACE 2-RBD complex (PDB ID: 6M17) and is predicted to move slightly towards the ACE2 side of the complex, as revealed by 50 ns molecular dynamics (MD) simulation. **[B]** The initial position of Withanone (shown in golden yellow at 0 ns) and its final positioning as predicted from MD simulation after 50 ns (shown in green) is depicted as a magnified view. **[C, D]** Withanone at 0 ns (C), binds in the pocket-forming three H-bonds, D30, N33, and Q96 of ACE 2, in addition to alkyl and van der Waals interactions (D). **[E, F]** Withanone at 50 ns, after MD simulation) with final trajectory zoomed-in (E) and interactions of Withanone within ACE 2-RBD complex as seen in the final trajectory (F). All atoms RMSD of Withanone between initial and final positions is 2.166 Å. **[G, H]** Salt bridge interaction at the binding interface of ACE 2-RBD in the final trajectory without Withanone (G) and with Withanone (H). **[I]** Percent occupancy of the salt bridge and long-range ion-pair modulated by Withanone incorporation as seen by analysis of the simulation trajectories. *[Courtesy:* (Balkrishna, Pokhrel, *et al.*, 2021); *Under CCBY License].*

Flexibility analysis showed a slight increase in RMSD in the presence of withanone. The electrostatic component of binding free energy of the ACE2-RBD complex was decreased in the simulation trajectories with Withanone (Fig. **1.3**). In simple words, this means Withanone prevented stabilization of the interaction between ACE 2 and RBD (**Balkrishna, Pokhrel,** ***et al.*****, 2021**).

We postulate that such an interruption of electrostatic interactions between the RBD and ACE-2 would block or weaken COVID-19 entry and its subsequent infectivity. It shows that natural phytochemicals could well be the viable options for controlling COVID-19 entry into host cells, and *W. somnifera* may be the first choice of herbs in this direction to curb the COVID-19 infectivity. Similarly, we found that the phytochemical tinocordiside from Giloy (*T. cardifolia*) also binds to the ACE-2-RBD complex with substantial binding affinities (**Balkrishna, Pokhrel, and Varshney, 2020**).

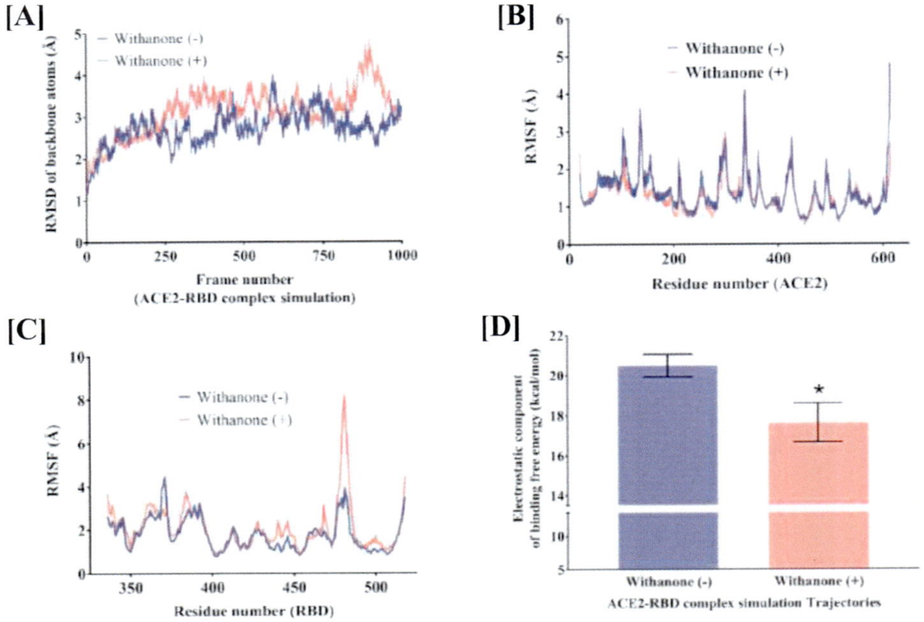

Fig. (1.3). Flexibility analysis of the ACE 2-RBD complex docked with Withanone. RMSD changes of backbone atoms (C, CA, N) of **[A]** the complex, **[B, C]** per residue RMSF (Cα atom only) of ACE 2 (C) and RBD (D) during 50 ns simulation time, as observed in the presence and absence of Withanone. **[D]** Comparison of electrostatic component of binding free energies in the ACE2-RBD complexes with and without Withanone. Statistical significance was analyzed through Welch's t-test and represented as * for $p < 0.05$. *[Courtsey:* (Balkrishna, Pokhrel, *et al.*, 2021)*;Under CCBY License].*

1.4.2. Scientific Rationale behind Pure Extract of Giloy (*T. cordifolia)* as Anti-SARS- CoV-2 Agent

T. cordifolia has been used as an excellent immuno-stimulant and serves as an excellent remedy against various microbial infections (Sinha *et al.*, 2004). This plant contains several important phytochemicals, like berberine, columbin, chasmanthin, jatrorhizine, palmarin, palmatine, tinocordifolioside, tinosporon, tinosporic acid, tinosporin, tinosporol, tinosporaside, tembeterine, tinosporic acid, tinosporal, and tinosporon (Mishra *et al.*, 2012; Sharma *et al.*, 2019). Giloy is extensively used for the treatment of several etiologies, like diabetes, dyspepsia, jaundice, rheumatoid arthritis, pyrexia, inflammations, gout, cardiac debility, excess mucus, urinary disorders, asthma, splenopathy, *etc.*

1.4.2.1. Pharmacological Perspective of Using Giloy

Clinical Evaluation against Tuberculosis: Rasayana drugs prepared from Guduchi (*T. cordifolia*), Ashwagandha (*W. somnifera*), Yastimadhu (*Glycyrrhiza glabra*) were found to be effective in the management of tuberculosis with anti-Koch's treatment (Vyas, *et al.*, 2012).

Immunomodulatory Activity: The isolated polysaccharide G1-4A from *T. cordifolia* was evaluated for immunomodulatory effects on *Mycobacterium tuberculosis* (MTB) infected murine macrophage cell line RAW 264.7 and in aerosol mouse models. G1-4A treatment modulated the levels of pro-inflammatory cytokines (TNF-α, IL-β, IL-6, IL-12, IFN-γ) in the cells infected with all the strains. Similarly, the treatment of G1-4A up-regulated the expression of TNF-α, INF-γ, and nitric oxide in the lungs of MTB-infected BALB/c mice. The results demonstrated that the Giloy compound G1-4A modulates the host immune responses and improves the therapeutic efficacy to control tuberculosis (Gupta, *et al.*, 2016).

1.4.2.2. Computational Evidence for T. cordifolia as Anti-SARS-CoV-2 Agent

The major phytocomponents reported in Giloy (*T. cordifolia*) are tinosporine, tinocordiside, diterpenoid furanolactone, tinosporaside, cordifolide, cordifol, syringin, clerodane furano diterpene, tinosporidine, columbin, heptacosanol, b-sitosterol, and tinosporide. Cordifolioside A and syringin have been reported to possess immunomodulatory activity. Tinosporin and furanolactone have been claimed especially for the treatment of the targeted viruses, including retroviruses (HIV-1, HIV-2) all subgroups, HTLV, Herpes Simplex Virus (HSV), and another viral disease.

We have tested all of the reported phytochemicals of Giloy through *in-silico* models. We have found that one of the Giloy compounds, tinocordiside, docks very well within the ACE-2-RBD complex, akin to withanone. The simulated state of tinocordiside also showed favourable binding poses within the ACE---RBD interface with several interacting sites (Fig. **1.4**) (Balkrishna, Pokhrel, and Varshney, 2020).

Based on this computational study, we suggest that tinocordiside rich extracts of Giloy would be one more viable option for controlling COVID-19 entry into host cells, and the general immunomodulatory nature of Giloy would enhance innate immunity against COVID-19 infections.

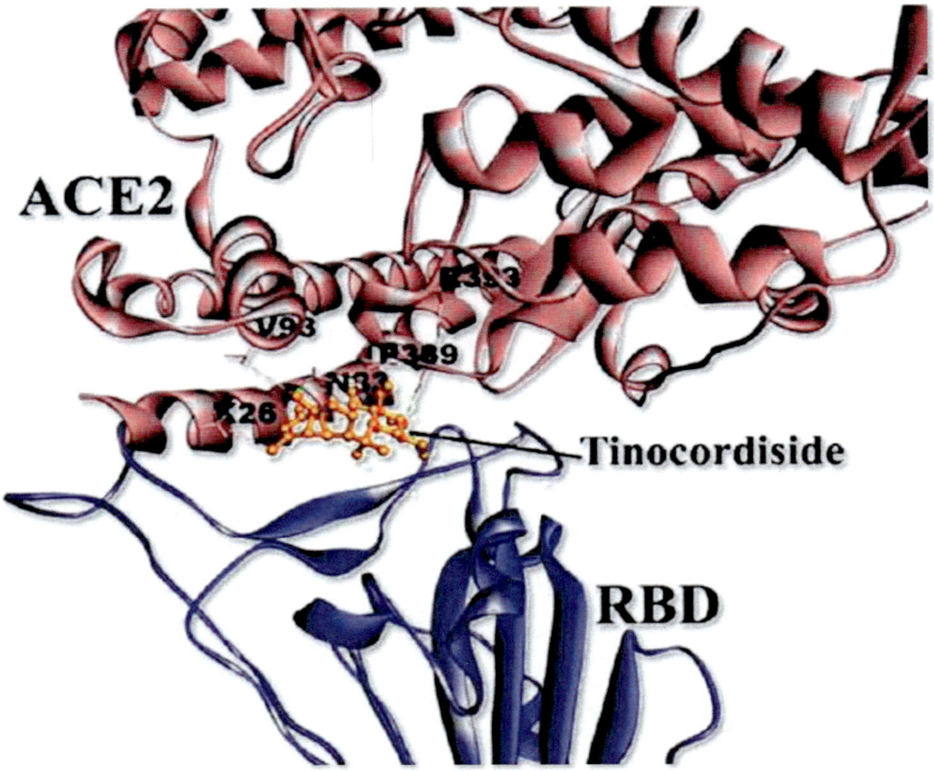

Fig. (1.4). Binding poses of tinocordiside (from *T. cordifolia*) in ACE-2-RBD complex. *Tinocordiside docks into the ACE-2-RBD complex and interacts at the interface of the ACE-2-RBD complex. [Courtsey* (Balkrishna, Pokhrel, and Varshney, 2020)*; Under CCBY License].*

In addition, Tulsi (*O. sanctum*) was also mined for its rich phytochemicals. We discovered that Scutellarein, a natural flavone found in Tulsi, docked well in the enzyme cavity of the RNA-dependent RNA polymerase (RdRp) enzyme of coronavirus. RdRp is the central enzyme needed by coronavirus for its multiplication and growth. Therefore, inhibition of RdRp provides an attractive means of controlling COVID-19 spread and its pathogenicity.

1.4.3. Scientific Rationale Behind Pure Extract of Tulsi (*O. sanctum)* as Anti-SARS-CoV-2 Agent

In Ayurveda, Tulsi is known as "Mother Medicine of Nature" and "The Queen of Herbs" for its medicinal properties and spiritual use. Tulsi has been adopted into spiritual rituals and lifestyle practices that provide a vast array of health benefits that are just beginning to be confirmed by modern science (Cohen, 2014).

The medicinal properties of Tulsi have been studied in hundreds of scientific studies, including *in vitro* animal and human models. These studies revealed that Tulsi has a unique combination of actions, including antimicrobial (including antibacterial, antiviral, antifungal, antiprotozoal, antimalarial, antihelmintic), antidiarrheal, antioxidant, anti-inflammatory, hepatoprotective, neuroprotective, cardioprotective, antidiabetic, analgesic, antipyretic, antiallergic, immunomodulatory, antiasthmatic, antitussive, adaptogenic, anti-stress activities (Pattanayak, *et al.*, 2010; Mahajan *et al.*, 2013).

1.4.3.1. Pharmacological Perspective of Tulsi and its Phytocomponents

Anti-asthmatic Activity: The anti-asthmatic activity of an ethanol extract of Tulsi leaves and the oils of *O. sanctum* has been shown to be effective against histamine-induced pre-convulsive dyspnea in guinea pigs. The anti-asthmatic activity of Tulsi was validated dose-dependently against histamine-induced bronchospasm (Singh and Agrawal, 1991).

Broncho-dilatory Activity: Bronchodilator activity of *O. sanctum* in mild and moderate asthma patients has been evaluated. Capsules of *O. sanctum* (200 mg, twice daily) were administered in 41 patients over one week, and a washout time of one week was allowed between the two drug schedules. FEV1 (representative of the amount of air that can be expelled in 1 min) and Peak Expiratory Flow Rate (PEFR) were recorded in these patients to assess the bronchodilator activity before the drug administration, on 4th and 7th day of administration of *O. sanctum* and the parameters obtained were compared with that of the standard drug, Salbutamol. *O. sanctum* produced significant improvement in both FEV1 and PEFR values and resolved symptoms of asthma. Results suggested that Tulsi (*O. sanctum*) exerts significant bronchodilator activity in mild and moderate bronchial asthma (Vinaya, *et al.*, 2017).

Immunomodulatory Activity: In the humoral immune responses, *O. sanctum* diminished levels of IgG1 and elevated the levels of IgG2a, which pointed towards the establishment of a protective immune response. The results were in line with the earlier studies on the immunomodulatory potential of *O. sanctum* in Swiss albino mice immunized with the sheep red blood cells and subsequently treated with the various doses of the OS extract for 2 weeks. This treatment brought about a significant rise in the antibody titer compared to the aqueous extract at the same dose. Many other studies have also supported the immunomodulatory activity of *O. sanctum*, like immuno-stimulation in cattle suffering from subclinical mastitis as well as an increased IL-2 gene expression and IL-2 production in male Wistar rats (Vinaya, *et al.*, 2017).

Pulmonary Disorders: Beneficial effect of *O. sanctum* against monocrotaline-induced pulmonary hypertension in rats has been assessed. *O. sanctum* (200 mg/kg) treatment ameliorated increased lung weight to body weight ratio, right ventricular hypertrophy, increased RVSP, and RVoTD/AoD ratio. Moreover, *O. sanctum* treatment decreased Nox-1 expression and increased Bcl2/Bax ratio caused by MCT. This study demonstrated that OS has therapeutic ability against MCT-induced PH in rats, attributed to its antioxidant effect (Bhalla *et al.*, 2017; Meghwani *et al.*, 2018).

1.4.3.2. Computational Evidence for O. sanctum as Anti-SARS-CoV-2 Agent

Tulsi extracts are a rich source of flavones and flavonoids. Flavones constitute a major class in the flavonoid family based on a 2-phenyl-1-benzopyran-4-one backbone. Natural flavones include apigenin, baicalein, chrysin, luteolin, Scutellarein, tangeritin, wogonin, and 6-hydroxyflavone. Scutellarein is one such flavone found in Tulsi (*O. sanctum*). The antiviral activity of flavones has been known since the 1990s when it was shown that the simultaneous application of apigenin with acyclovir resulted in an enhanced antiviral effect on herpes simplex virus types 1 and 2 (HSV-1 and HSV-2) in cell culture (Mucsi, Gyulai, and Béládi, 1992).

Naturally occurring phytochemicals are regarded as a great source of potential medications against various ailments. Studies have demonstrated that the selected naturally occurring flavonoids exhibit antiviral activities. There are multiple sources of evidence that myricetin and Scutellarein are strong chemical inhibitors of SARS-CoV helicase, and this effect is mediated through inhibition of ATPase activity (Yu *et al.*, 2012).

RNA-dependent RNA polymerase (RDRP), also called RNA replicase, catalyzes the replication of RNA from an RNA template and are essential proteins encoded in the genomes of all RNA- containing viruses with no intermediate DNA stage. These are essential for the survival of viruses. Hence, RNA-dependent RNA polymerase (RDRP) recently emerged as a promising target because of its key role in viral replication and its high conservation among viral strains. We also targeted the RDRP of SARS-CoV-2 in an *in-silico* study using Tulsi (*O. sanctum*) phytocomponents. Our study showed that a few phyto-compounds present in Tulsi might hit the catalytic cleft of the RDRP (Fig. **1.5**). Scutellarein might have an inhibitory effect on SARS-CoV-2 RdRp. This study has been made available in the public domain as a pre-print (unpublished data).

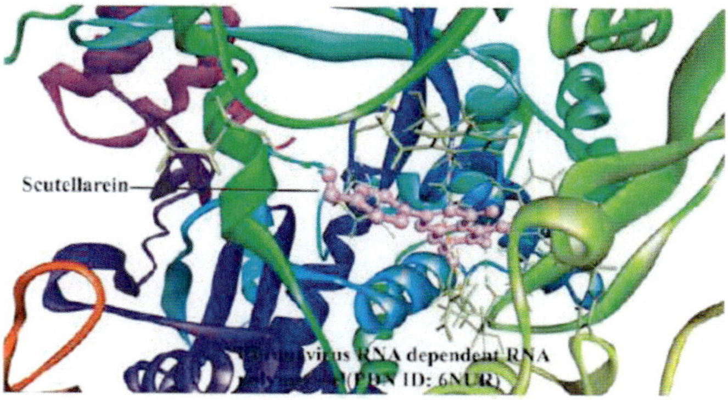

Fig. (1.5). Binding poses of Scutellarein (from *O. sanctum*) with SARS-CoV RDRP Scutellarein binds to SARS-CoV RDRP with high affinity.

Taken together, these studies showed that Ashwagandha, Giloy, and Tulsi would work well in tandem as effective prophylactics; and would also strengthen the innate immunity to fight off COVID-19 infections. Based on the observations from our computational studies, Coronil was formulated out of aqueous extracts of *W. somnifera*, *T. cordifolia,* and *O. sanctum*.

We continued to identify more such molecules, the most recent ones being columbin, nimbocinol, azadirachtin, cirsilineol, orientin, sungucine, and ergotamine from *O. sanctum* (Tulsi), *Azadirachta indica* (Neem), *T. cordifolia* (Giloy), *Salvia officinalis* (Tej Patta), and *Strychnos nux-vomica* (Kuchla), which were found to target PLpro and RdRP of SARS-CoV-2 required for virus replication within the host cell (Balkrishna, Mittal and Arya, 2020; Balkrishna, Pokhrel and Varshney, 2021) (Fig. **1.6**).

After our initial computational studies were made available publicly through pre-prints by Research Square on March 20th, 2020 (for the withanone study) and Authorea on April 16th, 2020 (for tinocordiside study), several articles on computation-based/ *in-silico* studies predicting potential anti-SARS-CoV-2 phytocompounds from different research groups appeared in the public domain in the following months, implicating the awareness that our pioneering studies generated. Notable ones among these are studies by Kumar *et al.* (Kumar, Dhanjal, Bhargava, *et al.*, 2020; Kumar, Dhanjal, Kaul, *et al.*, 2020), Sudeep *et al.* (Sudeep, 2020), and Shree et al. (Shree *et al.*, 2020). These studies showed that withanone targets SARS-CoV-2 main protease (Mpro) and host transmembrane TMPRSS2 (Kumar, Dhanjal, Bhargava, *et al.*, 2020). Likewise, withaferin A is reported to bind TMPRSS2 and GRP78 (Kumar, Dhanjal, Kaul, *et al.*, 2020; Sudeep, 2020). GRP78 receptor is the main target of the MERS-CoV spike protein interaction, similar to the ACE-2 receptor that is the target for SARS-

CoV-2 spike protein (Chu *et al.*, 2018). The study by Shree *et al.* (Shree *et al.*, 2020) identified withanoside and somniferine from *W. somnifera*, tinocordiside present in *T. cordifolia* and Vicenin, Isorientin 40-O-glucoside 200-O-p-hydroxybenzoate, and Ursolic acid from *O. sanctum* as potential inhibitors of SARS-CoV-2 Mpro (Main protease), the key enzyme of coronaviruses with a pivotal role in mediating viral replication and transcription (Jin *et al.*, 2020). Recently, a computational study by Vivek-Ananth *et al.* predicted 96 potential phytochemical inhibitors for TMPRSS2 and 9 such inhibitors for cathepsin L (Vivek-Ananth *et al.*, 2020). **TMPRSS2** and cathepsin L are two human proteases that play key roles in promoting SARS-CoV-2 entry into human host cells (Hoffmann, *et al.*, 2020; Wan *et al.*, 2020; X. Ou *et al.*, 2020). The plant sources of these identified phytochemicals are used in traditional medicines for their anti-viral and anti-inflammatory activities. Six out of the top nine of the predicted phytochemical inhibitors of **TMPRSS 2** are found in *Strychnos nux-vomica* (Kuchla) (Vivek-Ananth, *et al.*, 2020).

[A]

[B]

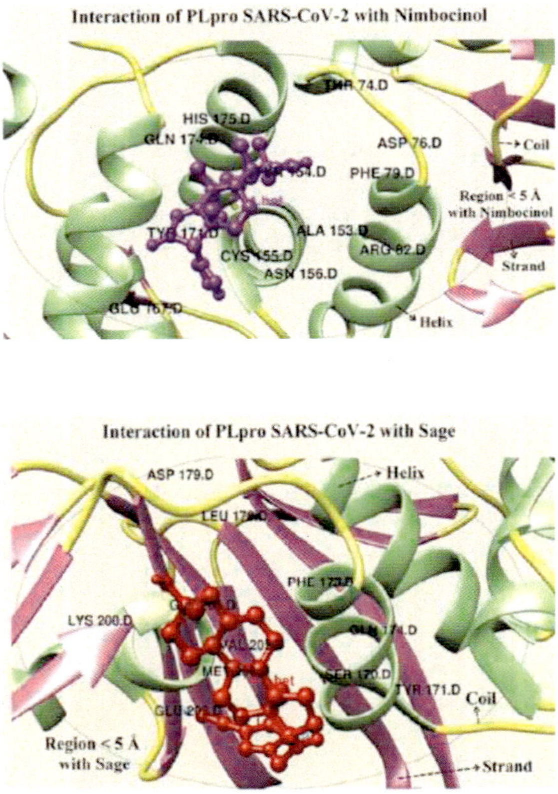

Fig. (1.6). Molecular interactions of Nimbocinol and Sage with PLpro SARS-CoV-2. Pictures representing the binding sites and molecular interactions of Nimbocinol and Sage with PLpro SARS-CoV-2. *[Courtsey:* (Balkrishna, Mittal and Arya, 2020)*; Under CCBY License].*

CONCLUDING REMARKS

In conclusion, computational biological studies helped us in identifying withanone and tinocordiside as major entry inhibitors for SARS-CoV-2. While continuing to bioprospecting, we move ahead, in parallel, to experimentally validate the computational outputs for obtaining a drug license so that the formulated phytotherapeutics could be used by modern medical practitioners.

CHAPTER 2

Formulation, Licensing, Chemical Characterization, and Validation of Ayurvedic Medicine

Abstract: This chapter, besides sharing the story behind the formulation and development of Ayurvedic medications acceptable in modern medicine, provides a detailed standard operating procedure for developing Ayurvedic drugs. To fight the COVID-19 infection, caused by the SARS-CoV-2 coronavirus, Patanjali Research Institute (PRI), Haridwar, developed the Divya Swasari Coronil kit. It contains Coronil Tablet, Divya Swasari Vati, and Divya Anu Taila. Divya Pharmacy, Haridwar, India, has obtained a manufacturing license from the Ayurvedic & Unani Department of Uttarakhand, Dehradun (License No.: 13-71-72/D-431/2020-2021) for Coronil and Swasari Vati tablets. Divya Coronil tablet has been formulated from a blend of Giloy, Ashwagandha, and Tulsi, whereas Divya Swasari Vati and Divya Anu Taila were prepared according to the classical recipe mentioned in traditional Ayurvedic texts. Analytical methods have been developed to identify and quantify the active phytoconstituents present in these blends and tablets. Sophisticated techniques are used in the manufacturing of these tablets, like liquid chromatography, equipped with single quadrupole, colloisan cell and time of light (UPLC/QToF MS), high-performance liquid chromatography (HPLC) equipped with PDA detector and high-performance thin layer chromatography (HPTLC) with automatic spotting, in which developing and scanning chambers are used for the identification and quantification of herbs. The methods have been validated in-house using ICH-Q2 (R1) and pharmacopoeia guidelines to demonstrate the repeatability, reproducibility, and reliability of the data generated. There are stringent quality checks for the authentication of raw material used in the manufacturing of the tablet, along with in-process checks and the final release of the batch. The herbs used during the manufacturing of these products have been authenticated, and voucher specimens have been stored in a government-approved depositary. The synergistic effect of these tablets has been studied by Patanjali Research Institute (PRI) for their immunity-boosting properties and the restoration of health of SARS-CoV-2 infected patients.

Keywords: CoP, HPTLC, Manufacturing license, Pharmacopoeia guidelines, Raw material selection and sampling, UPLC/QToF MS.

Acharya Balkrishna

SELECTION OF RAW MATERIAL

For any formulation, selecting the right quality raw material is of prime importance. In Ayurvedic preparations, raw material is mainly herbs or their standardized extracts. In the Coronil tablet, extracts of Ashwagandha, Tulsi, and Giloy were used. Likewise, Divya Swasari Vati is a traditional formulation comprising of 9 herbs.

Coronil tablet is a new formulation; therefore, all the three plants used for manufacturing went through stringent quality check parameters. However, Divya Swasari Vati, being a traditional formulation, already had its herbal constituents authenticated, and the quality check parameters were already established. The stringent quality parameters were applied for every batch of herbs procured from outside sources. Being a natural product, many factors are responsible for the selection of the right quality raw material. The below-listed factors are considered during the selection of the right quality of raw material:

i. Geographical location: It plays a major role in deciding product quality. Herbs grown at high altitudes will have different constituents compared to herbs grown in dry places like deserts or humid conditions that exist near a sea shore.
ii. Maturity period: The maturity period of the crop is another important criterion for selection.
iii. Season of harvesting.
iv. Drying condition: Sun drying, shade drying, air drying, drying under controlled temperature, *etc.*, play a major role in deciding the quality of the material.
v. Storage: Temperature, humidity, light, *etc.*, affect the quality of raw material.
vi. Protection from insects and pests.
vii. Supply chain: Herbal material may be forest collected or farm cultivated. The supply chain plays a major role not only in selecting the quality but also in ensuring contamination-free raw material. A schematic representation of the supply chain used in India is shown in Fig. (**2.1**).

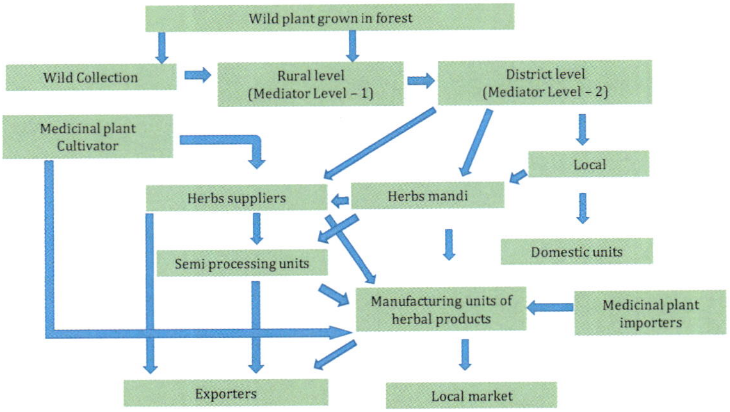

Fig. (2.1). Supply chain map used in India.

SAMPLING OF RAW MATERIAL

A sampling of raw material is one of the most important criteria for approving the right material quality. The reliability of any conclusions drawn from the analysis of a sample will depend upon how well the sample represents the whole batch. General recommendations for the sampling of pharmaceutical materials in connection with quality control are provided in the 39th report of the WHO Expert Committee on Specifications for Pharmaceutical Preparations.

Because of the specific characteristics of herbal materials, in particular their lack of homogeneity, special handling procedures are required in relation to sampling.

RECOMMENDED PROCEDURES OF SAMPLING

Sampling of Material in Bulk

As per WHO (WHO, WTR; 2005) guidelines, for bulk raw material, like herbs which consist of roots, stem, leaves, or whole plant, the first requirement is a physical inspection of each container or packaging material. The second step is to check if the label matches the specification, monograph, or other packaging and labelling criteria. Checking the condition of the package gives us information about the quality, quantity and stability of contents (loss during transportation, physical damage, increase in water content, *etc.*).

If the initial finding confirms that the batch is uniform, sampling should be initiated, and the whole material has to be quarantined to ensure that no unwanted insects or pests are being carried. As per the guidelines that detail the sampling procedure, if a batch consists of five or lesser containers or packaging units, a sample should be taken from each unit. From a batch of 6–50 units, a sample is taken from five units, but sampling should include the first, middle, and last unit. In the case of batches of over 50 units, the sample should be taken from 10% of the total number of units, rounding up the number of units to the nearest multiple of 10. For example, from a batch of 51 units, sampling should be done from six packages. Similarly, as per pharmacopoeia guidelines for articles of botanical origin, if the number of containers is between 1 and 10, all the containers should be sampled, but if the number is between 11 and 19, the containers sampled should be 11 and if the number of containers is more than 19, the formula n=10+(N/10) should be used where N is the number of containers in the supplied batch and n is the next highest whole number.

After opening, the container should be inspected, and sampling should be performed for:

- Organoleptic and physical characteristics like colour, texture, and odour.
- The correct part of the raw material like roots, stems, leaves, rhizomes, whole plant, *etc.*, if present.
- Physical characteristics of the material such as being whole, cut, crushed, compressed, *etc.*
- Nature of raw material like being dry, semi-dry, wet *etc.*
- Presence of foreign particles like sand, stone, glass particles, dirt, mould, or signs of decay.
- Presence of insects or pests.
- Presence of adulterants like other items of the same plant origin or from different plants.
- The presence of poor or degraded packaging material originated from the same or different containers.

From each container or package selected, samples should be taken from the top, middle and bottom of the container. In the case of sacks and packages, samples should be taken by hand or by scoop; first from the top, second from a depth of about 10 cm from the top, and the third and fourth from the middle and bottom of the package. The four original samples should then be pooled and mixed thoroughly.

An even, and square-shaped heap from the pooled homogenized sample is prepared and then divided diagonally into four equal parts. Two diagonally opposite parts are then removed and mixed carefully. The process is repeated until the required quantity necessary for performing three to five times complete testing is obtained. Any remaining material should be returned to the batch. The sample should be taken up to the lab for physical and chemical analysis as per specifications. Analysis should be performed as per in-house standard operation procedure (SOP) or as per the official monograph in duplicate, and any remaining sample should be stored for future reference. The portion of the test sample should be stored as reference material for at least one year after the shelf life of the final product so that it can be used for re-testing if needed.

For herbal raw material, the final samples should be tested initially for the following characteristics:

- Particle size (sieve test);
- Identity and level of impurities;
- Moisture and ash content;
- Level of active ingredients, where possible.

Sampling of Material in Retail Packages

For any retail package, each sampling unit should be physically examined to ensure if it is intact or damaged. If any damage is observed, the possible reason for damage should be investigated and if the damage could cause any quality issue to the products. The contents should be inspected for uniformity and tested for identity. Uniformity should be tested on selected layer samples at different points in the material without intermixing. However, if this procedure is not possible, a number of sampling units should be randomly selected for sampling. It is not recommended to open all containers of products, which are liable to deteriorate under the influence of light, temperature, moisture or oxygen when held in a transit warehouse. However, materials in damaged containers which affect the quality of the product or those found to be non-uniform should either be rejected or individually sampled for a complete quality check. Consignment of units without a label should be summarily rejected.

For random sampling, each sampling unit should be serially numbered, and the required number of random sampling units selected based on multiples of a random number.

The number of units to be sampled depends on different assumptions, and three possible plans are proposed by WHO, as shown in Table **2.1**.

Table 2.1. Values of N, P, or R for the N sampling units.

Values of n, p or r	Values of N		
	N plan	P plan	R plan
2	up to 3	up to 25	up to 2
3	4-6	25-56	3-4

(Table 2.1) cont.....

Values of n, p or r	Values of N		
	N plan	P plan	R plan
4	7-13	57-100	5-7
5	14-20	101-156	8-11
6	21-30	157-225	12-16
7	31-42	-	17-22
8	43-56	-	23-28
9	57-72	-	29-36
10	73-90	-	37-44

i). The N Plan

The *'N plan'* should be used only when the material to be sampled is uniform and supplied from an approved vendor. The selection and approval of vendors is a prime requirement of Good Manufacturing Practices (GMP). This can be done by physical auditing of the vendor or by desktop auditing depending upon the suitability and criticality of the product. Samples can be withdrawn from any part of the container (usually from the top, middle and bottom of the consignment). The n plan is based on the formula $n = 1 + \sqrt{N}$, where N is the number of sampling units in the consignment. The formula is applicable if the number of containers that need to be sampled is more than 4; if N is less than or equal to 4, then every container should be sampled.

ii). The P Plan

The *'P plan'* should be used when the material is uniform and received from an approved vendor and the main purpose is to establish the identity of the product. The p plan is based on the formula $p = 0.4 \div N$, where N is the number of sampling units. The figures for p are obtained by rounding up to the next highest integer.

iii). The R Plan

The *'R plan'* may be used when the material is either non-uniform and/or received from an unapproved vendor or if the vendor is not audited or the consignment is received from a source that is not well known. The r plan may usually be used for herbal products intended for use as starting materials and will be processed to get an intermediate product. This plan is based on the formula $r = (1.5/\text{N})$, where N is the number of sampling units. The figures for r are obtained by rounding up to the next highest integer.

Types of Sampling Tools

The herbal raw material is broadly divided into four categories: the whole plant chopped into a coarse powder, gum exudes, fine powder and liquid. Sample of each type of material requires different types of sampling tools. Some of the common sampling tools used in herbal industries are:

i. Scoops

Spatula or scoop is a container of solid material mostly made up of stainless steel. The scoop features a handle on one end for holding it and a curved opening on the other end for placing it inside the package to withdraw the sample. Fig. (**2.2**) shows the recommended designs of scoops, which should preferably be square or round in shape. It is used for sampling coarse or fine powder.

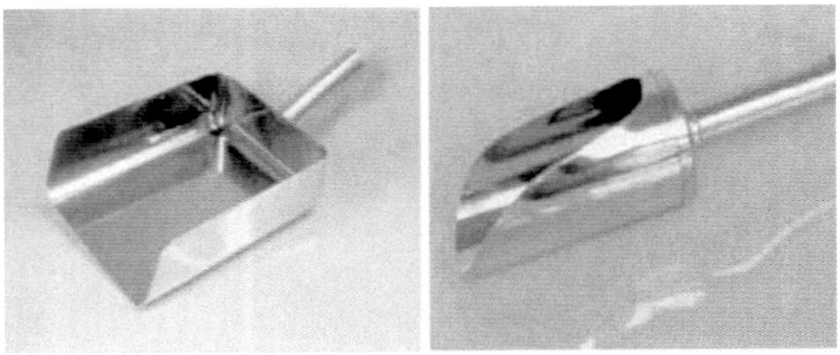

Fig. (2.2). Sampling scoops for solids.

ii. Dip Tubes

A dip tube is made up of non-reactive material like polypropylene or stainless steel. It is used for sampling liquid samples and topical products like oil and cream. Fig. (**2.3**) shows a typical design of a dip tube.

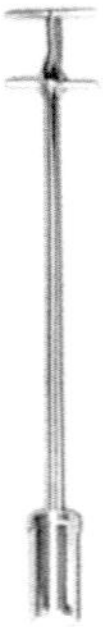

Fig. (2.3). Typical dip tube.

iii. Weighted Containers

For taking samples from large tanks and storage vessels or where physical contact is hazardous or if the product is highly volatile like a flavouring agent or a fragrance, weighted containers are used for sampling. A typical weighted container is shown in Fig. (**2.4**). The weighted container is designed in such a way that it can be opened at the required depth, and samples can be collected. Marks on the lowering cord of the container can be used to identify when the correct sampling depth has been reached.

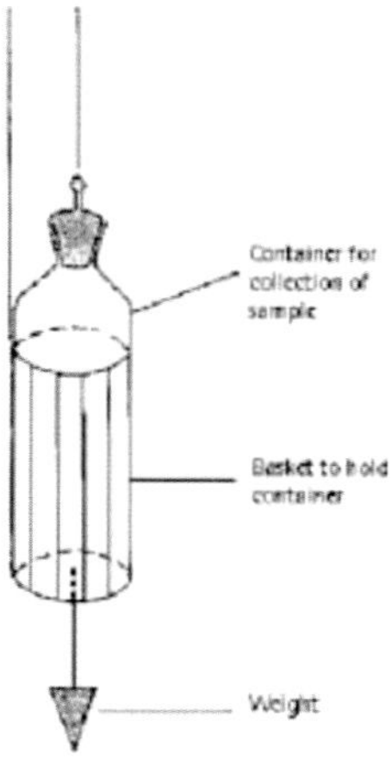

Fig. (2.4). Typical weighted container.

iv. Thieves

Sample thieves are usually made up of stainless steel or polypropylene and used for sampling fine powder. A sample thief consists of two tubes, a smaller one called the inner tube and the bigger one called the outer tube. The inner tube has a sampling slot, as shown in Fig. (**2.5 (i)**), which goes inside the outer tube and is used for collecting the sample. The outer tube has concentric holes, as shown in Fig. (**2.5 (ii)**). Both the inner and outer tubes are pointed to allow for easy sample penetration. During sampling, the inner tube is rotated so that the concentric holes on the outer tube are closed, and the thief easily enters inside the sample. After entering the desired sample depth, the inner tube is rotated so that the outer holes open and the sample gets collected inside the inner tube. Some thieves have a locking device that allows them to set the sample volume for reducing the weight variation in the sample population. Sampling thieves are also sometimes referred to as 'double-tube spears'.

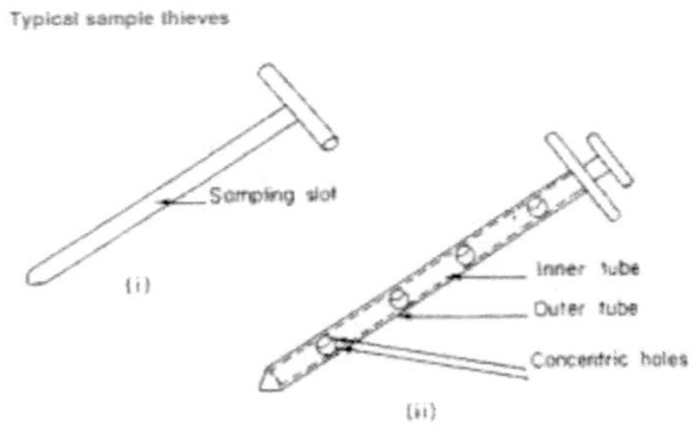

Fig. (2.5). Typical sample thieves.

Sampling thieves are designed in such a way that they can take samples at different positions in the bulk material. The concentric holes are made at different intervals so that sample gets withdrawn from different positions based on the total amount of the raw material, and a homogeneous amount of sample is withdrawn without disturbing the quality and wasting the sample.

v. Simple Bag-Sampling Spears

Simple bag-sampling spears are the most commonly used instruments for taking samples from bags because they are relatively cheap, simple and quick. There are various shapes and sizes of sampling spears available depending upon the usage. A closed spear for sampling large grains like maize, has a cut in the middle and pointed at one end to insert inside the sample and collect the sample from the middle (Fig. **2.6i**). For sampling small grains like wheat, a closed spear with a complete opening at one end is used to collect the sample (Fig. **2.6** (ii)). Generally, a spear has a maximum external diameter of about 12 mm but can be up to 25 mm in diameter. To obtain a good cross-sectional sample, the spear should be 40–45 cm in length. The tapered type of sampling spear penetrates bags easily. Other types of sampling spears are shown in Fig. (**2.6 ii, iii and iv**) depending upon their usage.

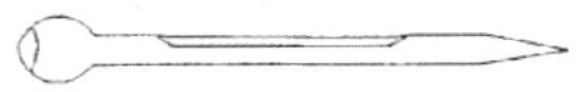

i: Closed spear for sampling large grains

ii: Closed spear for sampling small grains

iii: Open spear

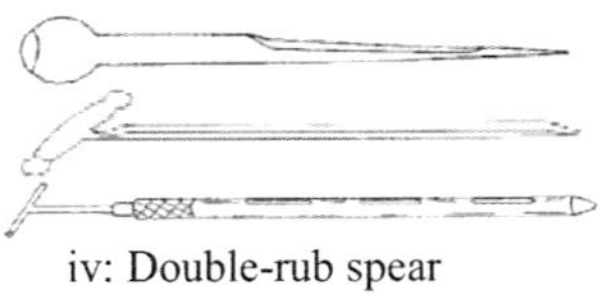

iv: Double-rub spear

Fig. (2.6). Typical sampling spears.

QUALITY CONTROL OF RAW MATERIALS AND FINISHED PRODUCTS

The quality control of both herbal raw materials and finished products is the fundamental requirement to ensure the quality of the product. It ensures that the product complies with the safety, efficacy and potency limits prescribed in the specification. Quality control assures that the product has gone through all the specified procedures like good agriculture and collection practices (GACP), good herbal processing practices (GHPP), good manufacturing practices (GMP), good laboratory practices (GLP) *etc.* and is safe for its intended use.

Regulatory bodies that govern herbal medicinal products vary with geography. For example, the Ministry of Ayurveda, Yoga and Naturopathy, Unani, Siddha and Homoeopathy (AYUSH) in India, Committee on Herbal Medicinal Products (HMPC) in Europe under Directive 2004/24/EC (Parliament, *et al.*, 2004), Food and Drug Administration (FDA) and the Dietary Supplements Health and Education Act (DSHEA) in the USA, and Therapeutic Good Administration (TGA) in Australia among others.

Quality control of herbal products is mainly divided into three broad categories:

Physical Parameters

i) *For powder*: Description, particle size (sieve test), bulk density, (tapped and untapped), *etc.*

ii) *Capsules*: Filled weight, average weight, weight variation, dissolution, disintegration, *etc.*

iii) *Tablet:* Average weight, weight variation, dissolution, disintegration, friability, hardness *etc.*

Chemical Parameters

As per ICH Q6A guidelines (Conference, *et al.*, 1999), the tests and acceptance criteria that should be considered for all new drug products are:

i. *Description*: A qualitative description of the dosage form should be provided (*e.g.* state, size, shape and colour). If any of these characteristics change during manufacture or storage, this change should be investigated and appropriate action taken. The acceptance criteria should include the final acceptable appearance. If the colour changes during storage, a quantitative procedure may be needed to identify the colour variation and its acceptance.

ii. *Identification*: Identification testing should establish the identity of the new drug product and the procedure should be able to discriminate the new product from other existing products. Identity tests should be specific for the new product. For example, Tools, like High Performance Liquid Chromatography (HPLC), High Performance Thin Layer Chromatography (HPTLC), Gas Chromatography (GC), Infrared (IR) Spectroscopy, Ultra Violet (UV) Visible Spectrophotometer or HPLC with mass, or GC with Mass Detector, are generally used for identification of the product. Either one or more of these procedures may be applied to authenticate the product.

iii. *Assay:* A specific stability-indicating assay to determine the strength (content) should be included for all new drug products. In many cases the same procedure *e.g.* HPLC, HPTLC, GC, or UV Visible Spectrophotometer *etc.* as used in identification, are also employed for assaying the new drug substance. Other supporting analytical procedures can also be used to determine the strength of the product. For example, Inductive Coupled Plasma (ICP), Atomic Absorption Spectroscopic (AAS), Gravimetric Analysis, Titration, Extractive Value, *etc.* can be used to determine the quantitative measure of the drug substance.

Contamination

This is a very critical parameter as far as herbal and dietary supplements are concerned. If unregulated, it can lead to life-threatening adverse effects. The parameters of the type of contaminant and its limit depends upon its usage and varies according to the geographical location. Contamination is broadly divided into:

Microbiological Contamination

This occurs due to environmental contamination or from the processing aids. Some of the basic microbiological parameters are:

a. Total plate count
b. Yeast and mould count
c. Detection of pathogenic bacteria such as *Escherichia coli*, *Salmonella* sp., *Pseudomonas aeruginosa*, *Staphylococcus* sp. among others.

Heavy Metals

This can occur due to soil, water and environmental contamination. Some of the basic heavy metals that need to be quantified and allowed are dependent upon daily acceptable dose. The USP < 232 > (United States Pharmacopoeia - USP, 2016) limit of components of drug products with 10 g maximum daily dose are listed in Table **2.2**.

Table 2.2. Acceptable maximum pharmacopoeia limits of heavy metal components for drug products.

Element	**Concentration Limits (µg/g) for Components Used in Oral Drug Products**	**Concentration Limits (µg/g) for Components Used in Parental Drug Products**	**Concentration Limits (µg/g) for Components Used in Inhalation Drug Products**
Cadmium	O.5	0.2	0.2
Lead	0.5	0.5	0.5
Inorganic arsenic	1.5	1.5	0.2
Inorganic mercury	3	0.3	0.1
Iridium	10	1	0.1
Osmium	10	1	0.1
Palladium	10	1	0.1
Platinum	10	1	0.1
Rhodium	10	1	0.1
Ruthenium	10	1	0.1
Chromium	1100	110	0.3
Molybdenum	300	150	1
Nickel	20	2	0.5
Vanadium	10	1	0.1
Copper	300	30	3

Residual Solvent

In pharmacopoeia < 467 > (United States Pharmacopoeia - USP, 2007) residual solvent is defined as organic volatile chemicals that are used or produced in the extraction, isolation, purification and manufacturing of herbal drug substances or products. Appropriate selection of the solvent for extraction, isolation or purification of a drug substance or an excipient may enhance the purity, yield or determine characteristics such as crystal form, purity and solubility. Therefore, the solvent is a critical element in the extraction process and may not be completely removed during the manufacturing process. Because residual solvents do not provide therapeutic benefit, they should be removed, to the extent possible to meet the safety based limits, ingredient and product specifications, good manufacturing practices, or other quality-based requirements. Concerning testing the herbal components or the final product, only certain solvents should be tested for, which are used during the manufacturing of the products. The Ayurvedic products are usually made by using herbal raw materials as such or their aqueous extracts. So testing of these products for residual solvent can be avoided provided that there is no possibility of cross-contamination during manufacturing or transportation. The term "permitted daily exposure" (PDE) is used to calculate the amount of residual solvent allowed. It is defined in the newer guidelines as a pharmaceutically acceptable intake of residual solvents to avoid confusion of differing values for ADI's (Acceptable Daily Intake) of the same substance.

Depending upon the risk, residual solvents are divided into three classes as described below.

a) *Class 1 solvents*: Solvents that should be avoided. They have known *carcinogens*, or strongly suspected as human carcinogens, and are environmental hazards. Table **2.3** defines the residual solvents and their allowed concentration limits and their concern:

Table 2.3. Acceptable maximum limits of residual Class-1 solvents.

Solvent	**Concentration Limit (ppm)**	**Concern**
Benzene	2	Carcinogen
Carbon tetrachloride	4	Toxic & environmental hazard
1,2-Dichloroethane	5	Toxic
1,1-Dichloroethane	8	Toxic
1,1,1-Trichloroethane	1500	Environmental hazard

b) *Class 2 solvents*: Non-genotoxic animal carcinogens or possible causative agents of other irreversible toxicity such as neurotoxicity or teratogenicity (Table **2.4**)

Table 2.4. Acceptable maximum residual limits of Class-2 solvents.

Solvent	**PDE (mg/day)**	**Concentration Limit (ppm)**
Acetonitrile	4.1	410
Chlorobenzene	3.6	360
Chloroform	0.6	60
Cumene	0.7	70

(Table 2.4) cont.....

Solvent	PDE (mg/day)	Concentration Limit (ppm)
Cyclohexane	38.8	3880
1,2-Dichloroethane	18.7	1870
Dichloromethane	6.0	600
1,2-Dimethoxyethane	1.0	100
N,N-Dimethylacetamide	10.9	1090
N,N-Dimethylformamide	8.8	880
1,4-Dioxane	3.8	380
2-Ethoxyethanol	1.6	160
Ethyleneglycol	6.2	620
Formamide	2.2	220
Hexane	2.9	290
Methanol	30.0	3000
2-Methoxyethanol	0.5	50
Methylbutyl ketone	0.5	50
Methylcyclohexane	11.8	1180
Methylisobutylketone	45	4500
N-Methylpyrrolidone	5.3	530
Nitromethane	0.5	50

c) *Class 3 solvents*: Solvents with low toxic potential, no health-based exposure limit is needed are defined in Table **2.5**. Class 3 solvents have PDEs of 50 mg or more per day i.e. 5000 ppm or 0.5%.

Table 2.5. List of Class-3 solvents allowed limit is 5000 ppm.

Acetic Acid	Acetone	Anisole	1-Butanol
2-Butanol	Butyl acetate	Tert-Butylmethyl ether	Dimethyl sulfoxide
Ethanol	Ethyl acetate	Ethyl ether	Ethyl formate
Formic acid	Heptane	Isobutyl acetate	Isopropyl acetate
Methyl acetate	3-Methyl-1-butaol	Methylethyl ketone	2-methyl-1-propanol
Pentane	1-Pentanol	1-Propanol	2-Propanol
Propyl acetate	Triethylamine	-	-

d) Solvent for which no adequate toxicological data was found are defined in Table **2.6** and are also of interest to the manufacturer of excipient, drug substances or drug products. The guidelines state that manufacturers should justify residual levels for these solvents.

Table 2.6. Solvents for which no adequate toxicological data is available.

1,1-Diethoxypropane	1,1-Dimethoxymethane	2,2-Dimethoxypropane
Isooctane	Isopropyl ether	Methylisopropyl ketone
Methyltetrahydrofuran	Petroleum ether	Trichliroacetic acid
Trifluoroacetic acid	-	-

RESIDUAL PESTICIDES

Pesticides are defined by the pharmacopoeia < 561 > (United States Pharmacopoeia - USP38) as any substance or mixture of substances intended to prevent, destroy, or control any pest, unwanted species of plants or animals causing harm during or otherwise interfering with the production, processing, storage, transport, or marketing of pure articles. The designation includes substances intended for use as growth regulators, defoliants or desiccants, and any substance applied to crops before or after harvest to protect the product from deterioration during storage and transport. As per the US pharmacopoeia, the list of pesticides and their allowed limits are defined in Table **2.7**.

Table 2.7. List of pesticides and their maximum allowed limit.

S. No	Substance	Limit (mg/kg)
1	Acephate	0.1
2	Alachlor	0.05
3	Aldrin and dieldrin (sum of)	0.05
4	Azinphos-ethyl	0.1
5	Azinphos-methyl	1
6	Bromide, inorganic (calculated as bromide ion)	125
7	Bromophos-ethyl	0.05
8	Bromophos-methyl	0.05
9	Brompropylate	3
10	Chlordane (sum of cis-,trans-, andoxychlordane)	0.05
11	Chlorfenvinphos	0.5
12	Chlorpyriphos-ethyl	0.2
13	Chlorpyriphos-methyl	0.1
14	Chlorthal-dimethyl	0.01

(Table 2.7) cont.....

S. No	Substance	Limit (mg/kg)
15	Cyfluthrin (sum of)	0.1
16	lambda-Cyhalothrin	1
17	Cypermethrin and isomers (sum of)	1
18	DDT (sum of o,p'-DDE, o,p'-DDT,p,p'-DDT, o,p'-TDE, and p,p'-TDE)	1
19	Deltamethrin	0.5
20	Diazinon	0.5
21	Dichlofluanid	0.1
22	Dichlorvos	1
23	Dicofol	0.5
24	Dimethoate and omethoate (sum of)	0.1
25	Dithiocarbamates (expressed as CS2)	2
26	Endosulphan (sum of isomers and endosulphan sulphate)	3
27	Endrin	0.05
28	Ethion	2
29	Etrimphos	0.05
30	Fenchlorophos (sum of fenchlorophos and fenchlorophos-oxon)	0.1
31	Fenitrothion	0.5
32	Fenpropathrin	0.03
33	Fensulfothion(sum of fensulfothion, fensulfothion-oxon, fensulfothion-oxonsulfon, and fensulfothion-sulfon)	0.05
34	Fenthion (sum of fenthion, fenthion-oxon, fenthion-oxon-sulfon, fenthion-oxo- -sulfoxid,fenthion-sulphon, and fenthion- sulpfoxid)	0.05
35	Fenvalerate	1.5
36	Flucytrinate	0.05
37	t-Fluvalinate	0.05
38	Fonophos	0.05
39	Heptachlor (sum of heptachlor, cis-heptachlorepoxide, and trans-heptachlorepoxide)	0.05
40	Hexachlorbenzene	0.1
41	Hexachlorocyclohexane (sum of isomers alpha-,beta-,gama- and delta-)	0.3
42	Lindan (-hexachlorocyclohexane)	0.6
43	Malathion and malaoxon (sum of)	1
44	Mecarbam	0.05
45	Methacriphos	0.05
46	Methamidophos	0.05
47	Methidathion	0.2

(Table 2.7) cont.....

S. No	Substance	Limit (mg/kg)
48	Methoxychlor	0.05
49	Mirex	0.01
50	Monocrotophos	0.1
51	Parathion-ethyl and Paraoxon-ethyl (sum of)	0.5
52	Parathion-methyl and Paraoxon-methyl (sum of)	0.2
53	Pendimethalin	0.1
54	Pentachloranisol	0.01
55	Permethrin and isomers (sum of)	1
56	Phosalone	0.1
57	Phosmet	0.05
58	Piperonyl butoxide	3
59	Pirimiphos-ethyl	0.05
60	Pirimiphos-methyl (sum of pirimiphos-methyl and N-desethyl- pirimiphos-methyl)	4
61	Procymidone	0.1
62	Profenophos	0.1
63	Prothiophos	0.05
64	Pyrethrum (sum of cinerin I, cinerin II, jasmolin I, jasmolin II, and pyrethrin II)	3
65	Quinalphos	0.05
66	Qunitozene (sum of quintozene, pentachloraniline, and methylpentachlorphenyksulphide)	1
67	S-421	0.02
68	Tecnazene	0.05
69	Tetradifon	0.3
70	Vinclozolin	0.4

Aflatoxins

As per the Department of Food Safety and Zoonoses of the World Health Organization, aflatoxins are poisonous substances produced by certain kinds of fungi (moulds) that are found naturally all over the world; they contaminate food crops and pose a serious health threat to humans and livestock. They pose a significant economic burden, causing an estimated 25% or more of the world's food crops to be destroyed annually.

Several types of aflatoxins (14 or more) occur in nature, but four aflatoxins B_1, B_2, G_1 and G_2 are particularly dangerous to humans and animals as they have been found in all major food crops. The limit defined by pharmacopoeia for a total of the four aflatoxins should be not more than 20 ppb and the limit for B_1 not be more than 5 ppb.

Other Contamination

As per the European Commission Regulation (EC) No. 1881/2006, many other contaminations need to be analyzed and are a great concern to human health. Some of the major contaminations are Ochratoxin-A, T-2 and HT-2 toxins, Dioxins and Polychlorinated Biphenyls (PCBs), Polycyclic Aromatic Hydrocarbons (PAH), Melamine and their structural analogues, *etc.*

RAW MATERIALS USED FOR MAKING CORONIL

Raw materials from three plants were used in making Coronil: *Ocimum sanctum* (Tulsi), *Withania somnifera* (Ashwagandha) and *Tinospora cordifolia* (Giloy). At Patanjali Research Institute, all the three materials were authenticated and standardized using sophisticated techniques like UPLC/QToF MS, HPLC, HPTLC, *etc.*

Chemical Characterization of Tulsi

The raw material used from Tulsi consists of dried whole plant of *Ocimum sanctum* (Family Lamiaceae) (Fig. **2.7**). It is an erect, 30-60 cm high, much-branched, annual herb, found throughout the country (API, Part-I, Volume-II, 2016). Tulsi is one of the most sacred plants of India and is also called "God Herself," "Holy Basil," "Queen of Herbs" and "The Medicine of Nature". For thousands of years, it is known for its healing properties. Ancient Sanskrit Ayurvedic texts like *Charak Samhita* and *Rigveda* written in about 5000 to 6000 BC have references to Tulsi. Holy texts from *Dhanvantari Nighantu* written in 1000 AD and *Raj Nighantu* in 1400 AD had references of Tulsi (Figs. **2.8** and **2.9**, respectively).

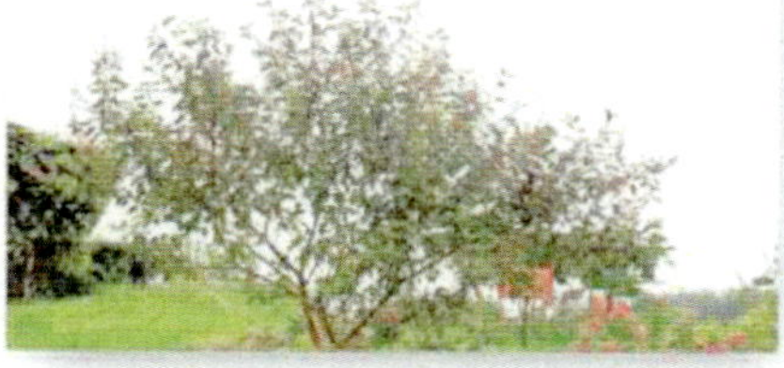

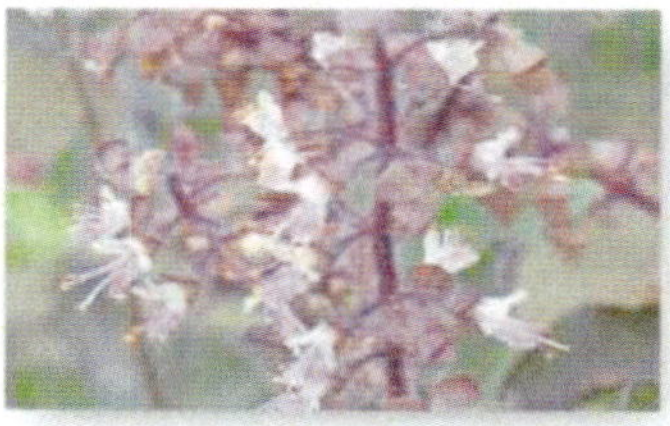

Fig. (2.7). Whole plant and flowers of *Ocimum sanctum* (Tulsi).

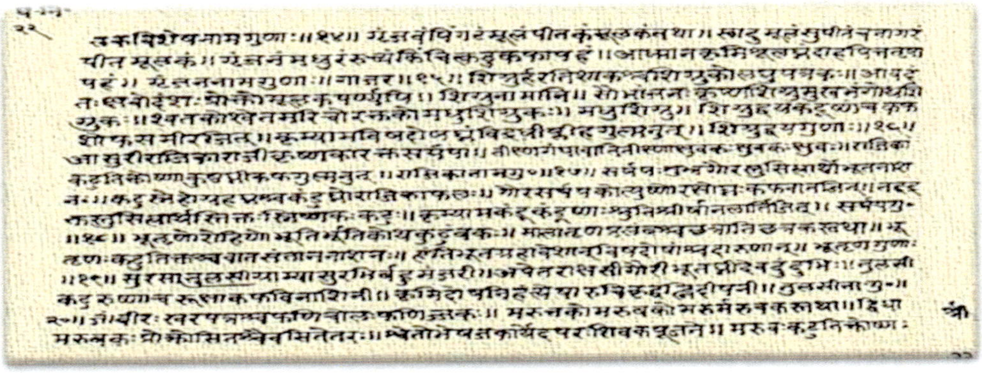

Fig. (2.8). Holy text about Tulsi in *Dhanvantari Nighantu* – 1000AD.

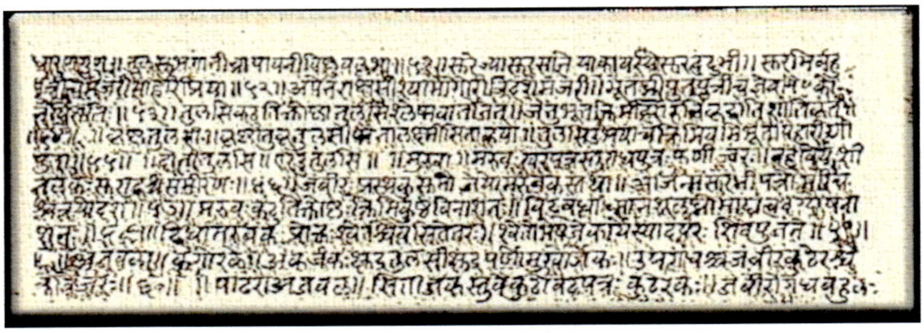

Fig. (2.9). Holy text about Tulsi in *Raj Nighantu* – 1400AD.

The identification of Tulsi should be authenticated from a reputed institution like CSIR – National Institute of Science Communication and Information Resources, Ministry of Science & Technology Govt. of India (Fig. **2.10**), Appendix 2.1).

UPLC/QToF MS Study of Tulsi

UPLC/QToF MS (Ultra High-Performance Liquid Chromatograph with Quadrupole Time of Flight) commonly known as LCMS-QToF is an analytical technique that advantageously combines the benefits of two different mass analyzers, one is quadrupole and the second is time-of-flight. QToF-MS instrumentation closely resembles that of a triple-quadrupole mass spectrometer, though the third quadrupole has been replaced by a time-of-flight tube. The first quadrupole (Q1) is capable of operating as a mass filter for the selection of specific ions based on their mass-to-charge ratio (*m*/*z*), where all ions are transmitted through the quadrupole. The second quadrupole (Q2) acts as a collision cell where ions are bombarded by neutral gas molecules such as nitrogen, resulting in the fragmentation of the ions. These ions reach into the time-of-flight analyzer, where mass separation occurs. Ions exhibiting a lighter mass will have a shorter time of flight, whereas heavier ions will take longer to traverse the flight path towards the detector.

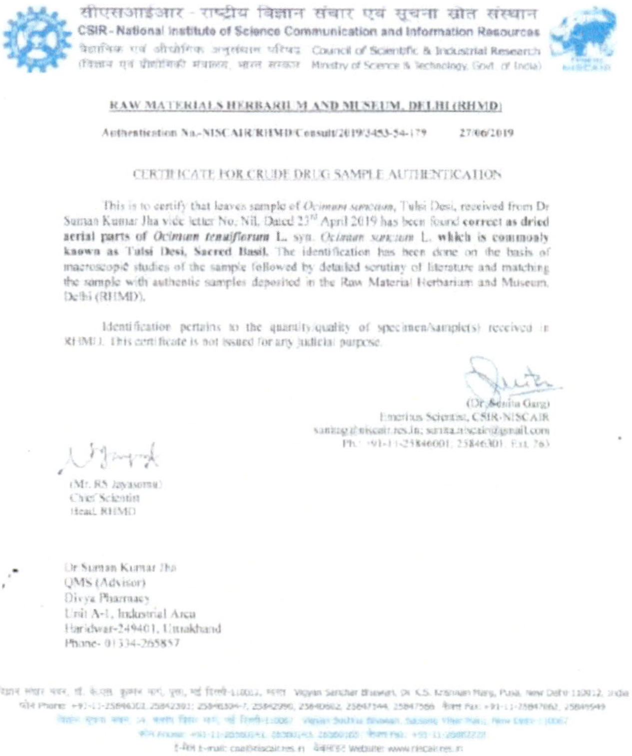

सीएसआईआर - राष्ट्रीय विज्ञान संचार एवं सूचना स्रोत संस्थान

CSIR - National Institute of Science Communication and Information Resources

Council of Scientific & Industrial Research

Ministry of Science & Technology, Govt. of India)

RAW MATERIALS HERBARIUM AND MUSEUM, DELHI (RHMD)

Authentication No.-NISCAIR/RHMD/Consult/2019/3453-54-179 27/06/2019

CERTIFICATE FOR CRUDE DRUG SAMPLE AUTHENTICATION

This is to certify that leaves sample of *Ocimum sanctum*, Tulsi Desi, received from Dr Suman Kumar Jha vide letter No. Nil, Dated 23rd April 2019 has been found **correct as dried aerial parts of *Ocimum tenuiflorum* L.** syn. *Ocimum sanctum* L. **which is commonly known as Tulsi Desi, Sacred Basil.** The identification has been done on the basis of macroscopic studies of the sample followed by detailed scrutiny of literature and matching the sample with authentic samples deposited in the Raw Material Herbarium and Museum, Delhi (RHMD).

Identification pertains to the quantity/quality of specimen/sample(s) received in RHMD. This certificate is not issued for any judicial purpose.

(Dr. Sunita Garg)
Emeritus Scientist, CSIR-NISCAIR
sunitag@niscair.res.in; sunita.niscair@gmail.com
Ph.: +91-11-25846001, 25846301, Ext. 263

(Mr. RS Jayasomu)
Chief Scientist
Head, RHMD

Dr Suman Kumar Jha
QMS (Advisor)
Divya Pharmacy
Unit A-1, Industrial Area
Haridwar-249401, Uttarakhand
Phone- 01334-265857

Vigyan Sanchar Bhawan, Dr. K.S. Krishnan Marg, Pusa, New Delhi 110012, India
E-mail: cae@niscair.res.in Website: www.niscair.res.in

Fig. (2.10). Authentication certificate of Tulsi from CSIR-NISCAIR.

UPLC/QToF MS is widely used for compound identification via spectral library matching and involves the comparison of mass spectra generated from unknown samples with a database containing spectra of known compounds. UPLC/QToF MS excels in the identification of ionizable species with high mass accuracy. This technique can identify exact masses to 4 decimal places, along with elemental compositions. The LC-MS/MS is a powerful tool for the detection of residual chemical compounds, confirmatory identification of organic molecules and quantitation of contaminants and adulterants in pharmaceutical and food samples at ppb or ppt levels.

Sample Preparation Method: Powdered Tulsi sample (100 mg) was dissolved in 10 ml of methanol: water (60:40) and sonicated for 30 min. The solution was centrifuged for 5 min at 10000 rpm and filtered through a 0.22 μm nylon filter.

UPLC/QToF MS analysis conditions: Analysis was performed on a Xevo G2-XS QToF of Waters with Acquity UPLC-I Class and Unifi software (Waters Corporation, Milford, MA, USA). Separation was carried out using Acquity UPLC HSS -T3 column (100 x 2.1 mm, 1.7 μm). The column was maintained at 40°C throughout the analysis and sample temperature was kept at 20°C during the analysis. Detection was carried out by Xevo G2-XS QToF. The elution was carried out at a flow rate of 0.4 ml/min using gradient elution of mobile phase (Table **2.8**), 0.1% formic acid in water (mobile phase A) and 0.1% formic acid in acetonitrile (mobile phase B). 1 μl of the test solution was injected during the analysis and the chromatogram was recorded for 45 min. The acquisition was performed at positive and negative modes whose analytical conditions are described in Table **2.9**. The chromatogram generated is illustrated in Fig. (**2.11**) in positive mode and Fig. (**2.12**) in negative mode. The compound observed based on their mass and fragmentation patterns are described in Tables **2.10** and **2.11**. Based on UPLC/QToF MS analysis, a total of 92 compounds were observed in Tulsi.

Table 2.8. Gradient elution program of mobile phase used in UPLC for Tulsi.

Time (min)	Flow (ml/min)	Mobile Phase A (%)	Mobile Phase (%)
0	0.4 ml/min	95	5
10	0.4 ml/min	85	15
20	0.4 ml/min	75	25
30	0.4 ml/min	50	50
45	0.4 ml/min	10	90
50	0.4 ml/min	10	90
51	0.4 ml/min	95	5
55	0.4 ml/min	95	5

Table 2.9. Xevo G2-XS QToF parameters for positive and negative modes used in identification of phytoconstituents in Tulsi.

Parameter	Polarity (+ve)	Polarity (-ve)
Ionisation type	ESI	ESI
Mode	MS^E	MS^E
Acquisition time	45 min	45 min
Mass range (m/z)	50-1200 m/z	50-1200 m/z

(Table 2.9) cont.....

Parameter	Polarity (+ve)	Polarity (-ve)
Cone Voltage	20 V	20 V
Capillary	1 kV	2 kV
Low CE	6.0 eV	6.0 eV
High CE	20-40 eV (ramp)	20-40 eV(ramp)
Source temperature	120 °C	120 °C
Desolvation Temperature	500 °C	500 °C
Cone gas flow	50 L/h	50 L/h
Desolvation gas flow	900 L/h	900 L/h
Lock Spray (Leucine Enkaphalin)	556.2766 m/z	554.2620 m/z

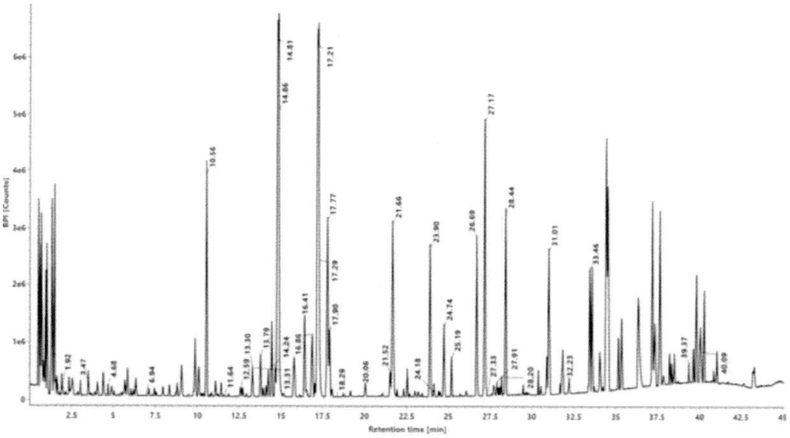

Fig. (2.11). UPLC/QToF MS Chromatogram of Tulsi in positive mode.

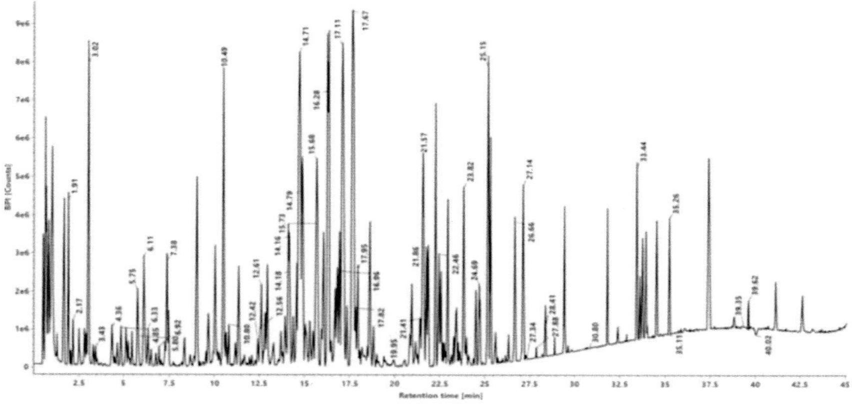

Fig. (2.12). UPLC/QToF MS Chromatogram of Tulsi in negative mode.

Table 2.10. Compounds identified in Tulsi extract with UPLC/QToF MS in positive mode.

Positive Mode							
S.No.	**Component Name**	**Formula**	**RT (min)**	**Observed m/z**	**Neutral Mass (Da)**	**Response**	**Adducts**
1.	Gallic acid	$C_7H_6O_5$	1.92	171.0283	170.0215	10169	+H
2.	Protocatechuic acid	$C_7H_6O_4$	3.47	155.0343	154.0266	5437	+H
3.	N-Methylcoclaurine	$C_{18}H_{21}NO_3$	4.68	300.1573	299.1521	119689	+H
4.	Vanillic acid	$C_8H_8O_4$	6.94	169.0493	168.0423	14279	+H
5.	Kaempferol-3-O- rutinoside	$C_{27}H_{30}O_{15}$	10.56	595.1680	594.1585	1912333	+H, +Na
6.	Vicenin 2	$C_{27}H_{30}O_{15}$	11.64	595.1680	594.1585	140016	+H, +Na
7.	Quercetin 3,4'- diglucoside	$C_{27}H_{30}O_{17}$	12.19	627.1586	626.1483	40363	+H, +Na
8.	Methyl eugenol	$C_{11}H_{14}O_2$	12.59	179.1061	178.0994	27712	+H
9.	Luteolin-7-O-glucoside	$C_{21}H_{20}O_{11}$	13.30	449.1067	448.1006	95212	+H, +Na
10.	Scutellarein	$C_{15}H_{10}O_6$	13.31	287.0534	286.0477	263995	+H
11.	Isovitexin	$C_{21}H_{20}O_{10}$	13.79	433.1116	432.1057	419672	+H
12.	Ellagic acid	$C_{14}H_6O_8$	14.05	303.0093	302.0063	43830	+H
13.	Isorhamnetin-3-O- glucoside	$C_{22}H_{22}O_{12}$	14.10	479.1151	478.1111	206621	+H, +Na
14.	Rutin	$C_{27}H_{30}O_{16}$	14.24	611.1643	610.1534	376773	+H, +Na
15.	Vitexin	$C_{21}H_{20}O_{10}$	14.25	433.1118	432.1057	219156	+H, +Na
16.	Quercetin-3-O-glucoside	$C_{21}H_{20}O_{12}$	14.65	465.1016	464.0955	185877	+H, +Na
17.	Morin	$C_{15}H_{10}O_7$	14.66	303.0483	302.0427	244728	+H
18.	Luteolin-7-O-glucuronide	$C_{21}H_{18}O_{12}$	14.81	463.0865	462.0798	4822852	+H, +Na
19.	Orientin	$C_{21}H_{20}O_{11}$	14.86	449.1069	448.1006	102135	+H
20.	5-Hydroxycoumarin	$C_9H_6O_3$	15.79	163.0388	162.0317	295781	+H
21.	(-)-Rabdosiin	$C_{36}H_{30}O_{16}$	16.41	741.1492	718.1534	266681	+Na
22.	Astragalin	$C_{21}H_{20}O_{11}$	16.61	449.1062	448.1006	48822	+H, +Na
23.	Citrusin C	$C_{16}H_{22}O_7$	16.86	349.1237	326.1366	560952	+Na
24.	Apigenin-7-O-glucoside	$C_{21}H_{20}O_{10}$	17.04	433.1114	432.1057	206417	+H
25.	Apigenin 7-glucuronide	$C_{21}H_{18}O_{11}$	17.21	447.0907	446.0849	4992918	+H, +Na
26.	luteolin 7-O-b-D-glucopyranosiduronic acid	$C_{27}H_{28}O_{17}$	17.29	313.0691	624.1327	19502	2x(+H)
27.	Ketocoumarin	$C_9H_6O_3$	17.77	163.0387	162.0317	927499	+H
28.	Chrysoeriol 7- glucuronide	$C_{22}H_{20}O_{12}$	17.90	477.1019	476.0955	632658	+H
29.	Eupalitin	$C_{17}H_{14}O_7$	18.29	331.0790	330.074	113907	+H
30.	N-feruloyltyramine	$C_{18}H_{19}NO_4$	20.06	314.1369	313.1314	185625	+H, +Na

(Table 2.10) cont.....

Positive Mode							
S.No.	**Component Name**	**Formula**	**RT (min)**	**Observed m/z**	**Neutral Mass (Da)**	**Response**	**Adducts**
31.	Quercetin	$C_{15}H_{10}O_{7}$	21.52	303.0483	302.0427	281945	+H
32.	Luteolin	$C_{15}H_{10}O_{6}$	21.66	287.0537	286.0477	1349581	+H
33.	Apigenin	$C_{15}H_{10}O_{5}$	23.90	271.0585	270.0528	961603	+H
34.	Kaempferol	$C_{15}H_{10}O_{6}$	24.18	287.0537	286.0477	36080	+H
35.	Chrysoeriol	$C_{16}H_{12}O_{6}$	24.42	301.0690	300.0634	95661	+H
36.	Isothymusin	$C_{17}H_{14}O_{7}$	24.74	331.0788	330.074	514378	+H
37.	Isothymonin	$C_{18}H_{16}O_{8}$	25.19	361.0894	360.0845	322006	+H
38.	Cirsimaritin	$C_{17}H_{14}O_{6}$	26.69	315.0841	314.079	876674	+H, +Na
39.	Cirsilineol	$C_{18}H_{16}O_{7}$	27.17	345.0943	344.0896	1763820	+H, +Na
40.	Glycyrrhizin	$C_{42}H_{62}O_{16}$	27.33	823.4189	822.4038	14292	+H, +Na
41.	Xanthomicrol	$C_{18}H_{16}O_{7}$	27.91	345.0940	344.0896	152419	+H, +Na
42.	7-Hydroxy-4-methoxyphenanthrene-2- O---D-glucoside	$C_{21}H_{22}O_{8}$	28.20	403.1359	402.1315	201304	+H, +Na
43.	4′,5-Dihydroxy-3′,7,8-trimethoxyflavone	$C_{18}H_{16}O_{7}$	28.44	345.0943	344.0896	1052485	+H, +Na
44.	Ganoderic acid S	$C_{30}H_{44}O_{3}$	29.84	453.3348	452.3291	115119	+H
45.	Arjunic acid	$C_{30}H_{48}O_{5}$	30.62	489.3574	488.3502	10009	+H
46.	Salvigenin	$C_{18}H_{16}O_{6}$	31.01	329.0997	328.0947	950683	+H, +Na
47.	5-Hydroxy-7,8,2’,3’-tetramethoxyflavone	$C_{19}H_{18}O_{7}$	32.23	359.1100	358.1053	216749	+H, +Na
48.	Stearidonic acid	$C_{18}H_{28}O_{2}$	32.85	277.2146	276.2089	111854	+H
49.	Dieugenol	$C_{20}H_{22}O_{4}$	33.46	349.1390	326.1518	840549	+Na, +H
50.	Linolenic acid	$C_{18}H_{30}O_{2}$	39.37	279.2299	278.2246	298262	+H
51.	Ursolic acid	$C_{30}H_{48}O_{3}$	39.50	457.3660	456.3604	20000	+H
52.	Oleanolic acid	$C_{30}H_{48}O_{3}$	40.09	457.3664	456.3604	44261	+H

Table 2.11. Compounds identified in Tulsi extract with UPLC/QToF MS in negative mode.

Negative Mode							
S.No	**Component Name**	**Formula**	**RT (min)**	**Observed m/z**	**Neutral Mass (Da)**	**Response**	**Adducts**
1.	Gallic acid	$C_7H_6O_5$	1.91	169.0136	170.0215	532854	-H
2.	Quinic acid	$C_{7}H_{12}O_{6}$	2.17	191.0554	192.0634	210746	-H

(Table 2.11) cont.....

Negative Mode							
S.No	**Component Name**	**Formula**	**RT (min)**	**Observed m/z**	**Neutral Mass (Da)**	**Response**	**Adducts**
3.	Syringic acid	$C_9H_{10}O_5$	3.02	197.0450	198.0528	1122689	-H, +HCOO
4.	Protocatechuic acid	$C_7H_6O_4$	3.43	153.0186	154.0266	84726	-H
5.	Caftaric acid	$C_{13}H_{12}O_9$	4.36	311.0405	312.0481	393857	-H
6.	Syringaldehyde	$C_9H_{10}O_4$	4.50	181.0497	182.0579	61193	-H, +HCOO
7.	4-Hydroxybenzoic Acid	$C_7H_6O_3$	4.85	137.0237	138.0317	177000	-H
8.	4',5-Dihydroxy-7,8-dimethoxyflavone	$C_{17}H_{14}O_6$	5.75	313.0710	314.079	472654	-H
9.	Methyl gallate	$C_8H_8O_5$	5.80	183.0292	184.0372	176132	-H
10.	o-Coumaric acid	$C_9H_8O_3$	6.11	163.0393	164.0473	164876	-H
11.	Veratric acid	$C_9H_{10}O_4$	6.33	181.0498	182.0579	212303	-H, +HCOO
12.	Vanillic acid	$C_8H_8O_4$	6.88	167.0339	168.0423	7054	-H
13.	Chlorogenic acid	$C_{16}H_{18}O_9$	6.92	353.0866	354.0951	28731	-H
14.	Caffeic acid	$C_9H_8O_4$	7.38	179.0343	180.0423	177551	-H
15.	Gallocatechin	$C_{15}H_{14}O_7$	8.34	305.0692	306.074	235874	-H
16.	Corilagin	$C_{27}H_{22}O_{18}$	9.54	633.0743	634.0806	218957	-H
17.	p-coumaric acid	$C_9H_8O_3$	10.17	163.0392	164.0473	124880	-H
18.	Salvianolic acid F	$C_{17}H_{14}O_6$	10.28	313.0707	314.079	181508	-H, +HCOO
19.	Kaempferol-3-O- rutinoside	$C_{27}H_{30}O_{15}$	10.49	593.1519	594.1585	2594749	-H, +HCOO
20.	5-Hydroxy-7-methoxyflavanone	$C_{16}H_{14}O_4$	10.56	269.0809	270.0892	205869	-H
21.	Citrusin F	$C_{22}H_{32}O_{14}$	10.80	519.1716	520.1792	409118	-H
22.	1,2,6-Tri-O-galloyl-b-D-glucose	$C_{27}H_{24}O_{18}$	10.82	635.0896	636.0963	138670	-H
23.	Vicenin 2	$C_{27}H_{30}O_{15}$	11.56	593.1512	594.1585	165285	-H
24.	5-Hydro-7,8,2'-Trimethoxyflavanone	$C_{18}H_{16}O_6$	11.68	327.0867	328.0947	183734	-H
25.	Quercetin 3,4'- diglucoside	$C_{27}H_{30}O_{17}$	12.10	625.1407	626.1483	196770	-H
26.	2-Methoxy-4- acetylphenol 1-O-α-L- rhamnopyranosyl-(1"→6')-β-D-glucopyranoside	$C_{21}H_{30}O_{12}$	12.42	473.1659	474.1737	318430	-H, +HCOO

(Table 2.11) cont.....

Negative Mode							
S.No	**Component Name**	**Formula**	**RT (min)**	**Observed m/z**	**Neutral Mass (Da)**	**Response**	**Adducts**
27.	1-Hydroxy-2,3,4,5-tetramethoxyxanthone	$C_{17}H_{16}O_{7}$	12.56	331.0814	332.0896	372886	-H
28.	Lithospermic acid	$C_{27}H_{22}O_{12}$	12.61	537.1042	538.1111	841816	-H
29.	Chicoric acid	$C_{22}H_{18}O_{12}$	12.76	473.0721	474.0798	239596	-H
30.	luteolin 7-O-b-D-glucopyranosiduronic Acid	$C_{27}H_{28}O_{17}$	13.17	623.1263	624.1327	143674	-H
31.	Luteolin-7-O- glucoside	$C_{21}H_{20}O_{11}$	13.22	447.0928	448.1006	156240	-H
32.	Isovitexin	$C_{21}H_{20}O_{10}$	13.71	431.0975	432.1057	379333	-H
33.	Isoquercetin	$C_{21}H_{20}O_{12}$	13.87	463.0873	464.0955	115597	-H
34.	Ellagic acid	$C_{14}H_{6}O_{8}$	13.94	300.9983	302.0063	466902	-H
35.	Citrusin B	$C_{27}H_{36}O_{13}$	14.01	567.2082	568.2156	156370	-H
36.	Isorhamnetin-3-O- glucoside	$C_{22}H_{22}O_{12}$	14.04	477.1013	478.1111	269437	-H
37.	Rutin	$C_{27}H_{30}O_{16}$	14.16	609.1463	610.1534	1296689	-H
38.	Vitexin	$C_{21}H_{20}O_{10}$	14.18	431.0971	432.1057	137782	-H
39.	Catechin-3-O-gallate	$C_{22}H_{18}O_{10}$	14.31	441.0818	442.09	143217	-H
40.	Quercetin-3-O- glucoside	$C_{21}H_{20}O_{12}$	14.56	463.0873	464.0955	867415	-H
41.	Luteolin-7-O- glucuronide	$C_{21}H_{18}O_{12}$	14.71	461.0718	462.0798	3177529	-H, +HCOO
42.	Orientin	$C_{21}H_{20}O_{11}$	14.79	447.0922	448.1006	147115	-H, +HCOO
43.	1-Hydroxy-2,3,4,7-tetramethoxyxanthone	$C_{17}H_{16}O_{7}$	15.31	331.0815	332.0896	387836	-H
44.	Methyl caffeate	$C_{10}H_{10}O_{4}$	15.68	193.0501	194.0579	1689096	-H
45.	Nonanedioic acid	$C_{9}H_{16}O_{4}$	15.73	187.0968	188.1049	180193	-H
46.	3,4′,5-Trihydroxy-3′,7-dimethoxyflavanone	$C_{17}H_{16}O_{7}$	16.05	331.0815	332.0896	900949	-H
47.	(-)-Rabdosiin	$C_{36}H_{30}O_{16}$	16.28	717.1480	718.1534	2148198	-H
48.	Astragalin	$C_{21}H_{20}O_{11}$	16.63	447.0916	448.1006	184242	-H
49.	Citrusin C	$C_{16}H_{22}O_{7}$	16.81	371.1337	326.1366	803328	+HCOO, -H
50.	Apigenin-7-O-glucoside	$C_{21}H_{20}O_{10}$	16.96	431.0976	432.1057	259621	-H
51.	Apigenin 7-glucuronide	$C_{21}H_{18}O_{11}$	17.11	445.0772	446.0849	2918998	-H, +HCOO
52.	Rosmarinic acid	$C_{18}H_{16}O_{8}$	17.67	359.0768	360.0845	4263827	-H, +HCOO

(Table 2.11) cont.....

Negative Mode							
S.No	**Component Name**	**Formula**	**RT (min)**	**Observed m/z**	**Neutral Mass (Da)**	**Response**	**Adducts**
53.	Chrysoeriol 7- glucuronide	$^{C}22^{H}20^{O}12$	17.82	475.0881	476.0955	598492	-H
54.	Monomethyl lithospermate	$^{C}28^{H}24^{O}12$	17.95	551.1197	552.1268	934880	-H
55.	Ferulaldehyde	$^{C}10^{H}10^{O}3$	19.95	177.0551	178.063	100293	-H
56.	N-feruloyltyramine	$^{C}18^{H}19^{NO}4$	19.98	312.1235	313.1314	83576	-H, +HCOO
57.	Quercetin	$^{C}15^{H}10^{O}7$	21.41	301.0348	302.0427	489520	-H
58.	Luteolin	$^{C}15^{H}10^{O}6$	21.57	285.0400	286.0477	1711541	-H
59.	Salvianolic acid A	$^{C}26^{H}22^{O}10$	21.86	493.1138	494.1213	613368	-H, +HCOO
60.	Formononetin	$^{C}16^{H}12^{O}4$	22.46	267.0655	268.0736	637833	-H, +HCOO
61.	Methyl rosmarinate	$^{C}19^{H}18^{O}8$	22.83	373.0920	374.1002	153484	-H, +HCOO
62.	Salvianolic acid C	$^{C}26^{H}20^{O}10$	23.14	491.0989	492.1057	137299	-H, +HCOO
63.	Apigenin	$^{C}15^{H}10^{O}5$	23.82	269.0450	270.0528	966320	-H
64.	Kaempferol	$^{C}15^{H}10^{O}6$	24.11	285.0397	286.0477	67379	-H
65.	Chrysoeriol	$^{C}16^{H}12^{O}6$	24.37	299.0552	300.0634	71165	-H
66.	Isothymusin	$^{C}17^{H}14^{O}7$	24.69	329.0661	330.074	518305	-H
67.	Isothymonin	$^{C}18^{H}16^{O}8$	25.15	359.0764	360.0845	172592	-H
68.	Cirsimaritin	$^{C}17^{H}14^{O}6$	26.66	313.0714	314.079	865563	-H
69.	Cirsilineol	$^{C}18^{H}16^{O}7$	27.14	343.0818	344.0896	1208569	-H
70.	Glycyrrhizin	$^{C}42^{H}62^{O}16$	27.34	821.3991	822.4038	134374	-H
71.	Xanthomicrol	$^{C}18^{H}16^{O}7$	27.88	343.0817	344.0896	180013	-H
72.	4′,5-Dihydroxy-3′,7,8-trimethoxyflavone	$^{C}18^{H}16^{O}7$	28.41	343.0815	344.0896	133597	-H
73.	Arjunic acid	$^{C}30^{H}48^{O}5$	30.80	533.3479	488.3502	143011	+HCOO,-H
74.	Dieugenol	$^{C}20^{H}22^{O}4$	33.44	325.1444	326.1518	1345730	-H
75.	2α-Hydroxyursolic Acid	$^{C}30^{H}48^{O}4$	35.11	517.3528	472.3553	105563	+HCOO,-H
76.	Ricinoleic acid	$^{C}18^{H}34^{O}3$	35.26	297.2427	298.2508	971653	-H
77.	Linolenic acid	$^{C}18^{H}30^{O}2$	39.35	277.2161	278.2246	34977	-H
78.	Ursolic acid	$^{C}30^{H}48^{O}3$	39.62	455.3525	456.3604	717117	-H, +HCOO
79.	Oleanolic acid	$^{C}30^{H}48^{O}3$	40.02	501.3579	456.3604	421377	+HCOO,-H

Conclusion: A total of 92 different phytoconstituents were identified in Tulsi extract. Some of these phytoconstituents were detected in both positive and negative modes, which were counted once.

HPLC-PDA Method Development for standardization of Tulsi

Experiment Methods: The quantification of marker compounds was performed on Waters HPLC equipped with Binary pump (1525), PDAD (Photo Diode Array Detector 2998) and auto-sampler (2707). The elution was carried out at a flow rate of 1.0 ml/min using gradient of the mobile phase A (0.1% orthophosphoric acid in water adjust pH 2.5 with diethylamine) and mobile phase B (0.1% orthophosphoric acid in a mixer of acetonitrile and water in the ratio of 88:12, adjust pH 2.5 with diethylamine) at a flow rate of 1.0 ml/min was used (Table **2.12**). This experiment was performed on Shodex C18-4E (4.6mm ID x 250 mm L) column and the column temperature was kept at 35°C during the analysis. 10 μl of test solution was injected during the analysis and chromatograph was recorded at 270 nm wavelength (for gallic acid, rutin, ellagic acid, isoquercetin, luteolin-7-O-β-glucuronide, luteolin and apigenin) and 325 nm (for rosmerinic acid, caffeic acid and methyl caffeate). The selection of wavelength depends upon the chromophore group present in the sample which absorbs a specific wavelength of light.

Table 2.12. HPLC gradient elution program of mobile phase of Tulsi.

Time (min)	Flow (ml/min)	Mobile Phase A (%)	Mobile Phase B (%)
0	1.0	95	5
12	1.0	90	10
25	1.0	85	15
35	1.0	75	25
50	1.0	60	40
60	1.0	30	70
61	1.0	95	5
65	1.0	95	5

Sample Preparation Method: 1.0 gm of powdered sample was diluted with 20 ml methanol: water (60:40) and sonicated for 30 min. This solution was centrifuged at 10000 rpm for 5 min and filtered using a 0.45 μm nylon filter (solution A) and this solution A was used for the analysis of Gallic acid, Caffeic acid. Rutin, Ellagic acid, Isoquercetin, Methyl caffeate, Luteolin and Apigenin. Solution A was further diluted to 10 times with the same solvent and used for the analysis of Luteolin-7-O-β-glucuronide and Rosmarinic acid.

Standard Preparation: A standard is defined as a highly pure molecule prepared and characterized at an in-house facility or purchased from an approved vendor with an authentic certificate confirming the molecule and its potency. Standards were dissolved in methanol to prepare the appropriate concentrations. A typical HPLC chromatogram of Tulsi extract and standard at different wavelengths are shown in Figs. (**2.13** and **2.14**).

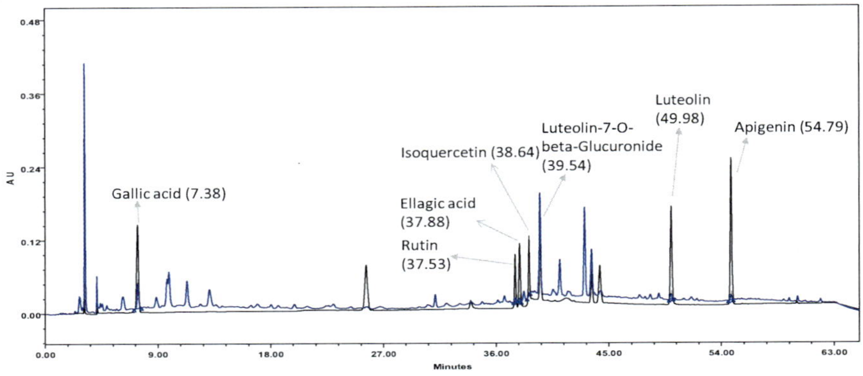

Fig. (2.13). Overlap chromatograph of standard mix in black font of Gallic acid (7.38min), Rutin (37.53 min), Ellagic acid (37.88 min), Isoquercetin (38.64 min), Luteolin-7-O-Beta-Glucoronide (39.54 min), Luteolin (49.98 min), Apigenin (54.79 min) and Tulsi raw material in Blue font at 270 nm.

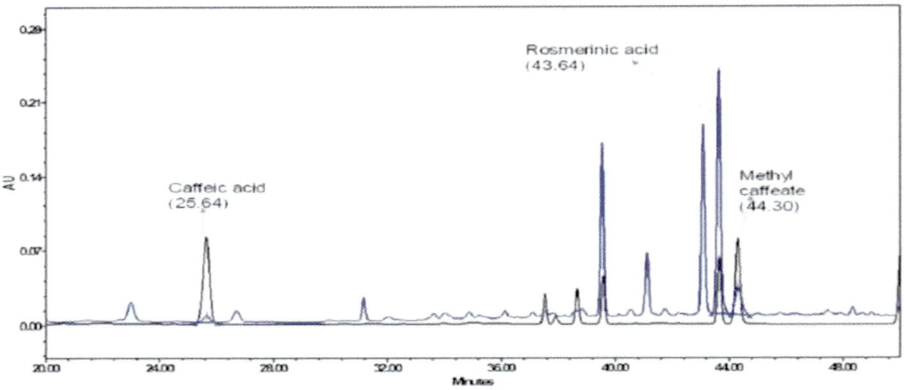

Fig. (2.14). Overlap chromatograph of the standard mix of Caffeic acid (25.64 min), Rosmarinic acid (43.64 min), Methyl caffeate (44.30 min) and Tulsi at 325 nm.

Quantitation of each compound is based on absorption at a specific wavelength of light using the Beer-Lambert law i.e concentration of the sample is directly proportional to absorption of light. The amounts of active constituents present in Tulsi extract are tabulated in Table **2.13**.

Table 2.13. Identity and quantities of marker phytoconstituents in Tulsi.

S. No.	Name of Marker Compound	Result (µg/mg)
1.	Gallic acid	0.227
2.	Caffeic acid	0.030
3.	Rutin	0.062
4.	Ellagic acid	0.048
5.	Isoquercetin	0.036
6.	Luteolin-7-O-Beta-Glucuronide	1.291
7.	Rosmarinic acid	1.374
8.	Methyl caffeate	0.164
9.	Luteolin	0.045
10.	Apigenin	0.033

HPLC-PDA Method Validation for Standardization of Tulsi

Analytical methods used for quantification of actives present in Tulsi are validated as per the ICH Q2R1 (Conference, *et al.*, 2005) and a summary of validation is tabulated in Table **2.14**.

Table 2.14. Summary of HPLC method validation of Tulsi.

S. No.	Parameters	Acceptance criteria	Result Obtained									
			Gallic acid	Caffeic acid	Rutin	Ellagic acid	Isoqu-ercetin	Luteolin 7-0 β glucuronide	Methyl caffate	Rosmarinic Acid	Luteolin	Apigenin
1	System Suitability	% RSD of Retention time - NMT 2.0%	0.03	0.23	0.12	0.11	0.23	0.01	0.11	0.21	0.14	0.16
		% RSD of area – NMT 2.0%	0.22	0.59	1.16	1.38	1.98	1.82	0.76	0.60	1.08	1.43
		USP trailing – NMT 2.0%	0.96	0.96	0.96	1.18	1.00	1.05	0.97	0.98	1.00	0.98
		Theoretical plates – NLT 2000	11848	64502	605348	444840	568747	548653	560753	323485	576336	795612
2	Specificity	No interfer-ence at retention time	Complies									

(Table 2.14) cont.....

S. No.	Parameters	Acceptance criteria	Result Obtained									
			Gallic acid	Caffeic acid	Rutin	Ellagic acid	Isoqu-ercetin	Luteolin 7-0 β glucuronide	Methyl caffate	Rosmarinic Acid	Luteolin	Apigenin
3	Linearity	Correlation coefficient NLT 0.99	1.0000	1.0000	1.0000	1.0000	0.9995	0.9999	1.0000	1.0000	1.0000	1.0000
4	Precision											
4.1	System	%RSD of area – NMT 2%	0.22	0.59	1.16	1.38	1.98	1.82	0.76	0.60	1.08	1.43
4.2	Inter mediate	%RSD of assay – NMT 3%	1.96	0.14	2.51	1.78	2.41	2.09	1.22	1.43	0.81	1.93
4.3	Method	%RSD of assay – NMT 3%	0.90	1.95	0.78	0.71	0.75	2.48	1.00	0.50	1.05	0.87
5	Limit of detection	%RSD of area – NMT 33%	2.43	3.09	3.90	2.83	0.28	2.74	1.20	0.53	1.33	4.34
6	Limit of Quanti-fication	%RSD of area – NMT 10%	0.22	0.59	1.16	1.38	2.04	1.82	0.76	0.60	1.08	1.43
7	Stability of solution after 24hours	Should be stable	Stable									

HPTLC Method Development for Standardization of Tulsi Experiment Methods

Preparation of sample: 1000 mg of sample was dissolved in 10 ml methanol: water (60: 40), sonicated and centrifuged to obtain a clear solution.

Chromatographic conditions: TLC plate: TLC plate with silica gel 60 F_{254}. (10 × 10 cm) (E. Merck, Darmstadt, Germany).

Mobile phase: Toluene: ethyl acetate: formic acid (9: 10:1)

Photo of developed TLC at 254 nm & 366nm is shown in Fig. (**2.15**) and overlay chromatogram of Sample & Standard at 280nm is shown in Fig. (**2.16**).

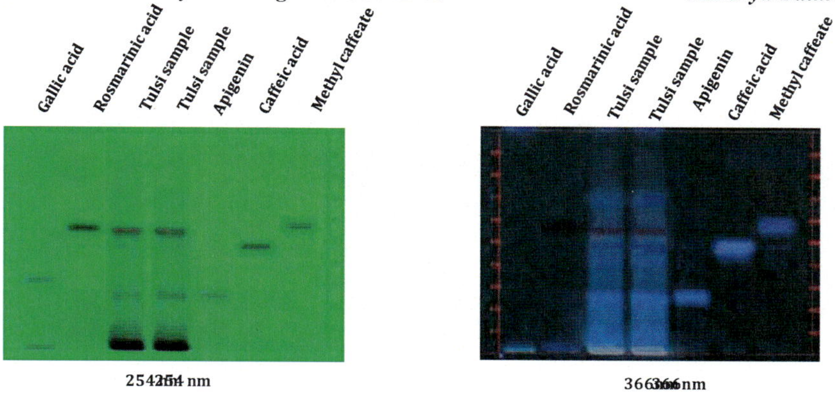

Fig. (2.15). HPTLC fingerprint of Tulsi. Track 1. Gallic acid, 2. Rosmarinic acid, 3 and 4. Tulsi sample, 5. Apigenin, 6. Caffeic acid, 7. Methyl caffeate.

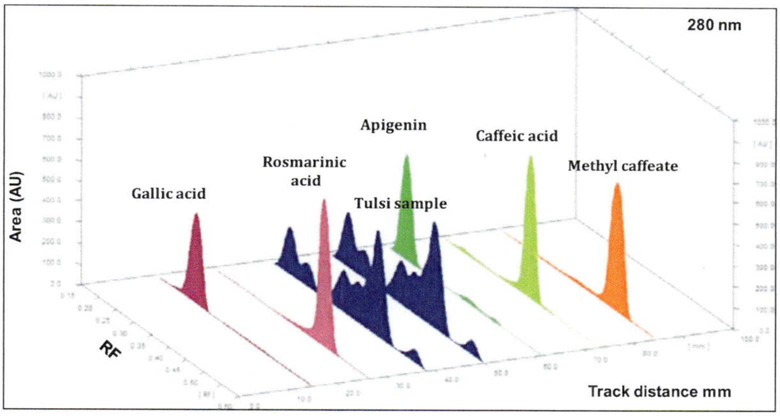

Fig. (2.16). Overlay chromatogram of Sample and Standard at 280 nm.

HPTLC Method Validation for Standardization of Tulsi Linearity for Rosmarinic Acid

A.1: Photo of developed TLC plate at 366 nm (Fig. **2.17**).

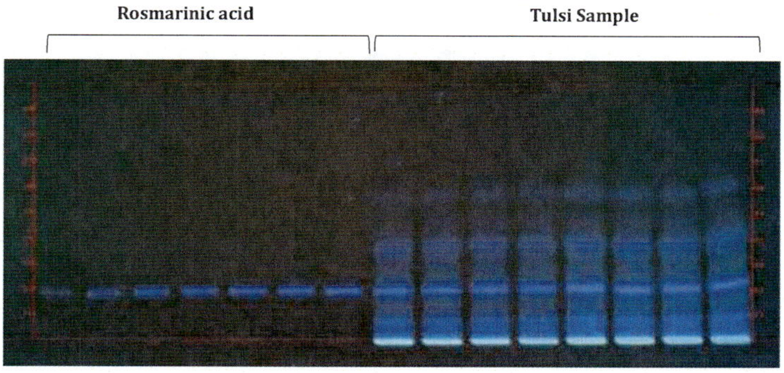

Fig. (2.17). Spotting of standard and sample for linearity study.

A.2 Calibration curve of Rosmarinic acid in Tulsi (Fig. **2.18**).

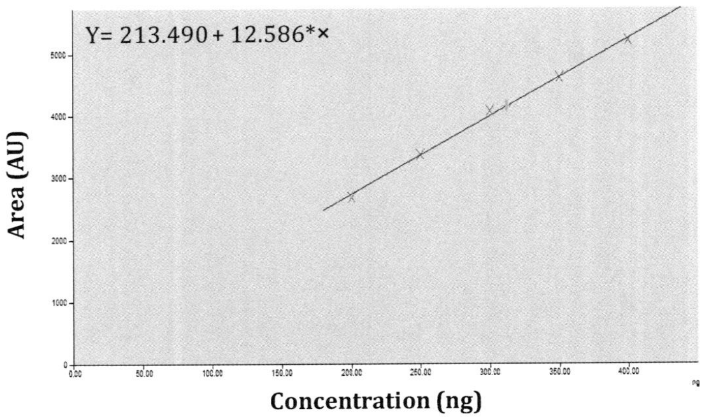

Fig. (2.18). Calibration curve Rosmarinic acid in Tulsi.

A.3 Chromatogram at 330 nm of Rosmarinic acid standard and Tulsi extract is shown in Fig. (**2.19**)

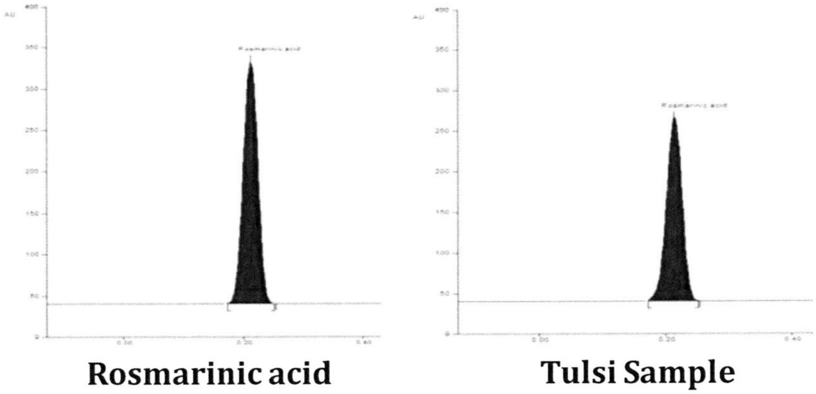

Fig. (2.19). Chromatogram of Rosmarinic acid and Tulsi at 330 nm.

B. Linearity of Luteolin 7- O-β-Glucuronide

B.1 Image of developed TLC plate for linearity study of Lute-line 7-0 Beta Glucoronide at 254 nm is shown in Fig. (**2.20**).

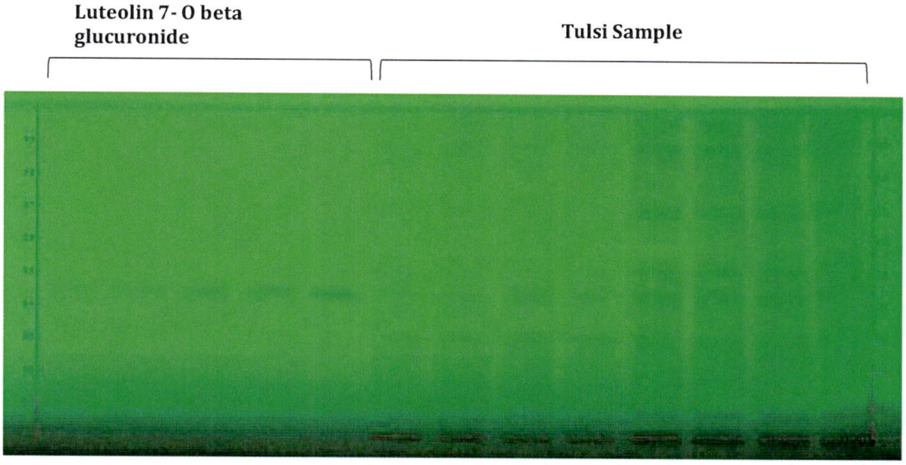

Fig. (2.20). Representative image of linearity study of Tulsi extract with standard Luteolin 7-O-β-Glucuronide.

B.2 Calibration curve of Luteloin 7- O-β-Glucuronide is shown in Fig. (**2.21**) and this is used to determine the amount of the compound in the Tulsi extract.

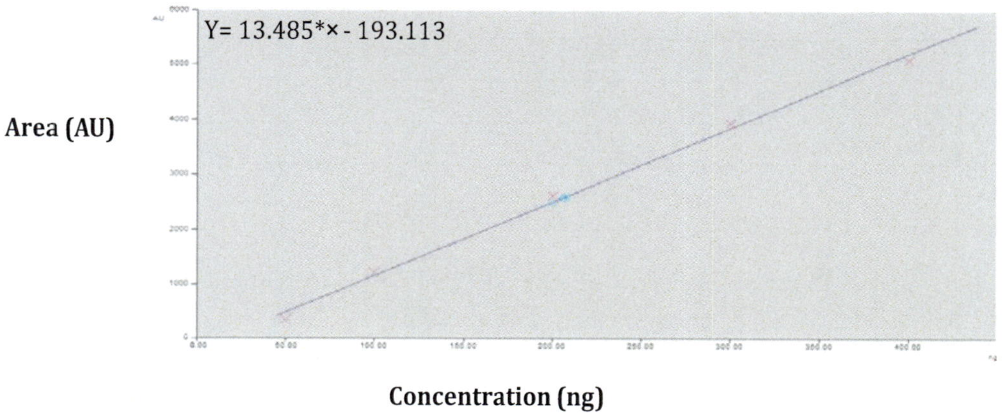

Fig. (2.21). Calibration curve of Luteolin 7- O-β -Glucuronide at 330 nm using HPTLC.

B.3 Chromatogram of standard Luteoline 7-O-β-Glucuronide and a sample of Tulsi extract at 330 nm is shown in Fig. (**2.22**).

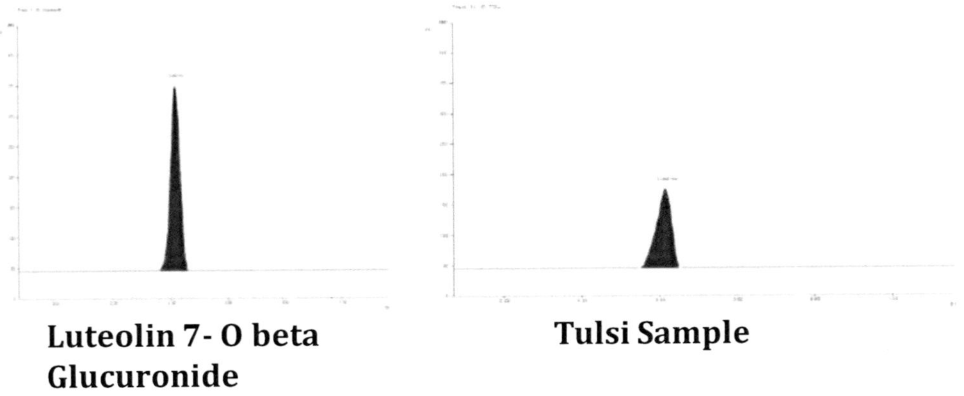

Fig. (2.22). Chromatogram of the standard and Tulsi extract using HPTLC at 330 nm.

C: Limit of detection (LOD), limit of quantification (LOQ), precision and recovery of Rosmarinic acid and Luteolin 7- O-β-Glucuronide is shown in Table **2.15**.

Table 2.15. Validation parameters used for method precision and a representative result obtained.

S. No.	**Parameter**	**Rosmarinic Acid**	**Luteline 7-O-β-Glucuronide**
1.	LOD (ng/spot)	0.40	1.11
2.	LOQ (ng/spot)	1.21	3.36
3.	Intra day precision (% RSD)	0.56	0.42
4.	Inter day precision (% RSD)	1.26	0.80
5.	Recovery (mean%)	94.23	98.18

D: Amount of phytoconstituents present in Tusli extract

The amount of Rosmarinic acid and Luteline 7-O-β-Glucuronide determined using the standard curve is shown in Table **2.16**.

Table 2.16. Amount of Rosmarinic acid and Luteline 7-O-β-Glucuronide in Tulsi extract.

S. No.	**Marker**	**Content (%w/w)**
1.	Rosmarinic acid	0.18%
2.	Luteolin 7- O-β-glucuronide	0.12%

Chemical Characterization of Ashwagandha

The sample of Ashwagandha used in Coronil consists of dried mature roots of *Withania somnifera* (API, Part-I, Volume-I, 2016) (Family Solanaceae), a perennial shrub, found in wastelands, cultivated fields and open grounds throughout India (Fig. **2.23**).

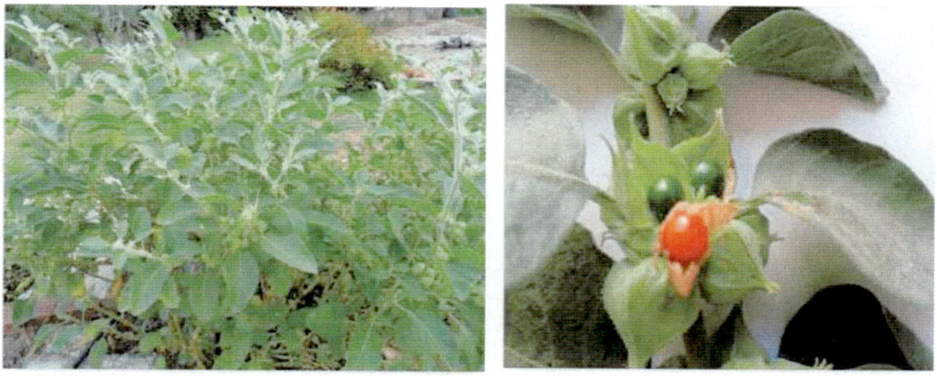

Fig. (2.23). Whole plant flower and fruit of *Withania somnifera* (Ashwagandha).

Roots are collected in winter, washed and cut into short pieces. The ancient Sanskrit Ayurvedic text like *Charak Samhita, Rigveda,* written about 5000 BC to 6000 BC, had references to Ashwagandha. The holy text from *Dhanvantari Nighantu* – written in 1000 AD (Fig. **2.24**) and *Raj Nighantu* – 1400 AD (Fig. **2.25**) had references to Ashwagandha.

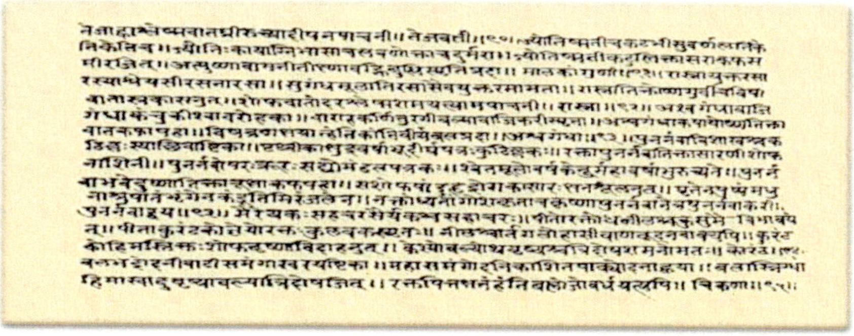

Fig. (2.24). Holy text about Ashwagandha in *Dhanvantari Nighantu* – 1000 AD.

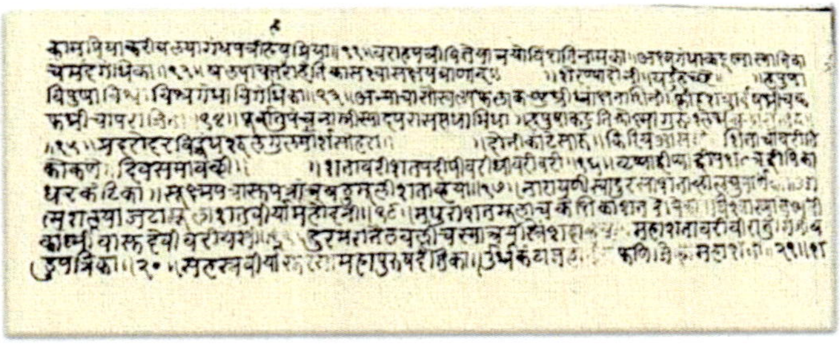

Fig. (2.25). Holy text about Ashwagandha in *Raj Nighantu* – 1400 AD.

The positive identification of Ashwagandha was authenticated by experts in the certified institutions designated by the Government of India, such as CSIR – National Institute of Science Communication and Information Resources, Ministry of Science and Technology, Govt. of India. The authentication certificate is shown in Fig. **(2.26)**, Appendix 2.1.

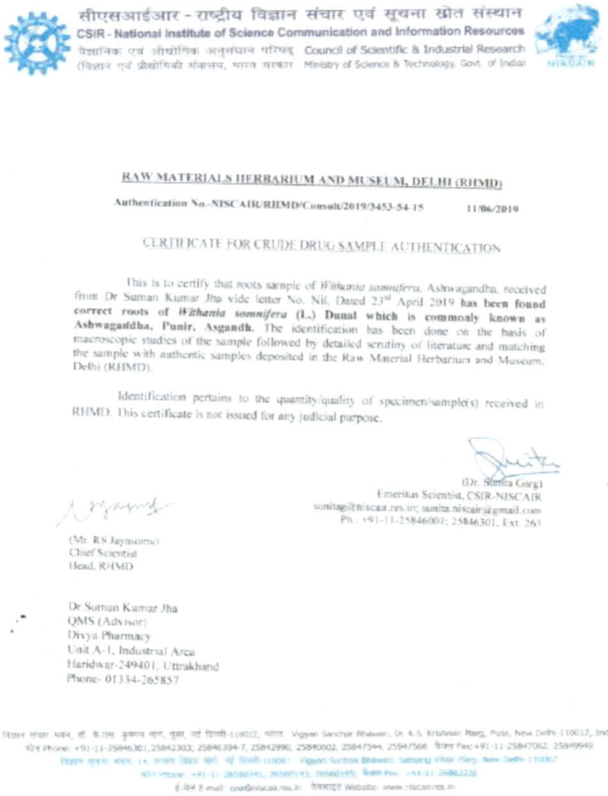

सीएसआईआर - राष्ट्रीय विज्ञान संचार एवं सूचना स्रोत संस्थान
CSIR - National Institute of Science Communication and Information Resources
वैज्ञानिक एवं औद्योगिक अनुसंधान परिषद् Council of Scientific & Industrial Research
(विज्ञान एवं प्रौद्योगिकी मंत्रालय, भारत सरकार Ministry of Science & Technology, Govt. of India)

RAW MATERIALS HERBARIUM AND MUSEUM, DELHI (RHMD)

Authentication No.-NISCAIR/RHMD/Consult/2019/3453-54-15 **11/06/2019**

CERTIFICATE FOR CRUDE DRUG SAMPLE AUTHENTICATION

This is to certify that roots sample of *Withania somnifera*, Ashwagandha, received from Dr Suman Kumar Jha vide letter No. Nil, Dated 23rd April 2019 **has been found correct roots of *Withania somnifera* (L.) Dunal which is commoaly known as Ashwagaddha, Punir, Asgandh.** The identification has been done on the basis of macroscopic studies of the sample followed by detailed scrutiny of literature and matching the sample with authentic samples deposited in the Raw Material Herbarium and Museum, Delhi (RHMD).

Identification pertains to the quantity/quality of specimen/sample(s) received in RHMD. This certificate is not issued for any judicial purpose.

(Dr. Sunita Garg)
Emeritus Scientist, CSIR-NISCAIR
sunitag@niscair.res.in; sunita.niscair@gmail.com
Ph.: +91-11-25846001; 25846301, Ext. 263

(Mr. RS Jaysumu)
Chief Scientist
Head, RHMD

Dr Suman Kumar Jha
QMS (Advisor)
Divya Pharmacy
Unit A-1, Industrial Area
Haridwar-249401, Uttrakhand
Phone- 01334-265857

Vigyan Sanchar Bhawan, Dr. K.S. Krishnan Marg, Pusa, New Delhi-110012, India
Phone: +91-11-25846301 ...
E-mail: coa@niscair.res.in Website: www.niscair.res.in

Fig. (2.26). Authentication certificate of Ashwagandha from CSIR-NISCAIR.

UPLC/QToF MS study of Ashwagandha

Sample Preparation Method: 10 ml methanol was added in about 50.0 mg of Ashwagandha sample and sonicated for 30 min. Then this solution was centrifuged for 5 min at 8000 rpm and filtered through a 0.22 µm nylon filter. The filtered solution was further diluted to 2 times with the same solvent and used for analysis.

UPLC/QToF MS Condition: Analysis was performed on a Xevo G2-XS QToF of Waters with Acquity UPLC- I Class and Unifi software. Separation was carried out using Acquity UPLC HSS -T3 column (100 x 2.1 mm, 1.7 µm). The column was maintained at 40°C throughout the analysis and sample temperature was kept at 20°C during the analysis. Detection was carried out by Xevo G2-XS QToF. The elution was carried out at a flow rate of 0.4 ml/min using gradient elution Table **2.17** of mobile phase 0.1% formic acid in water (mobile phase A) and 0.1% formic acid in acetonitrile (mobile phase B). 1 µl of test solution was injected during the analysis and chromatogram was recorded. The instrumental conditions for QToF are tabulated in Table **2.18**. The positive and negative mode chromatograms are shown in Fig. **(2.27)** and 2.28 respectively. The compounds identified in the Aswagandha samples were listed in Table **2.19**.

Table 2.17. Gradient elution program of mobile phase used in UPLC/QToF MS.

Time (min)	Flow (ml/min)	Mobile Phase A (%)	Mobile Phase B (%)
0	0.4	90	10
10	0.4	90	10
25	0.4	80	20
40	0.4	75	25
45	0.4	75	25
60	0.4	50	50
70	0.4	25	75
71	0.4	90	10
75	0.4	90	10

Table 2.18. List of parameters used in UPLC/QToF MS for identification of phytoconstituents.

Parameter	Polarity (+ve)	Polarity (-ve)
Ionization type	ESI	ESI
Mode	MS^E	MS^E
Acquisition time	65 min	65 min
Mass range (m/z)	50-1000 m/z	50-1000 m/z

(Table 2.18) cont.....

Parameter	**Polarity (+ve)**	**Polarity (-ve)**
Cone Voltage	40 V	40 V
Capillary	1 kV	2 kV
Low CE	6.0 eV	6.0 eV
High CE	15-40 eV (ramp)	15-40 eV(ramp)
Source temperature	120 °C	120 °C
Desolvation Temperature	500 °C	500 °C
Cone gas flow	50 L/h	50 L/h
Desolvation gas flow	900 L/h	900 L/h
Lock Spray (Leucine Enkaphalin)	556.2766 m/z	554.2620 m/z

Table 2.19. Compounds identified compounds in Ashwagandha extract using UPLC/QToF MS in positive and negative mode.

Positive Mode							
S. No.	**Component Name**	**Formula**	**RT (min)**	**Observed m/z**	**Neutral Mass (Da)**	**Response**	**Adducts**
1	Pseudotropine	$C_8H_{15}NO$	0.62	142.1227	141.1154	839740	+H
2	Quercetin-3- rhamnogentiobioside	$^{C}33^{H}40^{O}21$	9.64	773.2124	772.2062	155969	+H, +Na
3	Kaempferol-3-rutinoside- 7-glucoside	$^{C}33^{H}40^{O}20$	13.56	757.2169	756.2113	165110	+H, +Na
4	3-O-Feruloylquinic acid	$^{C}17^{H}20^{O}9$	14.00	391.0992	368.1107	42451	+Na, +H
6	Quercetin 3-O- robinobioside	$^{C}27^{H}30^{O}16$	21.51	611.1598	610.1534	147736	+H, +Na
7	3,5,7,2′, 6′-Hydroxy- flavone 5-2- -O-β-D- glucopyranoside	$^{C}21^{H}20^{O}12$	21.63	465.1021	464.0955	232414	+H
8	Rutin	$^{C}27^{H}30^{O}16$	22.16	611.1609	610.1534	286817	+H, +Na
9	Kaempferol 3-O-α-L- rhamnopyranosyl-(1→2)- β-- -glucopyranoside	$^{C}27^{H}30^{O}15$	23.60	595.1648	594.1585	124853	+H, +Na
10	Nicotiflorin	$^{C}27^{H}30^{O}15$	25.12	595.1653	594.1585	171903	+H, +Na
11	Astragalin	$^{C}21^{H}20^{O}11$	25.54	449.1072	448.1006	247652	+H, +Na
12	N-trans-Coumaroyltaramine	$^{C}17^{H}17^{NO}3$	28.78	284.1277	283.1208	131731	+H, +Na
13	N-feruloyltyramine	$^{C}18^{H}19^{NO}4$	30.82	314.1389	313.1314	3286237	+H, +Na
14	Quercetin	$^{C}15^{H}10^{O}7$	33.67	303.0498	302.0427	182096	+H
15	WithanosideVIII	$^{C}46^{H}72^{O}20$	37.39	967.4544	944.4617	614094	+Na, +H
16	Withanoside X	$^{C}40^{H}62^{O}15$	40.15	805.3975	782.4089	253679	+Na, +H
17	Cannabisin F	$^{C}36^{H}36^{N}2^{O}8$	40.94	625.2550	624.2472	1501958	+H, +Na

(Table 2.19) cont.....

18	2,3-Dihydrowithanolide E	$C_{28}H_{40}O_{7}$	43.28	489.2862	488.2774	5329781	+H, +Na
19	3-HDH-withanolide F	$C_{28}H_{40}O_{7}$	44.09	489.2854	488.2774	1512944	+H, +Na
20	(3β)-26-(β-D-Glucopyranosyloxy)-22-methoxyfurost-5-en-3-yl β-D-glucopyranoside	$C_{40}H_{66}O_{14}$	44.50	793.4366	770.4453	1330171	+Na, +H
21	Sitoindoside IX	$C_{34}H_{48}O_{11}$	44.55	655.3100	632.3197	358841	+Na
22	Viscosalactone B	$C_{28}H_{40}O_{7}$	44.98	489.2859	488.2774	11303149	+H, +Na
23	Withanoside IV	$C_{40}H_{62}O_{15}$	45.81	805.3988	782.4089	2081485	+Na, +H
24	Withastramonolide	$C_{28}H_{38}O_{7}$	46.53	487.2680	486.2618	103723	+H, +Na
25	Withafastuosin E	$C_{28}H_{40}O_{7}$	47.57	489.2848	488.2774	404687	+H, +Na
26	Withanoside VI	$C_{40}H_{62}O_{15}$	48.11	783.4170	782.4089	136625	+H, +Na
27	Physagulin D	$C_{34}H_{52}O_{10}$	48.92	643.3465	620.3561	327835	+Na, +H
28	2,3-didehydrosomniferícin	$C_{28}H_{40}O_{7}$	49.52	489.2848	488.2774	565497	+H, +Na
29	Coagulin Q	$C_{34}H_{52}O_{10}$	49.82	643.3467	620.3561	453312	+Na, +H
30	3α,6α-epoxy-4β,5β,27- trihydroxy-1- oxowitha- 24-enolide	$C_{28}H_{40}O_{7}$	50.02	489.2848	488.2774	706807	+H, +Na
31	2,3-Dihydrowithaferin-A	$C_{28}H_{40}O_{6}$	50.65	473.2902	472.2825	683870	+H, +Na
32	Viscosalactone A	$C_{28}H_{40}O_{6}$	51.82	473.2908	472.2825	1193666	+H, +Na
33	Withaferin A	$C_{28}H_{38}O_{6}$	52.22	471.2750	470.2668	2756345	+H, +Na
34	Grossamide	$C_{36}H_{36}N_{2}O_{8}$	52.73	625.2572	624.2472	2211645	+H, +Na
35	Quresimine A	$C_{29}H_{42}O_{7}$	52.96	503.3008	502.2931	1415363	+H, +Na
36	Grossamide_1	$C_{36}H_{36}N_{2}O_{8}$	53.04	625.2561	624.2472	1817455	+H
37	Withanoside V	$C_{40}H_{62}O_{14}$	54.09	789.4068	766.4140	1022972	+Na, +H
38	Withanolide A	$C_{28}H_{38}O_{6}$	54.63	493.2562	470.2668	194990	+Na, +H
39	24,25-Dihydrowithanolide D	$C_{28}H_{40}O_{6}$	56.42	473.2895	472.2825	473947	+H, +Na
40	Ashwagandhanolide	$C_{56}H_{78}O_{12}S$	58.20	975.5361	974.5214	3457982	+H, +Na
41	3-(2-O,3-O,4-O-Tribenzoyl- beta--xylopyranosyl)ole- ana-12-ene-28-oic acid ben- zyl ester	$C_{63}H_{74}O_{9}$	60.32	975.5350	974.5333	334974	+H, +Na
42	Withanolide B	$C_{28}H_{38}O_{5}$	60.75	477.2600	454.2719	131970	+Na, +H
Negative mode							
S. No.	**Component Name**	**Formula**	**RT (min)**	**Observed m/z**	**Neutral Mass (Da)**	**Response**	**Adducts**

(Table 2.19) cont.....

1	Gallic acid	$C_7H_6O_5$	1.19	169.0131	170.0215	28477	-H
2	Neochlorogenic acid	$^{C}16^{H}18^{O}9$	2.40	353.0863	354.0951	220268	-H
3	Chlorogenic acid	$^{C}16^{H}18^{O}9$	4.80	353.0866	354.0951	298621	-H
4	Cryptochlorogenic acid	$^{C}16^{H}18^{O}9$	5.61	353.0864	354.0951	335340	-H
5	Quercetin-3- rhamnogentiobioside	$^{C}33^{H}40^{O}21$	8.39	771.1980	772.2062	278982	-H, +HCOO
6	Kaempferol-3-rutinoside-7-glucoside	$^{C}33^{H}40^{O}20$	12.57	755.2037	756.2113	364083	-H, +HCOO
7	3-O-Feruloylquinic acid	$^{C}17^{H}20^{O}9$	13.65	367.1016	368.1107	147432	-H
8	3-O-Caffeoylshikimic acid	$^{C}16^{H}16^{O}8$	14.20	335.0753	336.0845	128354	-H
9	Quercetin 3-O-robinobioside	$^{C}27^{H}30^{O}16$	20.96	609.1466	610.1534	599631	-H
10	3,5,7,2′, 6′-Hydroxy- flavone 5-2--O- β-D- glucopyranoside	$^{C}21^{H}20^{O}12$	21.09	463.0875	464.0955	348933	-H, +HCOO
11	Rutin	$^{C}27^{H}30^{O}16$	21.64	609.1466	610.1534	996153	-H
12	Ferulic acid	$^{C}10^{H}10^{O}4$	21.76	193.0501	194.0579	320047	-H
13	Kaempferol 3-O-α-L-rhamnopyranosyl-(1→2)-β- D-glucopyranoside	$^{C}27^{H}30^{O}15$	23.11	593.1510	594.1585	534637	-H
14	Nicotiflorin	$^{C}27^{H}30^{O}15$	24.65	593.1509	594.1585	597617	-H
15	Astragalin	$^{C}21^{H}20^{O}11$	25.06	447.0925	448.1006	541538	-H, +HCOO
16	N-trans-Coumaroyltaramine	$^{C}17^{H}17^{NO}3$			283.1208		
17	N-feruloyltyramine	$^{C}18^{H}19^{NO}4$	30.25	312.1230	313.1314	2220031	-H, +HCOO
18	Quercetin	$^{C}15^{H}10^{O}7$	32.99	301.0339	302.0427	372796	-H
19	Withanoside III	$^{C}34^{H}52^{O}12$	33.31	697.3428	652.3459	22563	+HCOO
20	Luteolin	$^{C}15^{H}10^{O}6$	33.60	285.0386	286.0477	44496	-H
21	WithanosideVIII	$^{C}46^{H}72^{O}20$	36.84	989.4604	944.4617	2721783	+HCOO, -H
22	Withanoside X	$^{C}40^{H}62^{O}15$	39.59	827.4078	782.4089	1162617	+HCOO, -H
23	2,3-dihydro-3β-O-sulfate withaferin A	$^{C}28^{H}40^{O}10$ S	40.08	567.2266	568.2342	339474	-H
24	Cannabisin F	$^{C}36^{H}36^{N}2^{O}8$	40.31	623.2399	624.2472	1227146	-H, +HCOO
25	Kaempferol	$^{C}15^{H}10^{O}6$	41.24	285.0392	286.0477	394319	-H
26	2,3-Dihydrowithanolide E	$^{C}28^{H}40^{O}7$	42.58	533.2758	488.2774	12107888	+HCOO, -H

(Table 2.19) cont.....

27	3-HDH-withanolide F	$C_{28}H_{40}O_{7}$	43.34	533.2758	488.2774	2553359	+HCOO, -H
28	(3β)-26-(β-D-Glucopyranosyloxy)-22-methoxyfurost-5-en-3-yl β-D-glucopyranoside	$C_{40}H_{66}O_{14}$	43.78	815.4446	770.4453	6291180	+HCOO, -H
29	Sitoindoside IX	$C_{34}H_{48}O_{11}$	43.80	677.3182	632.3197	320001	+HCOO
30	Viscosalactone B	$C_{28}H_{40}O_{7}$	44.15	533.2762	488.2774	7927228	+HCOO, -H
31	Withanoside IV	$C_{40}H_{62}O_{15}$	44.98	827.4080	782.4089	16192332	+HCOO, -H
32	Withafastuosin E	$C_{28}H_{40}O_{7}$	45.73	531.2590	488.2774	221155	+HCOO, -H
33	Withafastuosin E	$C_{28}H_{40}O_{7}$	47.01	533.2753	488.2774	1071488	+HCOO
34	Withanoside VI	$C_{40}H_{62}O_{15}$	47.73	827.4077	782.4089	2132193	+HCOO, -H
35	Physagulin D	$C_{34}H_{52}O_{10}$	48.61	665.3549	620.3561	3423523	+HCOO, -H
36	2,3-didehydrosomnifericin	$C_{28}H_{40}O_{7}$	49.18	533.2750	488.2774	668927	+HCOO, -H
37	Coagulin Q	$C_{34}H_{52}O_{10}$	49.58	665.3538	620.3561	770004	+HCOO
38	3α,6α-epoxy-4β,5β,27- trihydroxy-1-oxowitha-24-enolide	$C_{28}H_{40}O_{7}$	49.73	533.2751	488.2774	1673972	+HCOO, -H
39	Viscosalactone A	$C_{28}H_{40}O_{6}$	51.59	517.2802	472.2825	1743987	+HCOO, -H
40	Withaferin A	$C_{28}H_{38}O_{6}$	52.40	469.2587	470.2668	288455	-H, +HCOO
41	Grossamide	$C_{36}H_{36}N_{2}O_{8}$	52.54	623.2407	624.2472	3396672	-H
42	Grossamide_1	$C_{36}H_{36}N_{2}O_{8}$	52.86	623.2407	624.2472	3702192	-H, +HCOO
43	Withanoside V	$C_{40}H_{62}O_{14}$	53.98	811.4134	766.4140	5559586	+HCOO, -H
44	Withanolide A	$C_{28}H_{38}O_{6}$	54.76	469.2577	470.2668	60500	-H
45	24,25-Dihydrowithanolide D	$C_{28}H_{40}O_{6}$	56.29	517.2800	472.2825	1085658	+HCOO, -H
46	Withanolide D	$C_{28}H_{38}O_{6}$	57.22	515.2645	470.2668	946054	+HCOO, -H
47	Ashwagandhanolide	$C_{56}H_{78}O_{12}S$	58.13	973.5137	974.5214	3864234	-H

(Table 2.19) cont.....

48	3-(2-O,3-O,4-O-Tribenzoyl- beta-D-xylopyranosyl)oleana- 12-ene- 28-oic acid ben-zyl ester	$C_{63}H_{74}O_{9}$	60.25	973.5156	974.5333	561295	-H

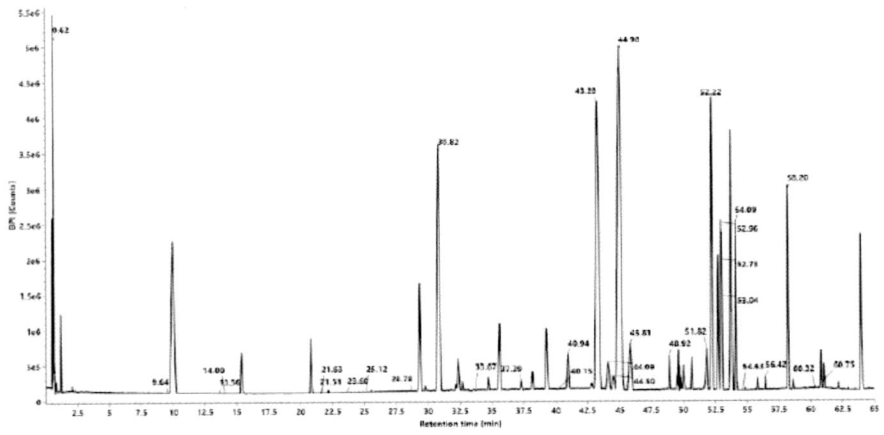

Fig. (2.27). Chromatogram of Ashwagandha extract in positive mode using UPLC/QToF MS.

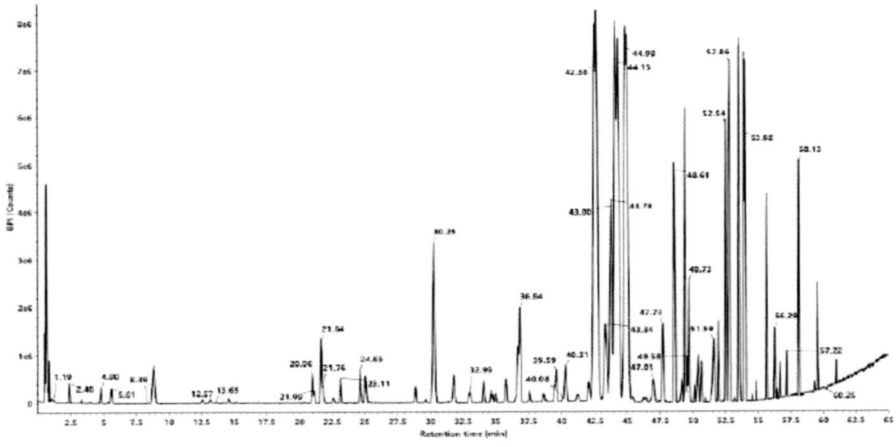

Fig. (2.28). Chromatogram of Ashwagandha extract in negative mode using UPLC/QToF MS.

Conclusion:

A total of 53 different phytoconstituents were identified in the Ashwagandha extract. Like in the case of Tulsi, some of these phytoconstituents were detected in both positive and negative modes and, therefore, they were counted once.

HPLC-PDA Method Development for Standardization of Ashwagandha Extract

Experiment Methods: The quantification of marker compounds was performed by HPLC (Prominence-i LC-2030c 3D Plus, Shimadzu, Japan). Separation was achieved using a Shodex C18-4E (4.6mm ID x 250 mm L) column subjected to binary gradient elution Table **2.20**. The elution was carried out at a flow rate of 1.5 ml/min using mobile phase A (0.14 g KH_2PO_4 was dissolved in 900 ml of water, 0.5 ml H_3PO_4 was added in this solution and made up to 1000 ml with water) and mobile phase B (Acetonitrile). The column temperature was kept at 27.0°C during the analysis. 10 µl of test solution was injected during the analysis and recorded the chromatograph at 227 nm wavelength.

Table 2.20. Details of gradient program used for HPLC method standardization for Ashwagandha.

Time (min)	Flow (ml/min)	A %	B%
0	1.5 ml/min	90	10
18	1.5 ml/min	70	30
23	1.5 ml/min	65	35
30	1.5 ml/min	65	35
35	1.5 ml/min	60	40
40	1.5 ml/min	50	50
45	1.5 ml/min	30	70
50	1.5 ml/min	20	80
51	1.5 ml/min	90	10
55	1.5 ml/min	90	10

Sample Preparation Method: About 1 gm of powdered sample was diluted with 25 ml methanol sonicated for 30 min. This solution was centrifuged at 10000 rpm for 5 min and filtered using a 0.45µm nylon filter and used for the analysis. A typical HPLC chromatogram of the sample is shown in Fig. **(2.29)**.

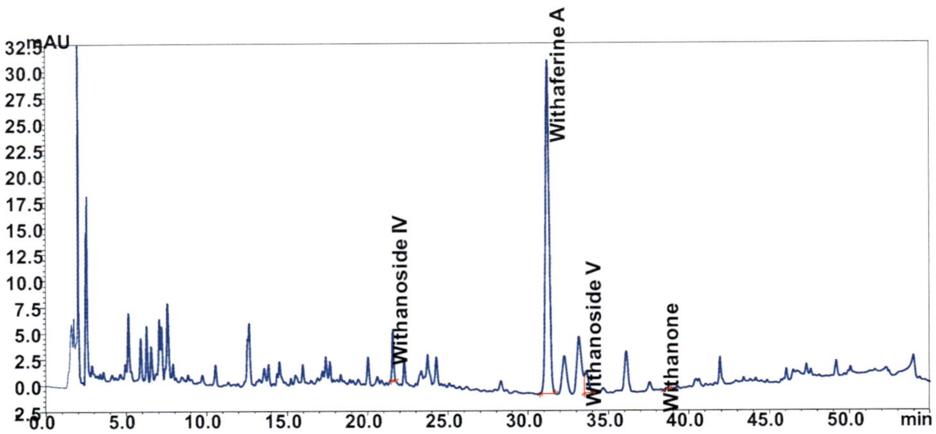

Fig. (2.29). Representative HPLC Chromatogram of Ashwagandha extract sample.

Standard Stock Solution

Standard Stock Solution: Standards Withanone (Potency-93.6%, Natural remedies), Withaferin A (Potency-98.0%, Natural remedies), Withanoside IV (Potency-96.2%, Natural remedies), Withanoside V (Potency-97.6%), Withanolide A (Potency-97.4%, Sigma Aldrich) and Withanolide B (Potency-96.31%, Tokyo chemical industries) and Betulinic acid (Potency-98.7%, Natural remedies) were dissolved in methanol to prepare 1000 ppm standard solution individually.

Standard Mix Working Standard: Take 0.05 ml of 1000 ppm from each standard stock solution and diluted it to 1 ml to prepare 50 ppm of standard mix working standard. A typical HPLC chromatogram of the standard is shown in Fig. **(2.30)**.

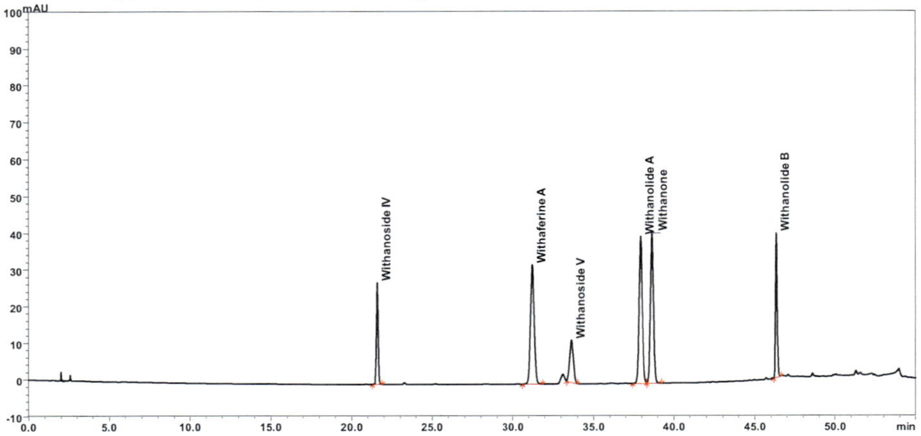

Fig. (2.30). Representative HPLC Chromatogram of mixed standards.

The amount of different phytoconstituents identified in Ashwagandha extract by HPLC using the standardized elution method is shown in Table **2.21**.

Table 2.21. Quantification of the different phytoconstituents in Ashwagandha extract using HPLC.

S. No.	Name of Marker Compound	Result in µg/mg
1	Withanoside IV	2.45
2	Withaferin A	12.27
3	Withanoside V	2.03
4	Withanone	0.04

HPLC-PDA Method Validation for Standardization of Ashwagandha Extracts

The analytical method used for quantification of actives present in Ashwagandha are validated as per ICH Q2R1 and a summary of method validation is shown in Table **2.22**.

Table 2.22. Summary of HPLC method Validation of Ashwagandha.

S. No.	Parameters	Acceptance Criteria	Result obtained					
			Withanoside IV	**Witha-ferine A**	**Withanoside V**	**Withanolide A**	**Withanone**	**Withanolide B**
1	System Suitability	% RSD of Retention time - NMT 2.0%	0.08	0.10	0.14	0.09	0.09	0.03
		% RSD of area – NMT 2.0%	1.72	1.24	0.56	0.89	1.12	1.33
		USP trailing – NMT 2.0%	1.08	1.06	1.06	1.03	1.06	1.21
		Theoretical plates – NLT 2000	165425	84156	99447	159697	189940	848596
2	Specificity	No interfere-ence at retention time of standard	Complies					
3	Linearity	Correlation coefficient NLT 0.99	0.9996	0.9994	0.9993	0.9994	0.9994	0.9993
4	**Precision**							

(Table 2.22) cont.....

S. No.	Parameters	Acceptance Criteria	Result obtained					
			Withano-side IV	Witha-ferine A	Withano-side V	Withano-lide A	Witha-none	Withan-olide B
4.1	System	RSD of area – NMT 2%	1.72	1.24	0.56	0.89	1.12	1.33
4.2	Intermediate	RSD of assay – NMT 2%	0.71	0.58	0.64	BDL	4.38	BDL
4.3	Method	RSD of assay – NMT 2%	0.25	0.84	1.04	BDL	3.57	BDL
5	Limit of detec tion	RSD of area – NMT 33%	2.51	2.70	2.57	1.26	1.46	1.71
6	Limit of Quantification	RSD of area – NMT 10%	1.51	1.47	0.76	1.39	1.23	1.25
7	Stability of solution 24hrs	Stable						

HPTLC Method Development for Standardization of Ashwagandha

Experiment Methods

Preparation of standard solution: The stock solution was prepared by dissolving 10 mg of each standard in 10 ml methanol and further 0.1 ml from stock solution diluted to 1 ml for making concentration 100 ppm.

Preparation of sample solution: 1 g of sample was dissolved in 10 ml methanol, sonicated for 20 minutes and centrifuged to obtain a clear solution.

Chromatographic Conditions

TLC plate: TLC plate with silica gel 60 F_{254}.

Mobile Phase

1. Toluene: ethyl acetate: formic acid (5: 5: 1) - for Withanone, Withaferin-A, Withanolide-A and Withanolide-B.

2. Ethyl acetate: formic acid: acetic acid: water (10: 1.1: 1.1: 2.6) - for Withanoside- IV and Withanoside-V.

HPTLC fingerprint of sample and standard is shown in Fig. **(2.31)**

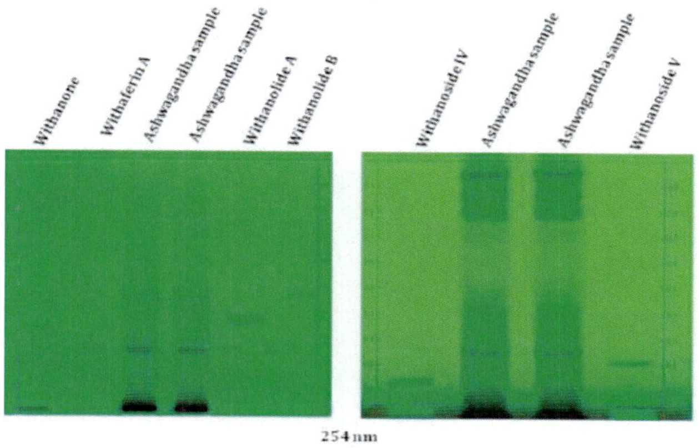

Fig. (2.31). Representative image of developed TLC at 254 nm Track 1. Withanone, 2. Withaferin-A, 3 and 4. Ashwagandha extract, 5. Withanolide-A, 6. Withanolide-B, 7. Withanoside-IV, 8 and 9. Ashwagandha extract, 10. Withanoside-V.

HPTLC Method Validation for Standardization of Ashwagandha Extract

A: Linearity determination - Linearity of Withanone is shown in Fig. **(2.32)** and correlation is shown in Table **2.23**.

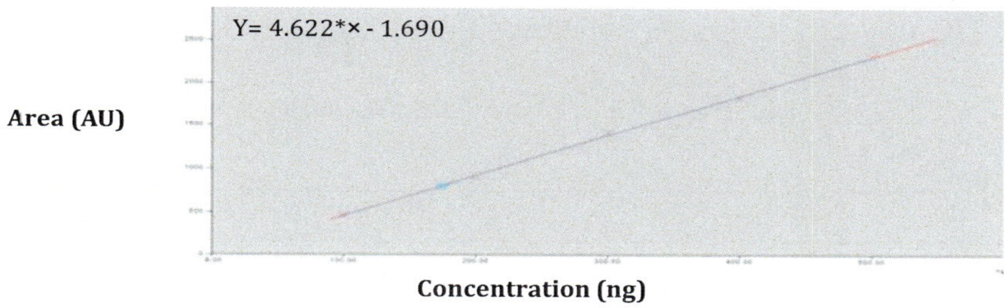

Fig. (2.32). Linearity curve of Withanone.

Table 2.23. Linearity correlation of Withanone using HPTLC.

Parameter	Withanone
Linearity range (ng)	100 – 500
Regression equation	4.622 *X – 1.690
Correlation coefficient	0.999

A.1 Detection of Withanone using HPTLC at 230 nm is shown in Fig. (**2.33**).

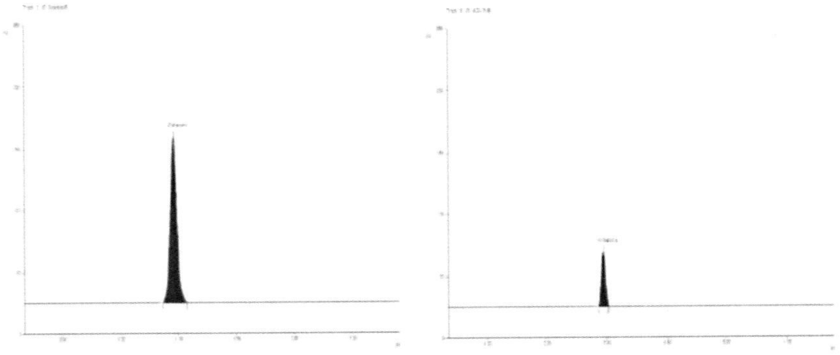

Withanone **Ashwagandha Sample**

Fig. (2.33). Chromatogram of Withanone standard and Ashwagandha extract sample at 230 nm as determined by HPTLC.

A.2 Limit of Detection and Limit of Quantification using the standardized method for HPTLC

The standardized method was used to identify the detection limit for Withanone using HPTLC. The identified limits for the method is shown in Table **2.24**.

Table 2.24. Limit of Detection and Quantification using the standardized HPTLC method for Withanone.

LOD	0.15 ng/spot
LOQ	0.44 ng/spot

A.3 Determination of method precision for Withanone identification using HPTLC

The variations seen in different extracts of Withanone using the standardized method were determined to ensure reproducibility of method is shown in Table **2.25**.

Table 2.25. Method precision to ensure reproducibility.

Precision	**% RSD**
Intraday	0.84%
Interday	0.64%

A.4 Percentage recovery of Withanone from Ashwagandha extract using HPTLC is shown in Table **2.26**.

Table 2.26. Recovery of Withanone from a representative batch of Ashwagandha extracts using the standardized method in HPTLC.

Recovery level	% Recovery	Mean Recovery %
80%	101.97%	96.23%
100%	94.99%	
120%	91.72%	

Result: Using the above-mentioned methods, the amount of Withanone was found to be 0.038% w/w in Ashwagandha extract.

B Determination of linearity of Withaferin A is shown in Fig. (**2.34**).

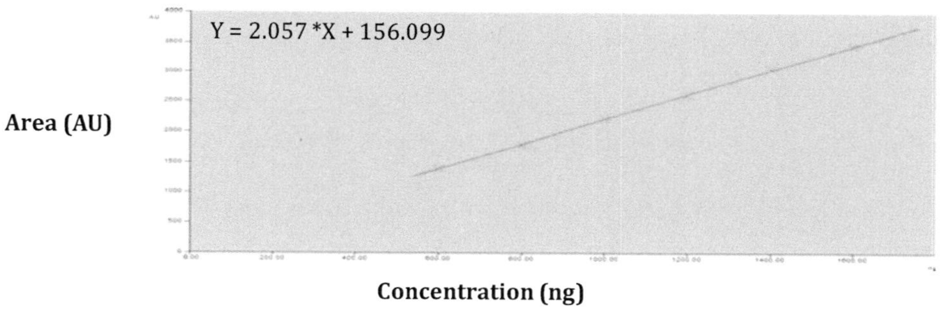

Fig. (2.34). Linearity curve of standard Withaferin A.

The linearity of different concentrations of Withaferin A using the standardized method for HPTLC was determined using the regression equation shown in Table **2.27**.

Table 2.27. Linearity correlation of Withaferin A using HPTLC.

Parameter	Withaferin A
Linearity range (ng)	600 – 1600
Regression equation	2.057 *X + 156.099
Correlation coefficient	0.999

B.1 Detection of Withaferin A at 230 nm using HPTLC is shown in Fig. (**2.35**).

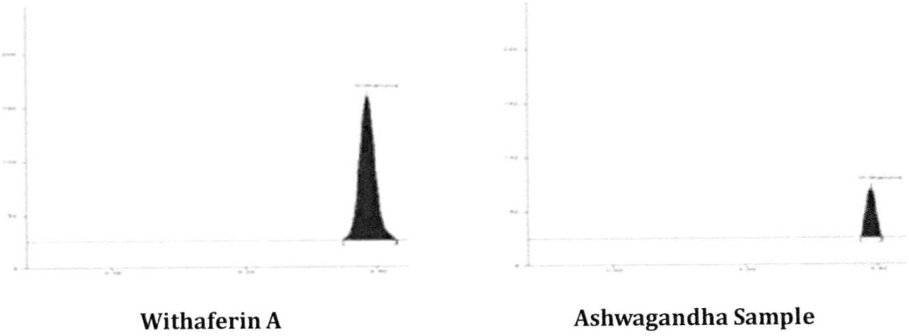

Fig. (2.35). Representative chromatogram of Withaferin A standard and a sample of Ashwagandha at 230 nm using HPTLC.

B.2 Limit of detection and limit of quantification using the standardized method for HPTLC

The limit of detection and quantitation of Withaferin A using the standardized method for HPTLC was quantified. The results obtained are shown in Table **2.28**.

Table 2.28. Limit of detection and quantification for Withaferin A using HPTLC method.

LOD	0.14 ng/spot
LOQ	0.41 ng/spot

B.3 Determination of method precision is shown in Table **2.29**

Table 2.29. Precision of the standardized method for detection of Withaferin A for HPTLC.

Precision	**% RSD**
Intraday	1.27%
Interday	1.27%

B.4 Observed recovery of Withaferin A by HPTLC is shown in Table **2.30**

Table 2.30. Percent recovery of Withaferin A using the standardized method for HPTLC.

Recovery Level	% Recovery	Mean Recovery %
80%	91.84%	93.37%
100%	93.96%	
120%	94.30%	

Result: Using the different quantification methods as described above, the amount of Withaferin-A was found to be 0.799% w/w in Ashwagandha extract.

C: Determination of linearity of standard Withanolide A is shown in Fig. **(2.36)**

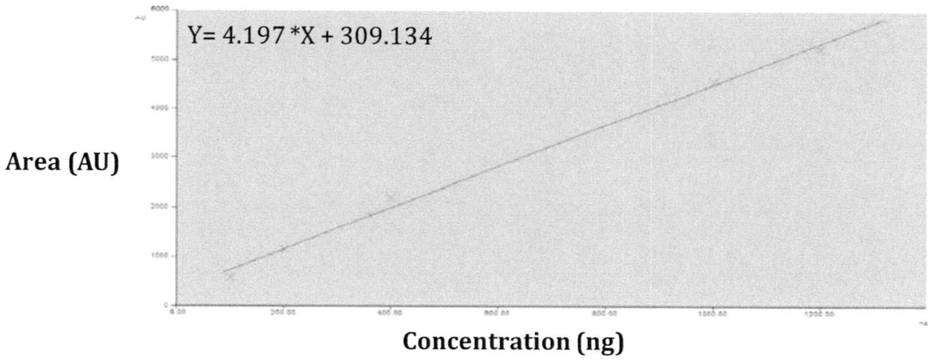

Fig. (2.36). Linearity curve of Withanolide A as determined by HPTLC.

The linearity of the HPTLC method for various concentrations of Withanolide A was determined by the regression equation shown in Table **2.31**.

Table 2.31. Determination of linearity correlation of standardized method used for Withanolide A in HPTLC.

Parameter	Withanolide A
Linearity range (ng)	100 – 1200
Regression equation	4.197 *X + 309.134
Correlation coefficient	0.998

C.1: Detection of Withanolide A at 230 nm using HPTLC is shown in Fig. (**2.37**).

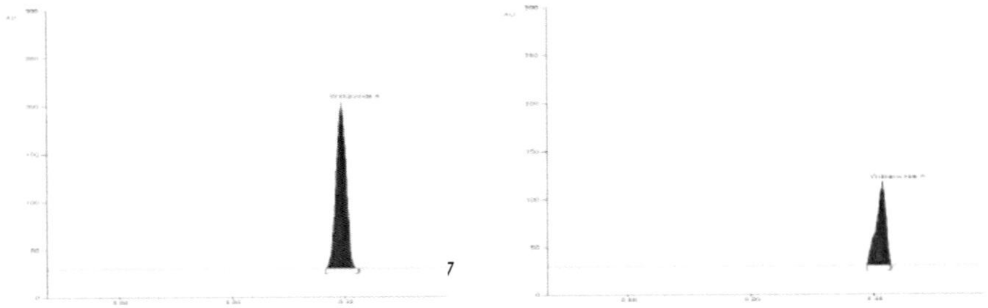

Withanolide A **Ashwagandha sample**

Fig. (2.37). Representative chromatogram of standard Withanolide A and a sample of Ashwagandha extract at 230 nm.

C.2: Limit of detection and limit of quantification of Withanolide A using HPTLC is shown in Table **2.32**.

Table 2.32. Limit of detection and quantification of Withaferin A using the standardized method in HPTLC.

LOD	3.94 ng/spot
LOQ	11.92 g/spot

C.3: Precision of HPTLC method for Withanolide A in HPTLC

The precision of the standardized method in HPTLC for the identification of Withanolide A is shown in Table **2.33**.

Table 2.33. Precision of standardized method for detection of Withanolide A in HPTLC.

Precision	**% RSD**
Intraday	0.69%
Interday	0.88

C.4: Percent recovery of Withanolide A using HPTLC is shown in Table **2.34**

Table 2.34. Recovery percentage of Withanolide A at different cut-off values using the standardized method in HPTLC.

Recovery Level	% Recovery	Mean Recovery %
80%	90.75%	94.32%
100%	96.60%	
120%	95.60%	

Result: The amount of Withanolide A was found to be 0.024% w/w in Ashwagandha extract.

D: Linearity of standard Withanolide B in HPTLC is shown in Fig. **(2.38)**

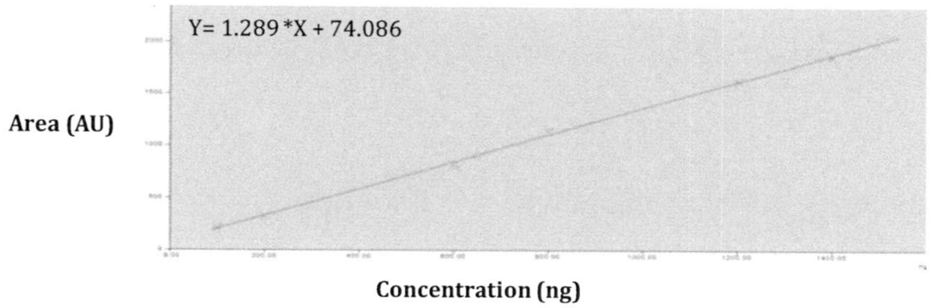

Fig. (2.38). Linearity curve of Withanolide B as determined by HPTLC.

The correlation coefficient of linearity was determined by the regression equation as shown in Table **2.35**.

Table 2.35. Linearity correlation of Withanolide B by HPTLC.

Parameter	Withanolide-B
Linearity range (ng)	100 – 1400
Regression equation	1.289 *X + 74.086
Correlation coefficient	0.999

D.1: Detection of Withanolide B by HPTLC at 230 nm is shown in Fig. (**2.39**)

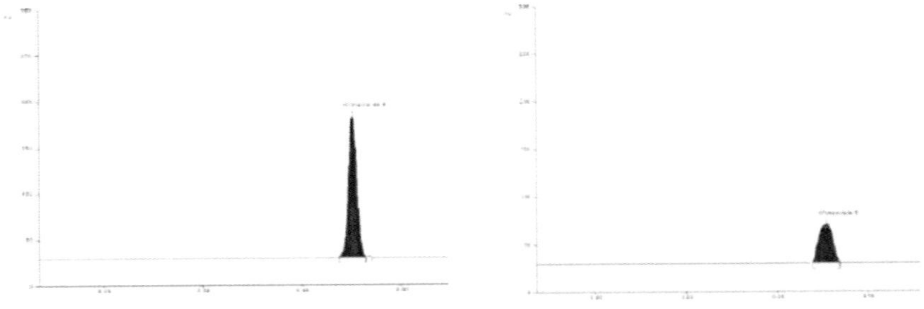

Withanolide B **Ashwagandha sample**

Fig. (2.39). Representative chromatogram of Withanolide B standard and Ashwagandha extract sample.

D.2: Limit of detection and limit of quantification of Withanolide B as determined by HPTLC.

The detection and quantification limits of the standardized method for Withanolide B using HPTLC is shown in Table **2.36**.

Table 2.36. Limits of detection and quantification of Withanolide B using the standardized method for HPTLC.

LOD	1.28 ng/spot
LOQ	3.89 g/spot

D.3: Method precision for detection of Withanolide B using HPTLC.

The precision of the standardized method for detection of Withanolide B was determined in different batches of Ashwagandha extract. The results are shown in Table **2.37**.

Table 2.37. Precision of the standardized HPTLC method in detection of Withanolide B.

Precision	**% RSD**
Intraday	1.08%
Interday	0.94

D.4: Recovery of Withanolide B in HPTLC

The percent recovery of Withanolide B using the standardized method in HPTLC is shown in Table **2.38**.

Table 2.38. Percent recovery of Withanolide B using HPTLC.

Recovery Level	% Recovery	Mean Recovery %
80%	91.88%	93.21%
100%	92.66%	
120%	95.10%	

Result: The amount of Withanolide B was found to be 0.108% w/w in Ashwagandha extract using the different methods mentioned above.

E: Linearity of Withanoside IV standard by HPTLC is shown in Fig. (**2.40**).

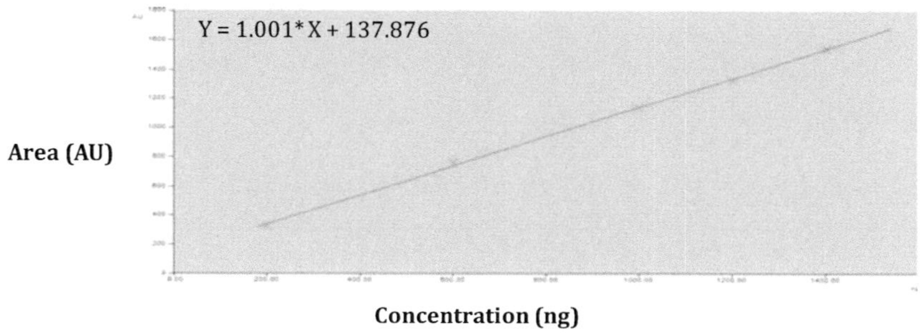

Fig. (2.40). Linearity curve of standard Withanoside IV as determined by HPTLC.

The linearity of the standardized method over different concentrations of Withanoside IV was determined using the regression equation shown in Table **2.39**.

Table 2.39. Linearity correlation of HPTLC method for different concentrations of Withanoside IV.

Parameters	Withanoside IV
Linearity range (ng)	200 – 1400
Regression equation	1.001* X + 137.876
Correlation coefficient	0.999

E.1: Detection of Withanoside IV at 230 nm using HPTLC is shown in Fig. (**2.41**).

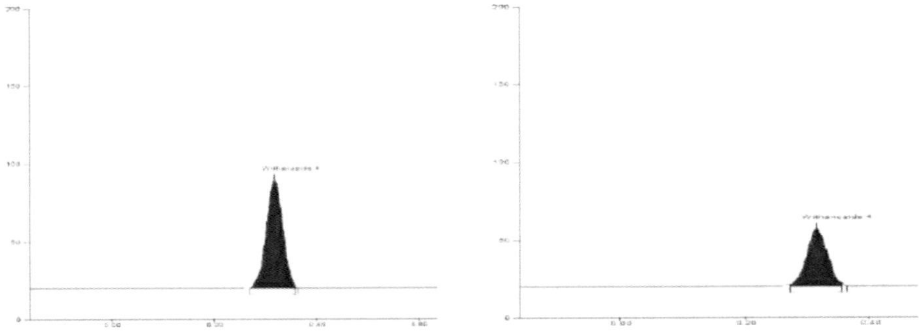

Withanoside IV **Ashwagandha sample**

Fig. (2.41). Representative chromatogram of Withanoside IV standard and Ashwagandha extract sample at 230 nm.

E.2: Limit of Detection and Limit of Quantification of Withanoside IV using HPTLC is shown in Table **2.40**.

Table 2.40. Minimum detection and quantification limits of Withanoside IV by HPTLC.

LOD	0.75 ng/spot
LOQ	2.27 g/spot

E.3: Precision of the standardized HPTLC method for detection of Withanoside IV

The precision of the standardized HPTLC method over different extracts of Ashwagandha was determined to account for reproducibility as shown in Table **2.41**.

Table 2.41. Precision of HPTLC method in detection of Withanoside IV using HPTLC method.

Precision	**% RSD**
Intraday	1.23%
Interday	0.66

E.4: Percent recovery of Withanoside IV using the standardized HPTLC method is shown in Table **2.42**.

Table 2.42. Percent recovery of Withanoside IV at various cut-off values using HPTLC.

Recovery Level	% Recovery	Mean Recovery %
80%	95.31%	94.40%
100%	94.67%	
120%	93.22%	

Result: Using the different methods described above, the amount of Withanoside IV was found to be 0.388% w/w in Ashwagandha extract.

F: Determination of linearity of Withanoside V using HPTLC

The linearity of the standardized method over different concentrations of Withanoside V was determined by HPTLC is shown in Fig. **(2.42)** and the linearity was correlated using the regression equation is shown in Table **2.43**.

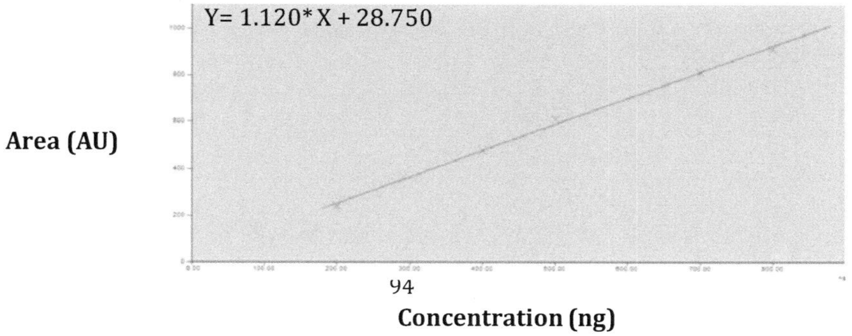

Fig. (2.42). Linearity curve of Withanoside V at different concentrations by HPTLC.

Table 2.43. Linearity correlation at different concentrations of Withanoside V by HPTLC.

Parameter	Withanoside V
Linearity range (ng)	200 – 800
Regression equation	1.120* X + 28.750
Correlation coefficient	0.998

F.1: Detection of Withanoside V at 230 nm by HPTLC is shown in Fig. (**2.43**).

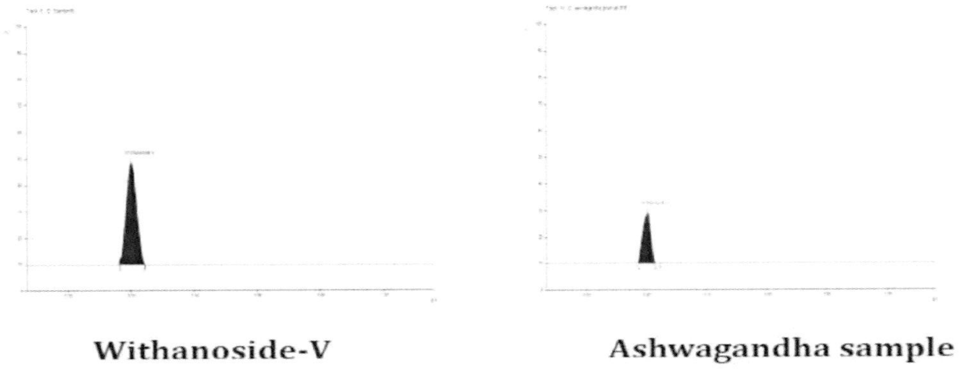

Fig. (2.43). Representative chromatogram of Withanoside V standard and Ashwagandha extract sample at 230 nm using HPTLC.

F.2: Limit of detection and limit of quantification of Withanoside V using HPTLC is shown in Table **2.44**.

Table 2.44. The limits of detection and quantification were determined for Withanoside V using the standardized method by HPTLC.

LOD	1.13 ng/spot
LOQ	3.98 g/spot

F.3: Precision of the standardized method for detection of Withanoside V using HPTLC

The reproducibility of the standardized method for Withanoside V was determined by HPTLC using different extracts of Ashwagandha. The results are shown in Table **2.45**.

Table 2.45. Precision of the standardized method for Withanoside V by HPTLC.

Precision	**% RSD**
Intraday	0.46%
Interday	1.13%

F.4: Percent recovery of Withanoside V using the standardized method by HPTLC

The recovery of Withanoside V at different cut-off values using the standardized method by HPTLC is shown in Table **2.46**.

Table 2.46. Recovery percentage of Withanoside V by HPTLC.

Recovery Level	% Recovery	Mean Recovery %
80%	90.38%	94.73%
100%	96.46%	
120%	97.36%	

Result: The amount of Withanoside V was found to be 0.066% w/w in Ashwagandha extract.

Conclusion:

The concentrations of the different Withanolides in the Ashwagandha extract are shown in Table **2.47**.

B.2 Limit of detection and limit of quantification using the standardized method for HPTLC

The limit of detection and quantitation of Withaferin A using the standardized method for HPTLC was quantified. The results obtained are shown in Table **2.28**.

Chemical Characterization of Giloy

Giloy or Guduci consists of dried mature pieces of the stem of *Tinospora cordifolia* (India, 2016) (Fam. Menispermaceae) Fig. (**2.44**), a perennial climber found throughout tropical India. The herb was collected during summer preferably in the month of May. Ancient Sanskrit Ayurvedic texts like *Charak Samhita, Rigveda,* written in about 5000 BC to 6000 BC, had references to Giloy. The holy text from *Dhanvantari Nighantu* was written in 1000 AD (Fig. **2.45**) and *Raj Nighantu* in 1400 AD (Fig. **2.46**).

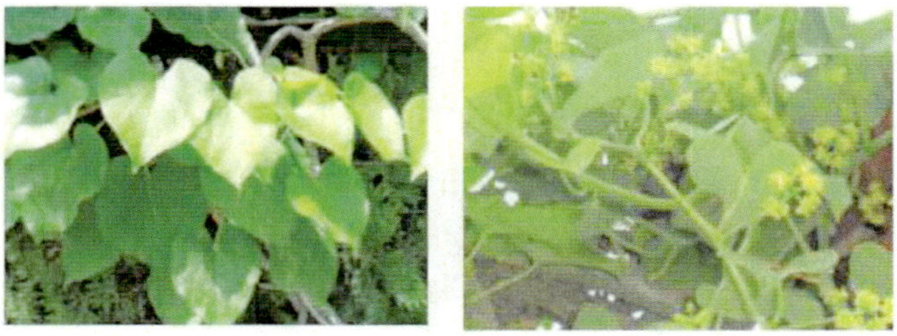

Fig. (2.44). Images of whole plant and flower of *Tinospora cordifolia* (Giloy).

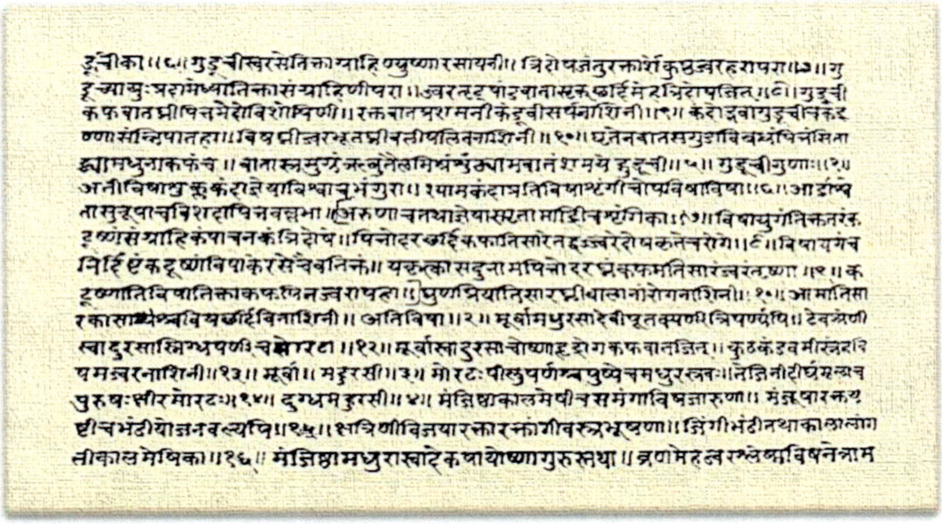

Fig. (2.45). Image of the holy text in *Dhanvantari Nighantu* – 1000 AD about Giloy.

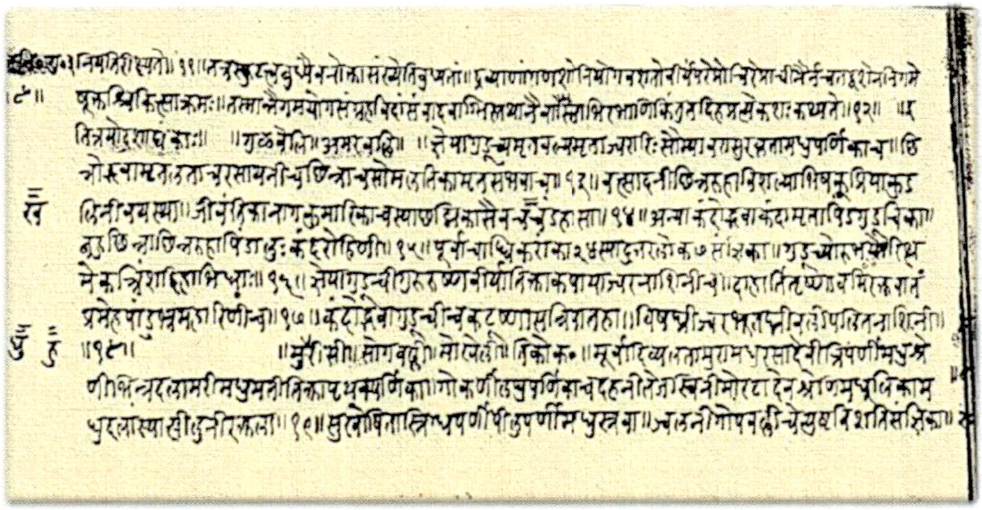

Fig. (2.46). Image of the holy text in *Raj Nighantu* – 1400 AD about Giloy.

The identification of Giloy should be authenticated from a reputed institution like CSIR – National Institute of Science Communication and Information Resources, Ministry of Science & Technology, Govt. of India (Fig. (**2.47**) (Appendix 2.3).

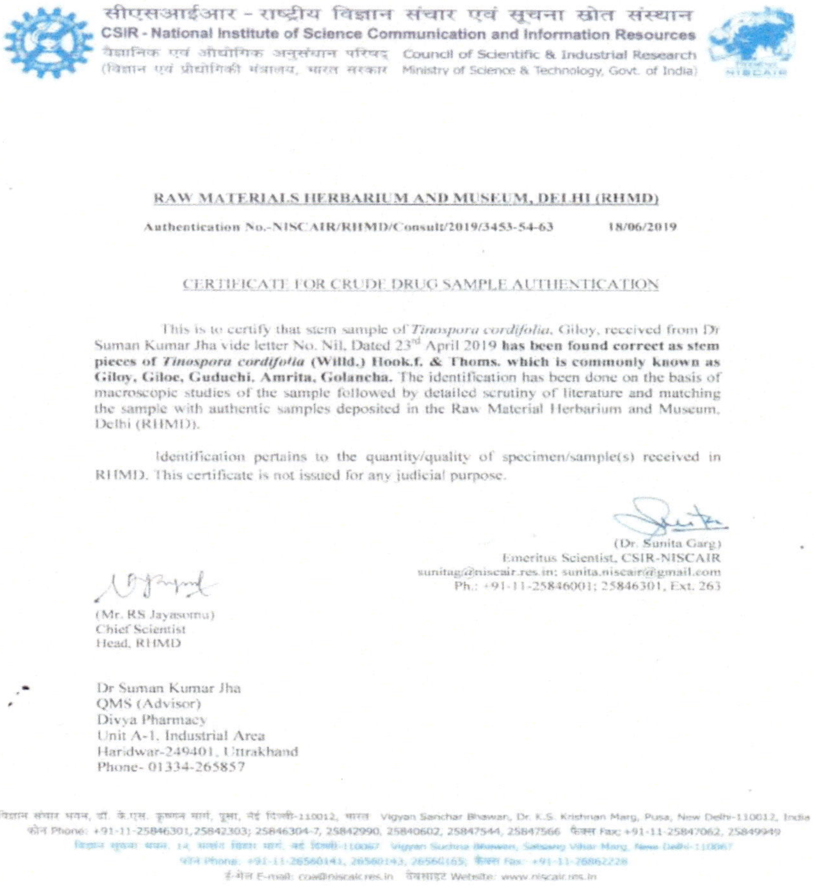

सीएसआईआर - राष्ट्रीय विज्ञान संचार एवं सूचना स्रोत संस्थान
CSIR - National Institute of Science Communication and Information Resources
वैज्ञानिक एवं औद्योगिक अनुसंधान परिषद Council of Scientific & Industrial Research
(विज्ञान एवं प्रौद्योगिकी मंत्रालय, भारत सरकार Ministry of Science & Technology, Govt. of India)

RAW MATERIALS HERBARIUM AND MUSEUM, DELHI (RHMD)

Authentication No.-NISCAIR/RHMD/Consult/2019/3453-54-63 18/06/2019

CERTIFICATE FOR CRUDE DRUG SAMPLE AUTHENTICATION

This is to certify that stem sample of *Tinospora cordifolia*, Giloy, received from Dr Suman Kumar Jha vide letter No. Nil, Dated 23rd April 2019 **has been found correct as stem pieces of *Tinospora cordifolia* (Willd.) Hook.f. & Thoms. which is commonly known as Giloy, Giloe, Guduchi, Amrita, Golancha.** The identification has been done on the basis of macroscopic studies of the sample followed by detailed scrutiny of literature and matching the sample with authentic samples deposited in the Raw Material Herbarium and Museum, Delhi (RHMD).

Identification pertains to the quantity/quality of specimen/sample(s) received in RHMD. This certificate is not issued for any judicial purpose.

(Dr. Sunita Garg)
Emeritus Scientist, CSIR-NISCAIR
sunitag@niscair.res.in; sunita.niscair@gmail.com
Ph.: +91-11-25846001; 25846301, Ext. 263

(Mr. RS Jayasomu)
Chief Scientist
Head, RHMD

Dr Suman Kumar Jha
QMS (Advisor)
Divya Pharmacy
Unit A-1, Industrial Area
Haridwar-249401, Uttrakhand
Phone- 01334-265857

Vigyan Sanchar Bhawan, Dr. K.S. Krishnan Marg, Pusa, New Delhi-110012, India
Phone: +91-11-25846301,25842303; 25846304-7, 25842990, 25840602, 25847544, 25847566 Fax: +91-11-25847062, 25849949
Vigyan Suchna Bhawan, Satsang Vihar Marg, New Delhi-110067
Phone: +91-11-26560141, 26560143, 26560165; Fax: +91-11-26862228
E-mail: coa@niscair.res.in Website: www.niscair.res.in

Fig. (2.47). Authentication certificate of Giloy from CSIR- NISCAIR.

UPLC/QToF MS Study of Giloy

Sample Preparation Method: 50.0 mg of *Tinospora cordifolia* hydromethanolic extract was dissolved in 10 ml of methanol: water (50:50) and sonicated for 30 min. This solution was centrifuged for 5 min at 10000 rpm and filtered through a 0.22 µm nylon filter.

UPLC/QToF MS Condition: Analysis was performed on a Xevo G2-XS QToF of Waters with Acquity UPLC- I Class and Unifi software. Separation was carried out using Acquity UPLC HSS -T3 column (100 x 2.1 mm, 1.7 µm). The column was maintained at 40°C throughout the analysis and sample temperature was kept at 20°C during the analysis. Detection was carried out by Xevo G2-XS QToF. The elution was carried out at a flow rate of 0.38 ml/min using gradient elution as shown in Table **2.48** of mobile phase 0.1% formic acid in water (mobile phase A) and 0.1% formic acid in acetonitrile (mobile phase B). 1 µl of test solution was injected during the analysis and the chromatograph was recorded for 48 min. The chromatogram obtained in positive mode is shown in Fig. **(2.48)** and negative mode in Fig. **(2.49)**.

Table 2.48. Details of gradient program used for UPLC/QToF MS of Giloy.

Time (Min)	Flow (ml/min)	Mobile Phase A (%)	Mobile Phase B (%)
0	0.4	95	5
5	0.4	90	10
10	0.4	85	15
30	0.4	80	20
40	0.4	65	35
55	0.4	20	80
60	0.4	20	80
61	0.4	95	5
65	0.4	95	5

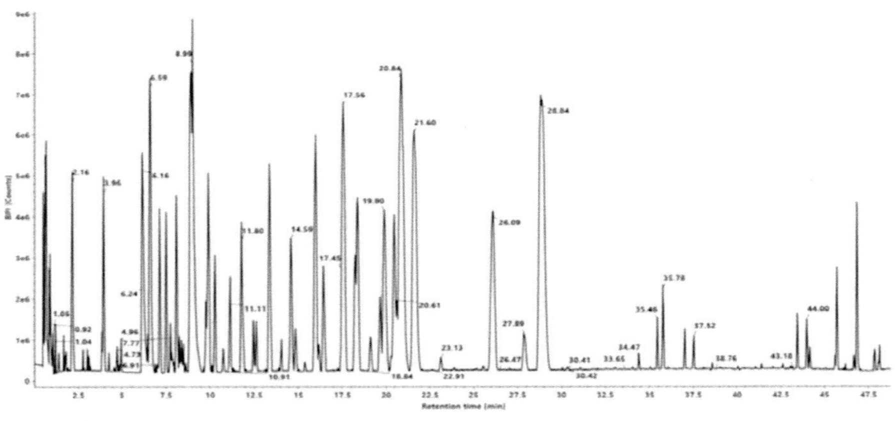

Fig. (2.48). Representative chromatograph of *Tinospora cordifolia* hydromethanolic extract in positive mode using UPLC/QToF MS.

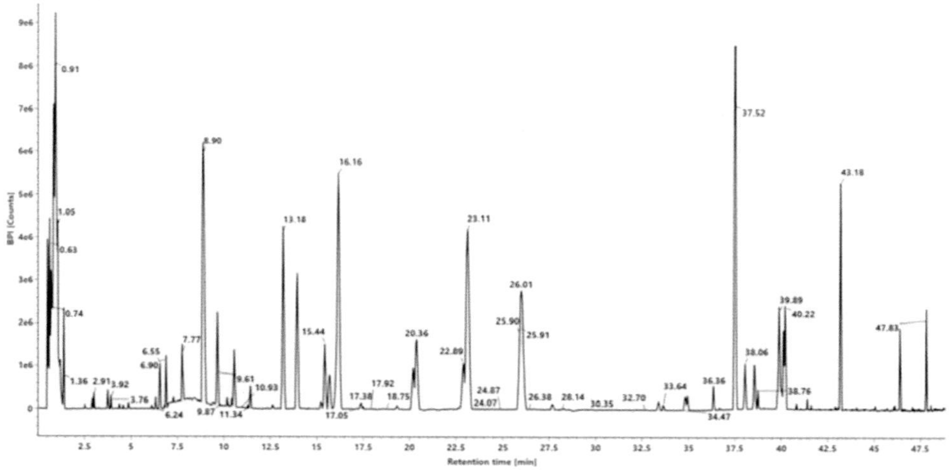

Fig. (2.49). Representative chromatograph of *Tinospora cordifolia* hydromethanolic extract in negative mode using UPLC/QToF MS.

<u>*Gradient Program:*</u>

Xevo G2-XS QToF Parameter: The different parameters used for the UPLC/QToF MS analysis of Giloy are shown in Table **2.49**.

Table 2.49. UPLC/QToF MS parameters used for analysis of Giloy.

Parameter	Polarity (+ve)	Polarity (-ve)
Ionisation type	ESI	ESI
Mode	MS^E	MS^E
Acquisition time	48 min	48 min
Mass range (m/z)	50-1200 m/z	50-1200 m/z
Cone Voltage	40 V	40 V
Capillary	1 kV	2 kV
Low CE	6.0 eV	6.0 eV
High CE	20-40 eV (ramp)	20-40 eV(ramp)
Source temperature	120 °C	120 °C
Desolvation Temperature	500 °C	500 °C
Cone gas flow	50 L/h	50 L/h
Desolvation gas flow	900 L/h	900 L/h
Lock Spray (Leucine Enkaphalin)	556.2766 m/z	554.2620 m/z

On the basis of UPLC/QToF MS analysis, Total 84 major compounds were found in *Tinospora cordifolia* hydromethanolic extract (methanol: water, 50:50) as shown in Table **2.50**.

Table 2.50. Identified compounds in Giloy extract using Positive and Negative modes of UPLC/QToF MS.

Positive Mode							
S.No	**Component name**	**Formula**	**RT (min)**	**Observed m/z**	**Neutral Mass (Da)**	**Response**	**Adducts**
1	Citric acid	$C_6H_8O_7$	0.92	215.0165	192.0270	188397	+Na, +H
2	Pyroglutamic acid	$C_5H_7NO_3$	1.04	130.0507	129.0426	204929	+H
3	N-Acetyl-glutamic acid	$C_7H_{11}NO_5$	1.05	212.0530	189.0637	96019	+Na, +H
4	Guanosine	$C_{10}H_{13}N_5O_5$	1.36	284.1000	283.0917	61913	+H
5	Dehydroheliamine	$C_{11}H_{13}NO_2$	2.16	192.1025	191.0946	1204359	+H, +Na
6	N-Methylcoclaurine	$C_{18}H_{21}NO_3$	3.96	300.1596	299.1521	1644553	+H
7	Higenamine	$C_{16}H_{17}NO_3$	4.73	272.1283	271.1208	287444	+H
8	Coclaurine	$C_{17}H_{19}NO_3$	4.96	286.1440	285.1365	336184	+H
9	Juzirine	$C_{17}H_{15}NO_3$	6.16	282.1131	281.1052	3095935	+H
10	8-O-tigloyldiderroside	$C_{22}H_{32}O_{13}$	6.24	527.1734	504.1843	43168	+Na
11	Syringin	$C_{17}H_{24}O_9$	6.32	395.1316	372.1420	214978	+Na
12	N-cis-Feruloyl typamine	$C_{18}H_{19}NO_4$	6.59	314.1393	313.1314	2272986	+H
13	Tinosinen	$C_{22}H_{32}O_{13}$	6.91	527.1735	504.1843	236605	+Na
14	Cordifolioside A	$C_{22}H_{32}O_{13}$	7.77	527.1730	504.1843	349771	+Na
15	Corchoionoside C	$C_{19}H_{30}O_8$	7.98	409.1820	386.1941	12079	+Na
16	L-Tetrahydrocolumbamine	$C_{20}H_{23}NO_4$	8.16	342.1700	341.1627	418200	+H
17	Longanine	$C_{19}H_{25}NO_6$	8.26	386.1600	363.1682	448843	+Na
18	Magnoflorine	$C_{20}H_{23}NO_4$	8.99	342.1706	341.1627	2894088	+H, +Na
19	Nictoflorin	$C_{27}H_{30}O_{15}$	9.63	595.1656	594.1585	118100	+H
20	Borapetoside A	$C_{26}H_{34}O_{12}$	10.43	561.1939	538.2050	93467	+Na
21	Cordioside	$C_{26}H_{34}O_{12}$	10.91	561.1939	538.2050	175906	+Na
22	(1R,2S,5R)-2-Isopropyl-5-methylcyclohexyl 4-O- β-D-glucopyranosyl-β-D-glucopyranoside	$C_{22}H_{40}O_{11}$	11.11	481.2616	480.2571	721672	+H
23	Menisperine	$C_{21}H_{25}NO_4$	11.80	356.1859	355.1784	2222250	+H
24	Tanegoside C	$C_{27}H_{36}O_{13}$	12.54	591.2032	568.2156	58230	+Na
25	Tinocordifolioside	$C_{21}H_{32}O_8$	12.62	413.2166	412.2097	76072	+H, +Na
26	1-deacetyltinosposide A	$C_{24}H_{34}O_{12}$	13.18	537.1938	514.2050	260384	+Na, +H
27	Tinosinenoside C	$C_{26}H_{36}O_{13}$	13.92	579.2038	556.2156	342088	+Na
28	Tetrahydrocoptisine	$C_{19}H_{17}NO_4$	14.59	324.1234	323.1158	1730055	+H

(Table 2.50) cont.....

Positive Mode							
S.No	**Component name**	**Formula**	**RT (min)**	**Observed m/z**	**Neutral Mass (Da)**	**Response**	**Adducts**
29	Tetrahydropalmatinee	$C_{21}H_{25}NO_4$	14.86	356.1862	355.1784	964944	+H
30	Borapetoside B	$C_{27}H_{36}O_{12}$	15.02	575.2077	552.2207	17969	+Na
31	Ecdysterone	$C_{27}H_{44}O_7$	15.38	481.3153	480.3087	161386	+H, +Na
32	Chasmanthin	$C_{20}H_{22}O_7$	15.70	375.1410	374.1366	55011	+H
33	Tinosineside A	$C_{26}H_{36}O_{13}$	16.19	579.2039	556.2156	993916	+Na, +H
34	N-methylstephisoferulin	$C_{28}H_{31}NO_7$	16.94	494.2169	493.2101	142931	+H
35	N-trans-Caffeoyltyramine	$C_{17}H_{17}NO_4$	17.45	300.1233	299.1158	178889	+H, +Na
36	6-Cinnamoylhernandine	$C_{29}H_{31}NO_8$	17.56	522.2127	521.2050	6368512	+H
37	Palmatosidea	$C_{26}H_{32}O_{12}$	18.00	559.1785	536.1894	49167	+Na
38	Tinoside	$C_{26}H_{32}O_{11}$	18.84	521.1984	520.1945	35479	+H
39	(S)-2,3,9,11-Tetramethoxytetrahydroprotoberberine	$C_{21}H_{25}NO_4$	19.12	356.1867	355.1784	877894	+H
40	Dihydroberberine	$C_{20}H_{19}NO_4$	19.90	338.1397	337.1314	3246237	+H
41	Tinocordiside	$C_{21}H_{32}O_7$	20.29	419.2044	396.2148	646903	+Na, +H
42	d-Corydaline	$C_{22}H_{27}NO_4$	20.61	370.2020	369.1940	1530070	+H
43	13,13a-Didehydro-9, 10-dimethoxy-2,3-(ethylenedioxy)-berbine	$C_{20}H_{19}NO_4$	20.84	338.1392	337.1314	8541309	+H
44	Columbamine	$C_{20}H_{19}NO_4$	21.60	338.1395	337.1314	6430180	+H
45	2-(3-Furyl)-7-(β-D-glucopyranosyloxy)-9-hydroxy-10b- methyl-- -oxododecahydro-2H-benzo[f]isochromen-10-yl acetate	$C_{26}H_{36}O_{12}$	22.91	563.2052	540.2207	404395	+Na, +H
46	Ligraminol B	$C_{28}H_{38}O_{14}$	23.13	621.2148	598.2262	899645	+Na, +H
47	Moupinamide	$C_{18}H_{19}NO_4$	26.09	314.1395	313.1314	4225794	+H, +Na
48	Berberine	$C_{20}H_{17}NO_4$	26.47	336.1231	335.1158	165566	+H
49	Pseudopalmatinee	$C_{21}H_{22}NO_4$	27.89	352.1550	352.1549	1466595	-e
50	Tinosporinenside C	$C_{26}H_{36}O_{12}$	28.16	563.2079	540.2207	61058	+Na
51	Palmatinee	$C_{21}H_{21}NO_4$	28.84	352.1549	351.1471	9848881	+H
52	Columbin	$C_{20}H_{22}O_6$	30.41	359.1488	358.1416	182025	+H
53	Cordifolide A	$C_{28}H_{38}O_{12}S$	30.42	621.1953	598.2084	41663	+Na
54	Tinosponinenside B	$C_{28}H_{38}O_{13}$	33.65	605.2194	582.2312	108506	+Na
55	(-)-Secoisolariciresinol-4-O-β-D-glucopyranoside	$C_{26}H_{36}O_{11}$	34.47	547.2136	524.2258	48647	+Na
56	Secoobaberine	$C_{38}H_{40}N_2O_8$	35.46	653.2853	652.2785	1001290	+H
57	Cannabisin H	$C_{28}H_{31}NO_8$	35.78	532.1971	509.2050	1173160	+Na
58	1-Acetyltinosinenoside D	$C_{38}H_{46}O_{17}$	37.52	797.2613	774.2735	900031	+Na
59	1-Acetyltinosinenoside E	$C_{38}H_{46}O_{17}$	38.76	797.2616	774.2735	261479	+Na
60	(3S)-1,7-Bis(3,4-dihydroxyphenyl)-5-oxo-3-heptanyl 6-O-benzoyl-β-D-glucopyranoside	$C_{32}H_{36}O_{12}$	43.18	613.227	612.2207	177957	+H, +Na

(Table 2.50) cont.....

S.No	Component name	Formula	RT (min)	Observed m/z	Neutral Mass (Da)	Response	Adducts
Positive Mode							
61	N-Formylannonaine	$C_{18}H_{15}NO_3$	44.00	294.1137	293.1052	552299	+H, +Na
Negative mode							
S.No.	**Component name**	**Formula**	**RT (min)**	**Observed m/z**	**Neutral mass (Da)**	**Response**	**Adducts**
1	D-Gluconic acid	$C_6H_{12}O_7$	0.63	195.0510	196.0583	521332	-H
2	Malic acid	$C_4H_6O_5$	0.74	133.0141	134.0215	683710	-H, +HCOO
3	Citric acid	$C_6H_8O_7$	0.91	191.0196	192.0270	3560714	-H
4	N-Acetyl-glutamic acid	$C_7H_{11}NO_5$	1.05	188.0563	189.0637	583097	-H
5	Guanosine	$C_{10}H_{13}N_5O_5$	1.36	282.0831	283.0917	43850	-H
6	Vanillic acid-4-O-β-D-glucopyranoside	$C_{14}H_{18}O_9$	2.91	329.0874	330.0951	103921	-H, +HCOO
7	3,4,5-Trimethoxyphenol-1-O-[β-D-apiofuranosyl-(1→6)]-β-D-glucopyranoside	$C_{20}H_{30}O_{13}$	3.76	477.1596	478.1686	158445	-H
8	N-Methylcoclaurine	$C_{18}H_{21}NO_3$	3.92	298.1448	299.1521	129590	-H
9	8-O-tigloyldiderroside	$C_{22}H_{32}O_{13}$	6.24	549.1818	504.1843	76434	+HCOO, -H
10	N-cis-Feruloyl typamine	$C_{18}H_{19}NO_4$	6.55	312.1243	313.1314	330962	-H, +HCOO
11	Tinosinen	$C_{22}H_{32}O_{13}$	6.90	549.1829	504.1843	519317	+HCOO, -H
12	Orcinol gentiobioside (Anacardoside)	$C_{19}H_{28}O_{12}$	7.30	447.1506	448.1581	195043	-H
13	Cordifolioside A	$C_{22}H_{32}O_{13}$	7.77	549.1829	504.1843	638414	+HCOO, -H
14	Corchoionoside C	$C_{19}H_{30}O_8$	8.00	431.1915	386.1941	43181	+HCOO
15	Kaempferol-3-gentiobioside	$C_{27}H_{30}O_{16}$	8.41	609.1457	610.1534	43492	-H
16	Magnoflorine	$C_{20}H_{23}NO_4$	8.90	340.1554	341.1627	2818196	-H, +HCOO
17	Nictoflorin	$C_{27}H_{30}O_{15}$	9.61	593.1513	594.1585	208453	-H
18	Decaffeoylacteoside	$C_{20}H_{30}O_{12}$	9.87	461.1663	462.1737	113401	-H
19	Borapetoside A	$C_{26}H_{34}O_{12}$	10.43	583.2020	538.2050	46834	+HCOO, -H
20	Cordioside	$C_{26}H_{34}O_{12}$	10.93	583.2019	538.2050	106745	+HCOO, -H
21	(-)-Lyoniresinol-3α-O-β-glucopyranoside	$C_{28}H_{38}O_{13}$	11.34	627.2287	582.2312	50408	+HCOO, -H
22	Neoeriocitrin dihydrochalcone	$C_{27}H_{34}O_{15}$	12.11	597.1822	598.1898	130029	-H
23	Tinocordifolioside	$C_{21}H_{32}O_8$	12.64	457.2081	412.2097	152938	+HCOO, -H
24	1-deacetyltinosposide A	$C_{24}H_{34}O_{12}$	13.18	513.1982	514.2050	2127129	-H
25	Borapetoside B	$C_{27}H_{36}O_{12}$	15.00	597.2184	552.2207	70551	+HCOO
26	Ecdysterone	$C_{27}H_{44}O_7$	15.44	525.3076	480.3087	1065742	+HCOO, -H
27	Tinosineside A	$C_{26}H_{36}O_{13}$	16.16	601.2144	556.2156	4088027	+HCOO, -H
28	Secoisolariciresinol monoglucoside	$C_{26}H_{36}O_{11}$	17.05	569.2233	524.2258	48899	+HCOO, -H

(Table 2.50) cont.....

Positive Mode							
S.No	Component name	Formula	RT (min)	Observed m/z	Neutral Mass (Da)	Response	Adducts
29	N-trans-Caffeoyltyramine	$C_{17}H_{17}NO_4$	17.38	298.1084	299.1158	209600	-H, +HCOO
30	Palmatosidea	$C_{26}H_{32}O_{12}$	17.92	581.1870	536.1894	89605	+HCOO
31	Borapetoside F	$C_{27}H_{34}O_{11}$	18.75	579.2075	534.2101	182051	+HCOO
32	Tinoside	$C_{26}H_{32}O_{11}$	18.97	565.1921	520.1945	90909	+HCOO, -H
33	Tinocordiside	$C_{21}H_{32}O_7$	20.36	441.2135	396.2148	1332972	+HCOO, -H
34	2-(3-Furyl)-7-(β-D-glucopyranosyloxy)-9-hydroxy-10b-methyl-4-oxododecahydro-2H-benzo[f]isochromen-10-yl acetate	$C_{26}H_{36}O_{12}$	22.89	585.2192	540.2207	1417389	+HCOO, -H
35	Ligraminol B	$C_{28}H_{38}O_{14}$	23.11	643.2246	598.2262	4553102	+HCOO, -H
36	Tincordin	$C_{19}H_{22}O_6$	24.07	345.1339	346.1416	97180	-H
37	Salvinicin A	$C_{25}H_{36}O_{12}$	24.87	527.2124	528.2207	48565	-H
38	Tinosporide	$C_{20}H_{22}O_7$	25.90	419.1349	374.1366	427767	+HCOO
39	5-Methoxybibenzyl-3,3′-di-O-β-D-glucopyranoside	$C_{27}H_{36}O_{13}$	25.91	567.2082	568.2156	201415	-H
40	Moupinamide	$C_{18}H_{19}NO_4$	26.01	312.1244	313.1314	2339942	-H, +HCOO
41	Tinosposinenside A	$C_{27}H_{36}O_{12}$	26.38	597.2181	552.2207	95504	+HCOO
42	Tinosposinenside C	$C_{26}H_{36}O_{12}$	28.14	585.2191	540.2207	313860	+HCOO, -H
43	Cordifolide A	$C_{28}H_{38}O_{12}S$	30.35	643.2070	598.2084	155391	+HCOO, -H
44	Borapetoside C	$C_{27}H_{36}O_{11}$	32.70	581.2223	536.2258	34372	+HCOO
45	Tinosposinenside B	$C_{28}H_{38}O_{13}$	33.64	627.2294	582.2312	301184	+HCOO
46	(-)-Secoisolariciresinol-4-O-β-D-glucopyranoside	$C_{26}H_{36}O_{11}$	34.47	569.2238	524.2258	93173	+HCOO
47	(2S,4aS,6aS,7R,9S,10R,10aR,10bS)-9-Acetoxy-2-(3-furyl)-4a,10-dihydroxy-10b-methyl-4- oxododecahydro-2H-benzo[f]isochromen-7-yl (2Z)-3-[4--β-D-glucopyranosyloxy)-3-methoxyphenyl]acrylate	$C_{36}H_{44}O_{16}$	36.36	731.2558	732.2629	510100	-H
48	1-Acetyltinosinenoside D	$C_{38}H_{46}O_{17}$	37.52	819.2731	774.2735	5204082	+HCOO, -H
49	Malyngic acid	$C_{18}H_{32}O_5$	38.06	327.2180	328.2250	397047	-H
50	1-Acetyltinosinenoside E	$C_{38}H_{46}O_{17}$	38.76	819.2732	774.2735	502988	+HCOO
51	Methyl 2,3,4-tri-O-acetyl-6-O-(3-O-allyl-2-O-benzyl-4,6-O-benzylidene-β-D-mannopyranosyl)-α-D-glucopyranoside	$C_{36}H_{44}O_{14}$	38.90	699.2655	700.2731	57362	-H, +HCOO
52	Tianshic acid	$C_{18}H_{34}O_5$	39.89	329.2338	330.2406	1380891	-H
53	Sanleng acid	$C_{18}H_{34}O_5$	40.22	329.2339	330.2406	913520	-H
54	(3S)-1,7-Bis(3,4-dihydroxyphenyl)-5-oxo-3-heptanyl 6-O-benzoyl-β-D-glucopyranoside	$C_{32}H_{36}O_{12}$	43.18	611.2138	612.2207	2464719	-H, +HCOO
55	7,8-Dihydroxyoctadecanoic acid	$C_{18}H_{36}O_4$	47.83	315.2544	316.2614	791547	-H

HPLC-PDA Method Development for Standardization of Giloy:

Experiment Methods: The quantification of marker compounds was performed by HPLC system (Prominenece i LC-2030C 3D+ from Shimadzu, Japan). A reverse phase column Shodex C18-4E (5 µm, 4.6 x 250 mm) was used and column temperature was maintained at 35.0°C. HPLC mobile phase A (0.1% orthophosphoric acid in water adjust pH 2.5 with diethylamine) and mobile phase

B (0.1% orthophosphoric acid in a mixer of acetonitrile and water in the ratio of 88:12, adjust pH 2.5 with diethylamine) the gradient program was shown in Table **2.51** at a flow rate of 1.0 ml/min were used. 10 µl of standard solutions and test solution was injected during the analysis. Chromatograph at 270 nm wavelength was recorded.

Table 2.51. HPLC Gradient program for Giloy.

Time (min)	Flow (ml/min)	A %	B%
0	1.0	90	10
10	1.0	90	10
20	1.0	85	15
45	1.0	60	40
50	1.0	10	90
55	1.0	10	90
56	1.0	90	10
60	1.0	90	10

Sample Preparation: 0.5 gm of powdered sample was diluted with 10 ml water: methanol (30:70) and sonicated for 30 min, centrifuged at 10000 rpm for 5 min and filtered using 0.45 µm nylon filter and used for the analysis.

The HPLC fingerprint of standard is shown in Fig. **(2.50)** and standard is shown in Fig. **(2.51)**.

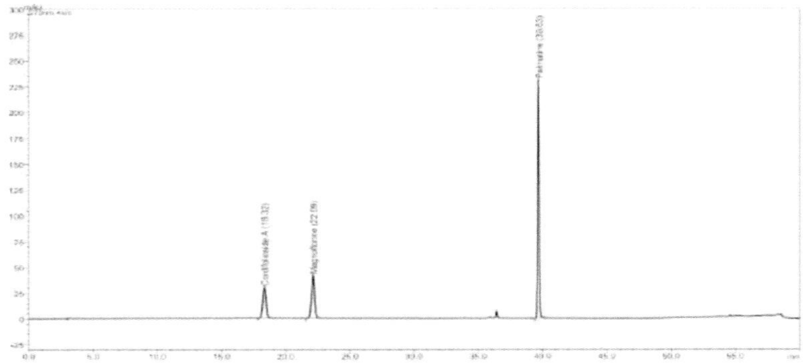

Fig. (2.50). Representative HPLC Chromatogram of mixed standards.

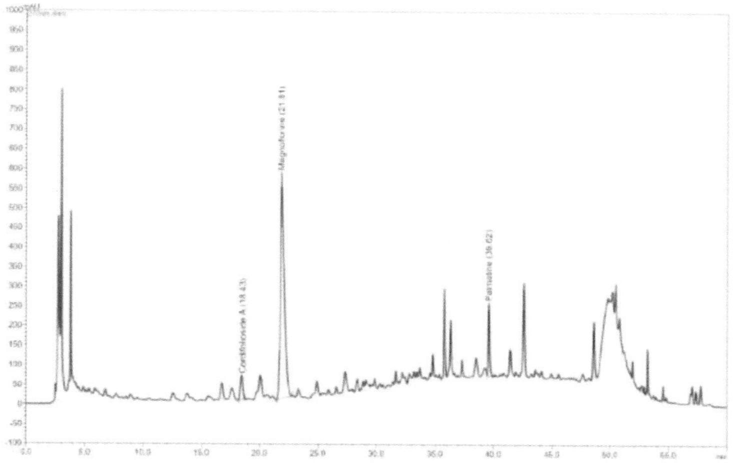

115

Fig. (2.51). Representative HPLC Chromatogram of Giloy extract sample.

Standard Preparation: Standards Palmatinee hydrochloride (Potency-75.1%, Sigma Aldrich), Cordifolioside A (Potency-98.0%, Chemfaces) and Magnoflorine (Potency-99.0%, Sigma Aldrich) were dissolved in methanol to prepare the appropriate concentrations.

Result: The amount of Cordifoliside A, Magnoflorine and Palmatinee in Giloy extract are found to be 1.664, 15.616 and 0.596 µg/mg respectively.

HPLC-PDA method validation for standardization of Giloy is shown in Table **2.52**.

Table 2.52. Summary of HPLC method validation of Giloy.

S. No.	Parameter	Acceptance Criteria	Result Obtained		
			Cordifolioside A	Magnoflorine	Palmatinee
1	System Suitability	% RSD of Retention time - NMT 2.0%	0.82	0.59	0.10
		% RSD of area – NMT 2.0%	1.32	0.72	1.22
		USP trailing – NMT 2.0%	1.80	1.17	1.38
		Theoretical plates – NLT 2000	22855	164476	392266
2	Specificity	No interference at retention time	Complies		
3	Linearity	Correlation coefficient NLT 0.99	0.9996	0.9998	0.9997

(Table 2.52) cont.....

S. No.	Parameter	Acceptance Criteria	Result Obtained		
			Cordifolioside A	Magnoflorine	Palmatinee
4	Precision				
4.1	System	%RSD of area – NMT 2%	1.32	0.72	1.22
4.2	Intermediate	%RSD of assay – NMT 2%	0.62	0.36	0.37
4.3	Method	%RSD of assay – NMT 2%	0.47	1.56	0.24
5	Limit of detection	%RSD of area – NMT 33%	0.62	0.88	0.79
6	Limit of Quantification	%RSD of area – NMT 10%	1.37	1.85	0.13

HPTLC Method Development for Standardization of Giloy *Experiment Methods*

Chromatographic Conditions: TLC plate: TLC plate with silica gel 60 F_{254}.

Mobile phase: chloroform: methanol: formic acid (6.5: 3.5: 1) ratio. Densitometric analysis: scanning was performed at a wavelength of 265 nm.

Quantification of Magnoflorine

Preparation of Standard Solution: The stock solution was prepared by dissolving 10 mg Magnoflorine in 10 ml of methanol. The working solution was prepared from stock solution by dissolving 0.1ml of stock solution in 1ml of methanol.

Preparation of Sample Solution: 500 mg of sample was dissolved in 10 ml of methanol: water (70: 30), it was then sonicated for 20 min and then centrifuged.

HPTLC fingerprint of Magnoflorine and samples are shown in Fig. (**2.52**).

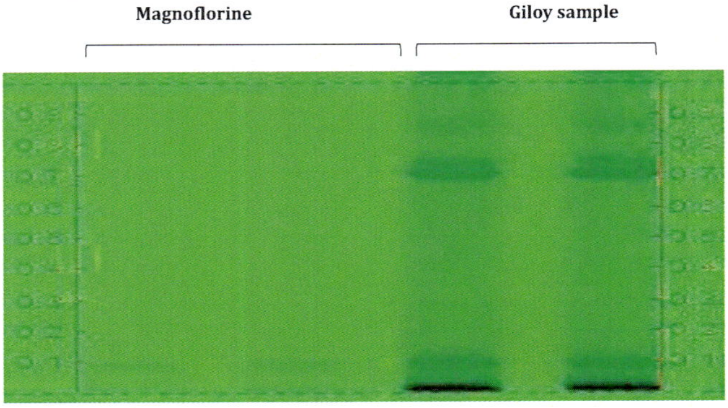

Fig. (2.52). HPTLC fingerprint of Giloy.

Results

HPTLC Method Validation for Standardization of Giloy

A Determination of linearity of Magnoflorine is shown in Fig. (**2.53**).

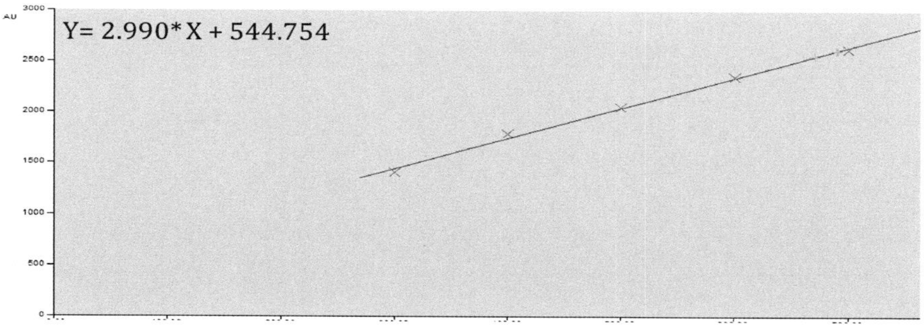

Fig. (2.53). Linearity curve of Magnoflorine as determined by HPTLC

The linearity of Magnoflorine was determined using the regression equation is shown in Table **2.53**.

Table 2.53. Linearity correlation of Magnoflorine by HPTLC.

Parameter	Magnoflorine
Linearity range	300 - 700 ng
Regression equation	2.990* X + 544.754
Correlation coefficient	0.99

A.1 Detection of Magnoflorine at 265 nm using HPTLC is shown in Fig. (**2.54**).

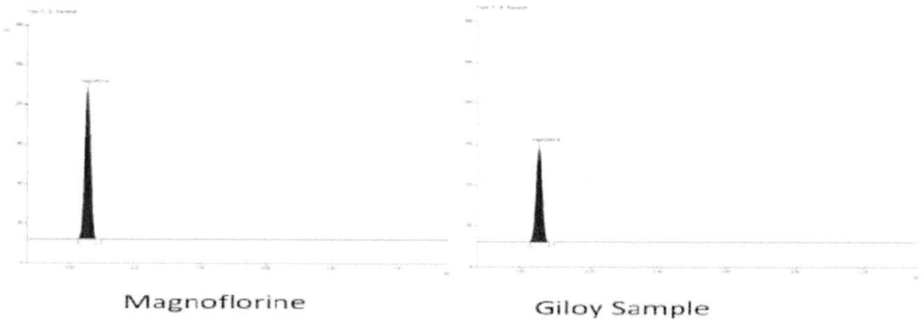

Fig. (2.54). Representative chromatogram of Magnoflorine standard and sample of Giloy extract.

The limit of detection and limit of quantification of magnoflorine from Giloy using HPTLC is shown in Table **2.54**.

Table 2.54. Limit of Detection and Quantification of Magnoflorine in Giloy by HPTLC.

LOD	1.34 ppm
LOQ	4.06 ppm

A.2: Precision of standardized method for HPTLC for detection of Magnoflorine using HPTLC is shown in Table **2.55**.

Table 2.55. Precision of HPTLC method determined with different batches of Giloy extract.

Precision	**% RSD**
Intraday	0.74%
Interday	0.59

A.3: Recovery of Magnoflorine at different cut-off values using HPTLC is shown in Table **2.56**.

Table 2.56. Recovery of Magnoflorine using the standardized method of HPTLC.

Recovery Level	**% Recovery**	**Mean Recovery %**
80%	96.26%	93.89%
100%	94.43%	
120%	90.98%	

Result: The amount of Magnoflorine was found to be 1.15% in giloy extract.

Coronil Tablet and Divya Swasari Vati

Coronil tablet and Divya Swasari Vati are manufactured at a GMP facility of Divya Pharmacy Unit-II, Khasra No. 210, 211, Patanjali food and herbal park, Laksar Road, Gram Padartha, Haridwar, Uttarakhand, India. The license was issued by Government (Fig. **2.55**) for the manufacturing of both these tablets. The COPP certificate for export of Coronil and Divya Swasari Vati is shown in Appendix 2.6 and 2.7, respectively.

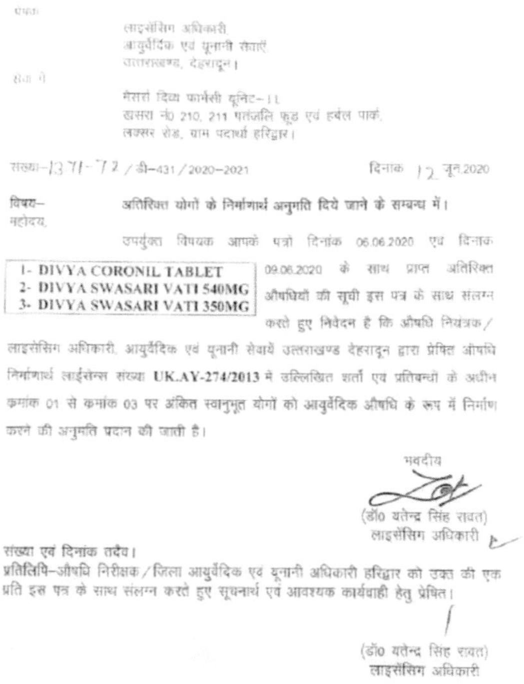

प्रेषक

लाइसेंसिग अधिकारी,
आयुर्वेदिक एवं यूनानी सेवाएँ
उत्तराखण्ड, देहरादून।

सेवा में

मैसर्स दिव्य फार्मेसी यूनिट–II,
खसरा नं0 210, 211 पतंजलि फूड एवं हर्बल पार्क,
लक्सर रोड, ग्राम पदार्था हरिद्वार।

संख्या–1371–72 / डी–431 / 2020–2021 दिनांक 12 जून 2020

विषय– अतिरिक्त योगों के निर्माणार्थ अनुमति दिये जाने के सम्बन्ध में।

महोदय,

उपर्युक्त विषयक आपके पत्रो दिनांक 06.06.2020 एवं दिनांक 09.06.2020 के साथ प्राप्त अतिरिक्त औषधियों की सूची इस पत्र के साथ संलग्न करते हुए निवेदन है कि औषधि नियंत्रक/लाइसेंसिग अधिकारी, आयुर्वेदिक एवं यूनानी सेवायें उत्तराखण्ड देहरादून द्वारा प्रेषित औषधि निर्माणार्थ लाईसेन्स संख्या **UK.AY-274/2013** मे उल्लिखित शर्तो एवं प्रतिबन्धो के अधीन क्रमांक 01 से कमांक 03 पर अंकित स्वानुभूत योगों को आयुर्वेदिक औषधि के रूप में निर्माण करने की अनुमति प्रदान की जाती है।

1- **DIVYA CORONIL TABLET**
2- **DIVYA SWASARI VATI 540MG**
3- **DIVYA SWASARI VATI 350MG**

भवदीय

(डॉ0 यतेन्द्र सिंह रावत)
लाइसेंसिग अधिकारी

संख्या एवं दिनांक तदैव।
प्रतिलिपि–औषधि निरीक्षक/जिला आयुर्वेदिक एवं यूनानी अधिकारी हरिद्वार को उक्त की एक प्रति इस पत्र के साथ संलग्न करते हुए सूचनार्थ एवं आवश्यक कार्यवाही हेतु प्रेषित।

(डॉ0 यतेन्द्र सिंह रावत)
लाइसेंसिग अधिकारी

Fig. (2.55). Image of the license certificate for the manufacture of Coronil tablet and Divya Swasari Vati.

To obtain a license the procedure followed is the submission of a formula sheet to the Drug Inspector of the district like in our case drug formula sheet was submitted to Drug Inspector Ayurveda at Haridwar. The Formula sheet contains - Hindi name of the drug, Latin or chemical name, part used, form, properties and action, Book reference along with Page No. in which this particular herb is defined, and quantity used. Along with this, the formula sheet should contain the manufacturing method, Indication, Dosage, Method of use, Presentation, Shelf life and Side effect. The Drug Inspector will review the formula along with all the details and if found satisfactory, forward it to Licensing authority, Ayurvedic and Unani services, in our case it at Dehradun.

The formula will be discussed with a panel of experts of a government body for approval. If the formula, references and other details are found to be satisfactory, the license is issued. The whole procedure for review and discussion after submitting the formula to the government authority will take about one month.

Chemical Characterization of Coronil Tablet

UPLC/QToF MS Study of Coronil

Sample Preparation Method: 10 ml methanol: water (80:20) was added in 101.1 mg of powdered sample and sonicated for 30 min. Then this solution was centrifuged for 5 min at 8000 rpm and filtered through a 0.22 μm nylon filter.

UPLC/QToF MS Condition: Analysis was performed on a Xevo G2-XS QToF of Waters with Acquity UPLC- I Class and Unifi software. Separation was carried out using the Nucleodur C18 Gravity column (100 x 2.0 mm, 1.8 μm). The column was maintained at 35°C throughout the analysis and sample temperature was kept at 20°C during the analysis. Detection was carried out by Xevo G2-XS QToF. The elution was carried out at a flow rate of 0.3 ml/min using gradient elution shown in Table **2.57** of mobile phase 0.1% formic acid in water (mobile phase A) and 0.1% formic acid in acetonitrile (mobile phase B). 2μl of test solution was injected during the analysis and recorded the chromatograph for 70 min.

Gradient Program

Table 2.57. Details of the gradient program used for UPLC/QToF MS.

Time (min)	Flow (ml/min)	Mobile Phase A (%)	Mobile Phase B (%)
0	0.3	95	5
5	0.3	90	10
15	0.3	80	20
35	0.3	70	30
45	0.3	65	35
60	0.3	20	80
65	0.3	10	90
66	0.3	95	5
70	0.3	95	5

Xevo G2-XS QToF Parameters is shown in Table **2.58**.

Table 2.58. List of parameters used for UPLC/QToF MS analysis.

Parameter	Polarity (+ve)	Polarity (-ve)
Ionisation type	ESI	ESI
Mode	MS^E	MS^E

(Table 2.58) cont.....

Parameter	**Polarity (+ve)**	**Polarity (-ve)**
Acquisition time	70 min	70 min
Mass range (m/z)	50-1200 m/z	50-1200 m/z
Cone Voltage	40 V	40 V
Capillary	1.5 kV	2 kV
Low CE	6.0 eV	6.0 eV
High CE	20-40 eV (ramp)	20-40 eV(ramp)
Source temperature	120 °C	120 °C
Desolvation Temperature	500 °C	500 °C
Cone gas flow	50 L/h	50 L/h
Desolvation gas flow	900 L/h	900 L/h
Lock Spray (Leucine Enkaphalin)	556.2766 m/z	554.2620 m/z

UPLC Chromatogram of Coronil tablet in positive mode is shown in Fig. (**2.56**) and negative mode is shown in Fig. (**2.57**). different phyto-constituents identified in both the positive and negative modes by UPLC/QToF MS in Coronil are shown in Table **2.59**.

Table 2.59. Identified compounds in Coronil tablet in positive and negative mode.

Positive Mode							
S.No.	**Component name**	**Formula**	**RT (min)**	**Observed m/z**	**Neutral Mass (Da)**	**Response**	**Adducts**
1	N-Methylcoclaurine	$C_{18}H_{21}NO_{3}$	2.60	300.1592	299.1521	312537	+H
2	Magnoflorine	$C_{20}H_{23}NO_{4}$	6.58	342.1704	341.1627	1391071	+H
3	Kaempferol-3-gentiobioside	$C_{27}H_{30}O_{16}$	12.96	611.1605	610.1534	303850	+H, +Na
4	Columbamine	$C_{20}H_{19}NO_{4}$	13.32	338.1385	337.1314	305004	+H
5	Ecdysterone	$C_{27}H_{44}O_{7}$	13.46	481.3149	480.3087	95249	+H, +Na
6	Dihydroberberine	$C_{20}H_{19}NO_{4}$	13.61	338.1388	337.1314	268053	+H
7	kaempferol-3-O-rutino- side (Nictoflorin)	$C_{27}H_{30}O_{15}$	13.98	595.1659	594.1585	123970	+H, +Na
8	kaempferol 5-O-β-D-glucoronopyranoside	$C_{21}H_{18}O_{12}$	14.01	463.0877	462.0798	1434459	+H, +Na
9	Astragalin	$C_{21}H_{20}O_{11}$	15.66	449.1082	448.1006	63918	+H
10	Palmatinee	$C_{21}H_{21}NO_{4}$	15.87	352.1548	351.1471	440694	+H
11	Baicalein-6-glucuronide	$C_{21}H_{18}O_{11}$	16.56	447.0927	446.0849	1243947	+H, +Na
12	Moupinamide	$C_{18}H_{19}NO_{4}$	19.70	314.1398	313.1314	1173694	+H, +Na
13	Quercetin	$C_{15}H_{10}O_{7}$	21.98	303.0497	302.0427	63101	+H

(Table 2.59) cont.....

14	Luteolin	$^{C}15^{H}10^{O}6$	22.21	287.0551	286.0477	200607	+H
15	Withanoside IV	$^{C}40^{H}62^{O}15$	26.95	783.4173	782.4089	220549	+H, +Na
16	Withanolide D	$^{C}28^{H}38^{O}6$	26.96	471.2747	470.2668	332882	+H
17	Viscosalactone B	$^{C}28^{H}40^{O}7$	28.12	489.2861	488.2774	2111414	+H, +Na
18	Kaempferol	$^{C}15^{H}10^{O}6$	28.47	287.0548	286.0477	57512	+H
19	Dehydroisoandrosterone	$^{C}19^{H}28^{O}2$	33.56	289.2165	288.2089	209778	+H
20	24,25-Dihydrowithanolide D	$^{C}28^{H}40^{O}6$	33.66	473.2911	472.2825	887318	+H, +Na
21	Withaferin A	$^{C}28^{H}38^{O}6$	36.63	471.2762	470.2668	4774338	+H, +Na
22	Withanolide A	$^{C}28^{H}38^{O}6$	39.28	471.2738	470.2668	115020	+H, +Na
23	Withanolide B	$^{C}28^{H}38^{O}5$	41.02	455.2787	454.2719	197817	+H, +Na
24	Withanoside V	$^{C}40^{H}62^{O}14$	41.53	767.4230	766.4140	342048	+H, +Na
25	Withanone	$^{C}28^{H}38^{O}6$	42.35	471.2723	470.2668	28012	+H, +Na
26	Cirsimaritin	$^{C}17^{H}14^{O}6$	44.05	315.0862	314.0790	283160	+H
27	Methyl rosmarinate	$^{C}19^{H}18^{O}8$	44.73	375.1068	374.1002	156358	+H
28	5-Hydroxy-7,8-dimethoxyflavone	$^{C}17^{H}14^{O}5$	50.77	299.0917	298.0841	1014772	+H
29	Withanolide G	$^{C}28^{H}38^{O}5$	51.75	455.2804	454.2719	155535	+H, +Na

Negative Mode							
S.No.	**Component name**	**Formula**	**RT (min)**	**Observed m/z**	**Neutral Mass (Da)**	**Response**	**Adducts**
1	Citric acid	$C_6H_8O_7$	1.08	191.0183	192.0270	955462	-H
2	Cordifolioside A	$^{C}22^{H}32^{O}13$	6.49	549.1796	504.1843	9760	+HCOO, -H
3	Magnoflorine	$^{C}20^{H}23^{NO}4$	6.56	340.1516	341.1627	142618	-H, +HCOO
4	3-O-trans- Feruloylquinic acid	$^{C}17^{H}20^{O}9$	9.72	367.1003	368.1107	617706	-H
5	Kaempferol-3-gentiobioside	$^{C}27^{H}30^{O}16$	13.01	609.1485	610.1534	1228467	-H
6	Ecdysterone	$^{C}27^{H}44^{O}7$	13.47	525.3068	480.3087	812518	+HCOO, -H
7	Kaempferol-3-O- rutino-side (Nictoflorin)	$^{C}27^{H}30^{O}15$	14.03	593.1529	594.1585	436009	-H
8	Kaempferol 5-O-β-D-glucoronopyranoside	$^{C}21^{H}18^{O}12$	14.09	461.0708	462.0798	1195779	-H, +HCOO
9	(-)-Rabdosiin	$^{C}36^{H}30^{O}16$	15.53	717.1501	718.1534	612346	-H

(Table 2.59) cont.....

10	Astragalin	$^{C}21^{H}20^{O}11$	15.72	447.0910	448.1006	124056	-H, +HCOO
12	Baicalein-6- glucuronide	$^{C}21^{H}18^{O}11$	16.64	445.0753	446.0849	1231457	-H
13	Rosmarinic acid	$^{C}18^{H}16^{O}8$	16.84	359.0738	360.0845	669327	-H
14	3,4-Dicaffeoylquinic acid	$C_{25}H_{24}O_{12}$	16.98	515.1182	516.1268	314301	-H
15	Tinosporide	$C_{20}H_{22}O_{7}$	19.62	419.1318	374.1366	206203	+HCOO
16	Moupinamide	$C_{18}H_{19}NO_{4}$	19.76	312.1210	313.1314	787736	-H, +HCOO
17	Tinocordiside	$C_{21}H_{32}O_{7}$	20.92	395.2046	396.2148	3998514	-H
18	Tanegoside C	$C_{27}H_{36}O_{13}$	21.95	567.2087	568.2156	163639	-H
19	Quercetin	$C_{15}H_{10}O_{7}$	22.09	301.0316	302.0427	87181	-H
20	Luteolin	$C_{15}H_{10}O_{6}$	22.31	285.0371	286.0477	226485	-H
21	Withanoside IV	$C_{40}H_{62}O_{15}$	26.97	827.4129	782.4089	5232836	+HCOO, -H
22	Viscosalactone B	$C_{28}H_{40}O_{7}$	28.15	533.2761	488.2774	3207838	+HCOO, -H
23	Kaempferol	$C_{15}H_{10}O_{6}$	28.59	285.0371	286.0477	94070	-H
24	Withanolide E	$C_{28}H_{38}O_{7}$	29.07	531.2571	486.2618	58235	+HCOO, -H
25	Withaferin A	$C_{28}H_{38}O_{6}$	36.64	515.2630	470.2668	30854	+HCOO, -H
26	Withanoside V	$C_{40}H_{62}O_{14}$	41.54	811.4182	766.4140	5577478	+HCOO, -H
27	Withanone	$C_{28}H_{38}O_{6}$	42.05	515.2553	470.2668	10648	+HCOO, -H
28	Methyl rosmarinate	$C_{19}H_{18}O_{8}$	44.79	373.0889	374.1002	102157	-H
29	Betulinic acid	$C_{30}H_{48}O_{3}$	60.15	455.3503	456.3604	115339	-H, +HCOO
30	Ursolic acid	$C_{30}H_{48}O_{3}$	60.62	501.3570	456.3604	150407	+HCOO, -H

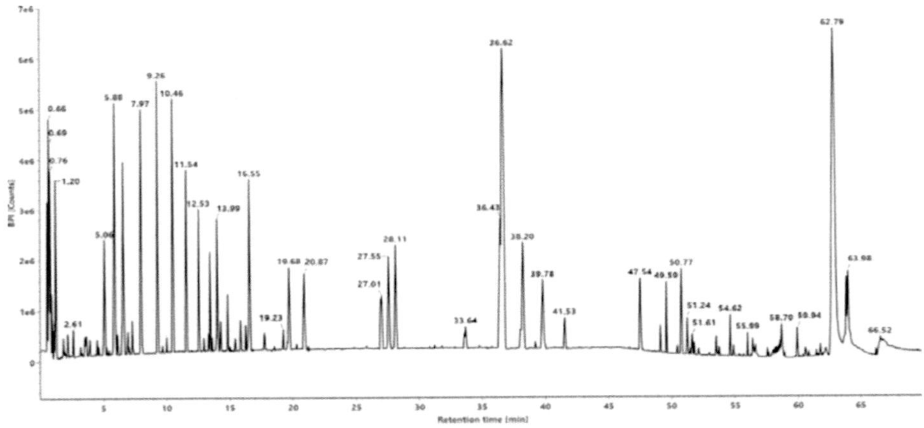

Fig. (2.56). Representative chromatograph of Coronil in positive mode using UPLC/QToF MS.

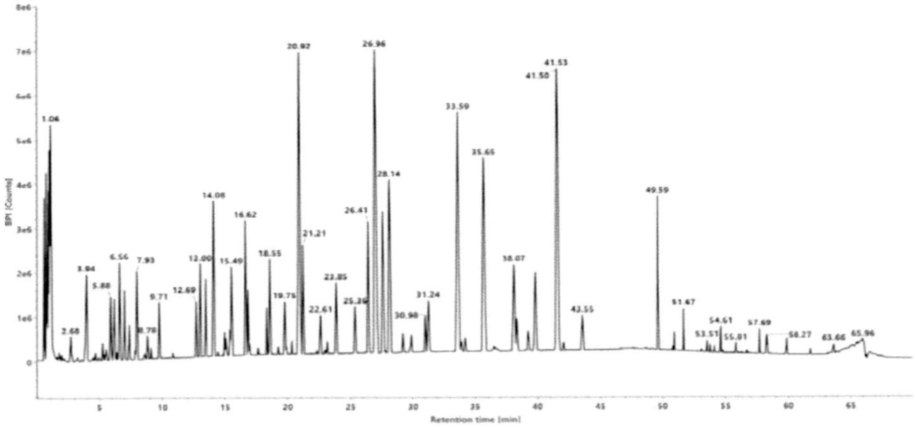

Fig. (2.57). Representative chromatograph of Coronil in negative mode using UPLC/QToF MS.

Conclusion: A total of 41 compounds were identified in the Coronil tablet and this analysis also confirmed the presence of Ashwagandha, Giloy and Tulsi in the medicinal formulation.

HPLC-PDA Method Development for Standardization of Coronil Tablet

Method development, validation, identification and quantification of marker compounds in Coronil tablet by HPLC.

HPLC Condition

Analysis was performed by Prominence-XR UHPLC system (Instrument ID: CHI-056) (Shimadzu, Japan) equipped with Quaternary pump (Nexera XR LC-20AD XR), DAD detector (SPD-M20 A), Auto-sampler (Nexera XR SIL-20 AC XR), Degassing unit (DGU-20A 5R) and Column oven (CTO-10 AS VP). Separation was achieved using a Shimadzu Shim pack GIST-HP C18 (3μm, 3 X 100 mm) column (Serial No.-20A00104) subjected to binary gradient elution. The two solvents used for the analysis consisted of water containing 0.1% orthophosphoric acid, adjust pH 2.5 with diethylamine (solvent A) and Acetonitrile (solvent B). Gradient programming of the solvent system was initially at 5% B for 0-10 min, 5-15% B from 10-20 min, 15-25% B from 20-40 min, 25-65% B from 40-60 min, 65-90% B from 60-65 min, 90-5% B from 65-66min, 5% B from 66-70 min, with a flow rate of 0.7 ml/min. 10 μl of standard and test solution were injected and the column temperature was maintained at 30 °C. Wavelengths were set 227 nm (for Withanone, Withaferin A, Withanoside IV, Withanoside V, Codifolioside A and Magnoflorine), 325 nm (for Rosmarinic acid and Palmatinee) and 210 nm for Ursolic acid and Betulinic acid).

Standard Preparation

Standard stock solution: Standards Palmatinee Hydrochloride (Potency-75.1%, Sigma Aldrich), Cordifolioside A (Potency-98.0%, Chemfaces), Magnoflorine (Potency-99.0%, Sigma Aldrich), Withanone (Potency-93.6%, Natural remedies), Withaferin A (Potency-98.0%, Natural remedies), Withanoside IV (Potency-96.2%, Natural remedies), Withanoside V (Potency-97.6%), Rosmarinic acid (Potency-98.0%, Sigma Aldrich), Ursolic acid (Potency-97.30%, Tokyo chemical industries) and Betulinic acid (Potency-98.7%, Natural remedies) were dissolved in methanol to prepare 1000 ppm standard solution individually.

Standard mix working standard: Take 0.05 ml of 1000 ppm from each standard stock solution and diluted it to 1 ml to prepare 50 ppm of standard mix working standard.

Sample Preparation: 0.5 gm of powdered Coronil tablet sample was diluted with 10 ml water: methanol (20:80) and sonicated for 30 min, centrifuged at 10000 rpm for 5 min and filtered using 0.45 μm nylon filter and used for the analysis.

A typical HPLC chromatogram of the sample is shown in Fig. (**2.58**).

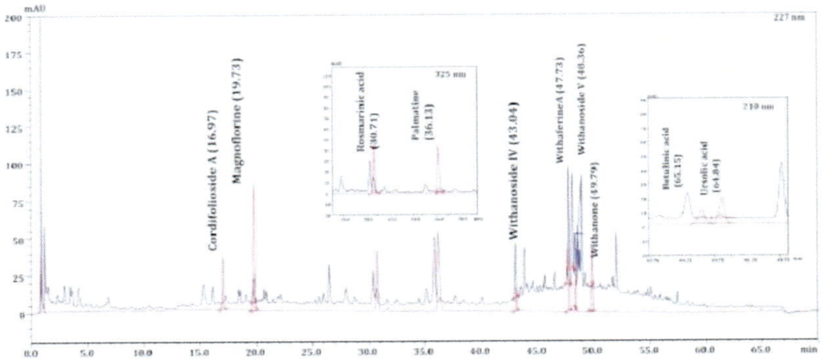

Fig. (2.58). Overlap HPLC chromatograph of the standard mix (in Purple) and Coronil (in Blue). Cordifolioside A, Magnoflorine, Withanoside IV, Withaferin A, Withanoside V and Withanone was quantified at 227 nm wavelength. Rosmarinic acid and Palmatinee were quantified at 325 nm wavelength. Betulinic acid and Ursolic acid were quantified at 210 nm wavelength.

Based on HPLC analysis the compounds identified and quantified are listed in Table **2.60**.

Table 2.60. Results of marker compounds in Coronil.

S.No.	Name Of Marker Compound	Retention time (in min.)	Result in (µg/mg)	Plant Species
1	Cordifolioside A	16.97	Below quantification limit	*Tinospora cordifolia*
2	Magnoflorine	19.73	0.238	*Tinospora cordifolia*
3	Rosmarinic acid	30.71	0.242	*Ocimum sanctum*
4	Palmatinee	36.12	0.051	*Tinospora cordifolia*
5	Withanoside IV	43.09	3.160	*Withania somnifera*
6	Withaferin A	47.75	2.016	*Withania somnifera*
7	Withanoside V	48.33	1.200	*Withania somnifera*
8	Withanone	49.79	0.010	*Withania somnifera*
9	Betulinic acid	64.55	0.063	*Ocimum sanctum*
10	Ursolic acid	64.86	0.125	*Ocimum sanctum*

Table 2.61. Summary of validation report of Coronil using HPLC.

S. N	Parameter	Acceptance criteria	Result obtained									
			Cordifo-lioside A	**Magnofo-rine**	**Rosmarinic acid**	**Palmatinee**	**Withano-side IV**	**Withaferin**	**Withano-side V**	**Withanone**	**Betulinic acid**	**Ursolic acid**
1	System Suitability	% RSD of Retention time - NMT 2.0%	0.54	0.47	0.32	0.76	0.86	0.82	0.88	0.56	0.22	0.43
		% RSD of area – NMT 2.0%	1.43	0.41	1.67	1.09	1.75	1.80	0.58	1.20	1.28	0.58
		Theoretical plates – NLT 2000	86501	120046	163214	123608	712718	1050356	1589022	964666	1932327	1906177
2	Specificity	No interference at retention time	Complies									
		Peak purity – NLT 0.980	0.997	0.99	0.987	0.991	0.994	0.985	0.986	0.982	0.998	0.983
3	Linearity	Correlation coefficient NLT 0.99	0.999	0.999	0.999	0.999	0.999	0.999	0.999	0.999	0.999	0.999
4	Precision											
4.1	System	%RSD of area – NMT 4%	BLQ	0.78	0.85	1.68	0.78	0.97	1.13	3.89	2.26	1.51
4.2	Intermediate	%RSD of assay – NMT 3%	BLQ	0.53	2.89	3.01	0.81	0.51	2.93	1.48	2.67	1.16
5	Limit of detection	%RSD of area – NMT 33%	3.59	1.78	1.29	0.76	1.60	2.01	2.86	5.41	8.53	2.68
6	Limit of Quantification	%RSD of area – NMT 10%	1.63	2.65	1.59	2.58	1.23	2.35	3.77	1.10	2.23	2.29
7	Stability	60°C for 24 hours	Stable									
		80 °C for 24 hours										
		366nm for 24 hours										
		257nm for 24 hours										
		White light for 24 hours										
		Solution in methanol for 48 hours										

To study the consistency of the manufacturing process, batch to batch analysis of the product was studied on 14 samples and results in μg/mg are shown in Table **2.62**.

Table 2.62. Batch analysis of Coronil tablet.

S. No.	Batch Number	Magnoflorine	Rosmarinic Acid	Palmatinee	Withanoside IV	Withaferin A	Withanoside V
1	#A CNT001	0.238	0.242	0.051	3.160	2.016	1.200
2	#A CNT002	0.272	0.199	0.033	2.404	2.339	0.485
3	#A CNT003	0.279	0.207	0.035	2.437	2.441	0.653
4	#A CNT004	0.283	0.121	0.012	1.977	1.794	0.647
5	#A CNT005	0.271	0.218	0.013	2.009	1.658	0.627
6	#A CNT006	0.217	0.211	0.018	2.409	1.184	0.723
7	#A CNT007	0.077	0.180	0.009	1.780	0.815	0.675
8	#A CNT008	0.076	0.171	0.009	1.768	0.769	0.642
9	#A CNT009	0.075	0.182	0.010	1.964	0.895	0.723
10	#A CNT010	0.076	0.178	0.010	1.927	0.848	0.659
11	#A CNT092	0.576	0.198	0.030	1.836	0.644	0.452
12	#A CNT110	0.101	0.131	0.015	1.973	0.788	0.656
13	#A CNT111	0.115	0.135	0.015	2.202	1.048	0.734
14	#A CNT112	0.095	0.125	0.015	1.895	0.736	1.453
	Limit (Not Less Than)	0.05	0.15	0.01	1.5	0.75	0.60

HPTLC Method Development for Standardization of Coronil Tablet

Experiment Methods

reparation of Sample Solution: 500 mg of sample was dissolved in 6 ml methanol: water (80: 20), sonicated, and centrifuged to obtain a clear solution.

Preparation of Standard Solution: The stock solution was prepared by dissolving 10 mg of Withaferin A, Rosmarinic acid, Ursolic acid, Withanoside IV, Palmatinee and Magnoflorine in 10 ml of methanol. The working solution was prepared from stock solution by dissolving 0.1ml of stock solution in 1ml of methanol.

Chromatographic Conditions

TLC plate: TLC plate with silica gel 60 F_{254}. (10 × 10 cm) (E. Merck, Darmstadt, Germany).

Mobile phase

A. For Withaferin A, Rosmarinic acid and Ursolic acid Toluene: ethyl acetate: formic acid (5: 5:1)

B. For Withanoside IV, Palmatinee and Magnoflorine

Ethyl acetate: formic acid: acetic acid: water (10: 1.1: 1.1: 2.6) Derivatization: Anisaldehyde sulphuric acid reagent.

Results

A: Results of Withanoside IV in Coronil

A.1: Representative image of developed TLC at 254 nm, Whit light after derivatization, 366nm and scan chromatogram at 530 and 254nm is shown in Fig. (**2.59**).

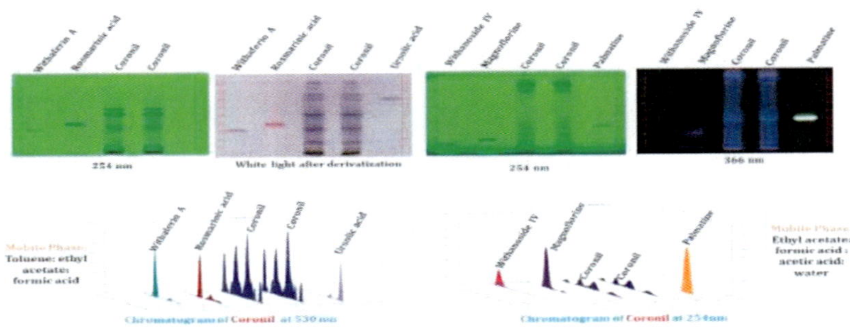

Fig. (2.59). HPTLC fingerprinting of Coronil tablet at 254 nm, White light after derivatization and 366nm with standards Withaferin A, Rosmarinic acid, Ursolic acid, Withanoside IV and Magnoflorine, and Palmatinee along with scan chromatogram at 530 and 254 nm.

HPTLC Method Validation for Standardization of Ashwagandha

A: Determination of linearity of Withanoside IV for application in Coronil is shown in Fig. **(2.60)**.

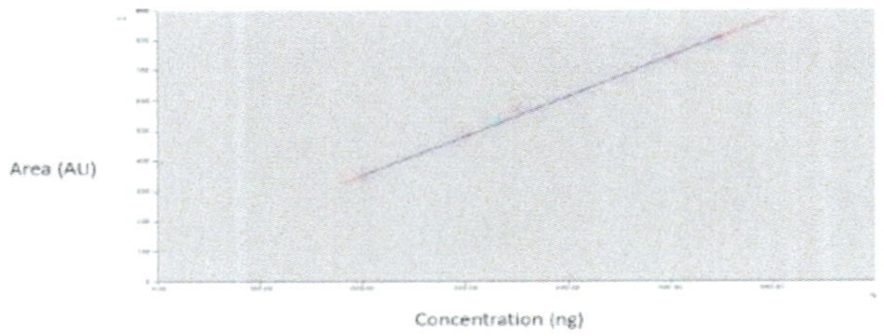

Fig. (2.60). Linearity of Withanoside IV as determined by HPTLC.

The linearity correlation coefficient was determined using the regression equation given in Table **2.63**.

Table 2.63. Correlation coefficient as determined by HPTLC for Withanoside IV.

Parameter	**Withanoside IV**
Linearity range (ng/spot)	200 – 600
Regression equation	1.309 *X + 89.031
Correlation coefficient	0.997
RF	0.25

A.1: Detection of Withanoside IV at 230 nm is show in in Fig. **(2.61)**.

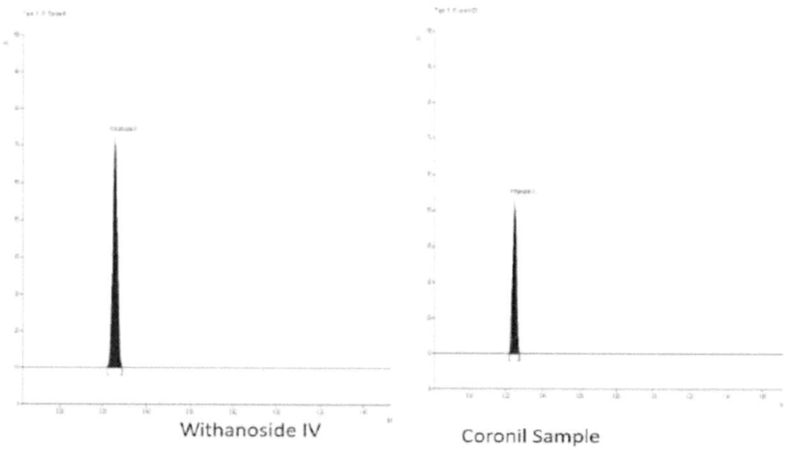

Fig. (2.61). HPTLC chromatogram of Withanoside IV standard and Coronil sample.

A.2: Limit of detection (LOD) and limit of quantification(LOQ) for Withanoside IV is shown in Table **2.64**.

Table 2.64. Determination of LOD and LOQ for Withanoside IV using HPTLC.

LOD	1.73 ppm
LOQ	5.26 pm

A.3: Precision of the method used for detecting Withanoside IV using HPTLC is shown in Table **2.65**.

Table 2.65. HPTLC standardized method precision for detection of Withanoside IV.

Precision	**% RSD**
is Intra day	0.94%
Inter day	0.80

A.4: Percent recovery of Withanoside IV using HPTLC is shown in Table **2.66**.

Table 2.66. Recovery percentage of withanoside IV using HPTLC.

Recovery Level	% Recovery	Mean Recovery %
80%	101.18%	98.89%
100%	94.91%	
120%	100.55%	

Result: Amount of Withanoside IV was found to be 0.245% in Coronil sample.

B Linearity of Withaferin A for analysis of Coronil is shown in Fig. (**2.62**).

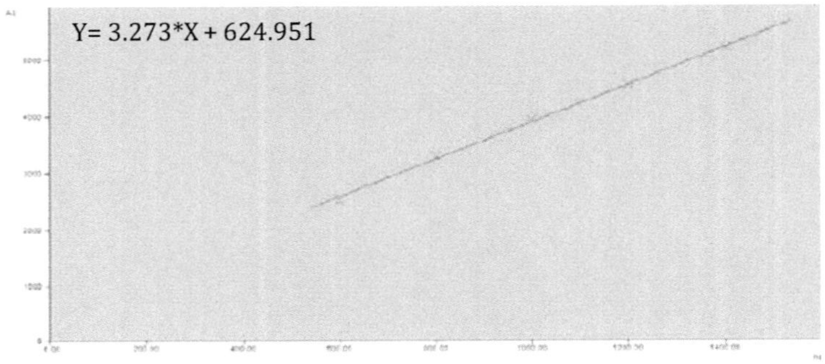

Fig. (2.62). Linearity of Withaferin A as determined by HPTLC.

The correlation coefficient of linearity was determined by the regression equation is shown in Table **2.67**.

Table 2.67. Regression equation used for determining the linearity of Withaferin A by HPTLC.

Parameter	Withaferin A
Linearity range (ng)	600 – 1400
Regression equation	624.951+3.273*X
Correlation coefficient	0.999
RF	0.38

B.1: Detection of Withaferin A at 230 nm is shown in Fig. (**2.63**).

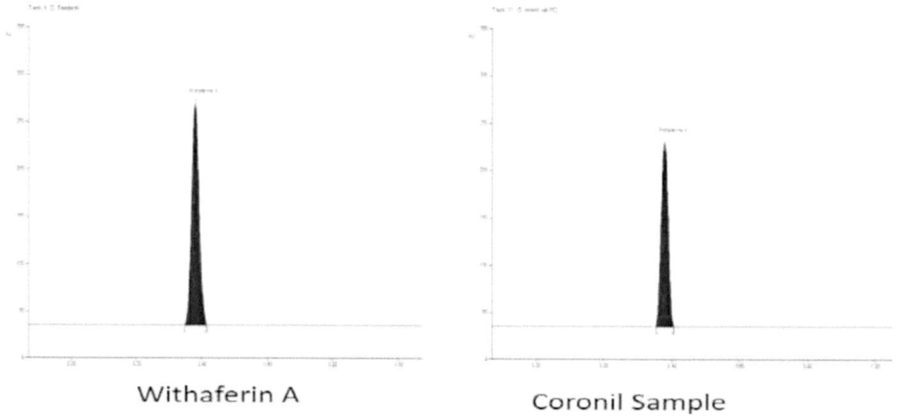

Fig. (2.63). Representative HPTLC chromatogram of standard and Coronil sample.

B.2: Limit of detection and limit of quantification of Withaferin A is shown in Table **2.68**.

Table 2.68. LOD and LOQ of Withaferin A as determined by HPTLC.

LOD	0.87 ppm
LOQ	2.63 pm

B.3: Precision of the standardized method for HPTLC in detection of Withaferin A is shown in Table **2.69**

Table 2.69. Method precision used in the detection of Withaferin A using HPTLC.

Precision	**% RSD**
Intraday	1.04%
Interday	0.94%

B.4: Recovery of Withaferin A using HPTLC is shown in Table **2.70**.

Table 2.70. Recovery of Withaferin A using HPTLC method.

Recovery level	% Recovery	Mean Recovery %
80%	95.81%	93.91%
100%	94.42%	
120%	91.51%	

Result: The amount of Withaferin A was found to be 0.243% in the Coronil sample.

C. Linearity of Magnoflorine in Coronil tablet is shown in Fig. **(2.64)**.

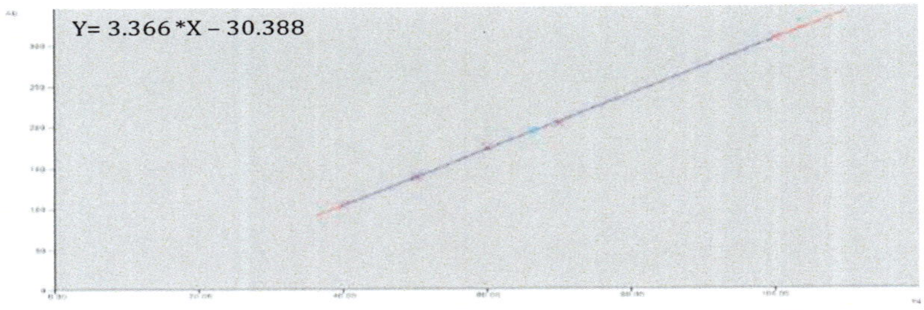

Fig. (2.64). Linearity of Magnoflorine using HPTLC method.

The correlation coefficient of linearity was determined by the regression equation is shown in Table **2.71**.

Table 2.71. Regression equation of Magnoflorine using HPTLC method.

Parameter	Magnoflorine
Linearity range (ng)	40 – 100
Regression equation	3.366 *X – 30.388
Correlation coefficient	0.999
RF	0.21

C.1: Detection of Magnoflorine at 265 nm is shown in Fig. **(2.65)**.

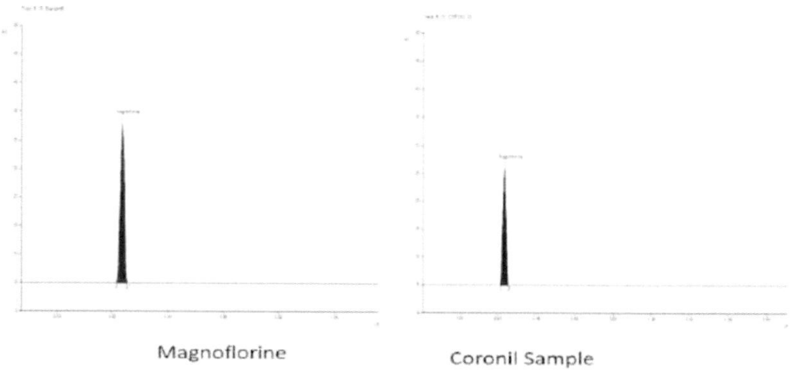

Fig. (2.65). HPTLC chromatogram of Magnoflorine standard and Coronil Sample.

C.2: Limit of detection and Limit of quantification of Mgnoflorine is shown in Table **2.72**.

Table 2.72. LOD and LOQ of Coronil tablet.

LOD	8.81 ppm
LOQ	26.71 pm

C.3: Precision of Coronil for Magnonoflorine is shown in Table **2.73**.

Table 2.73. Precision of Coronil tablet.

Precision	**% RSD**
Intraday	0.97%
Interday	1.05

C.4: Recovery of Magnoflorine in Coronil tablet is shown in is Table **2.74**.

Table 2.74. Recovery of Coronil tablet.

Recovery Level	**% Recovery**	**Mean Recovery %**
80%	100.32%	99.43%
100%	98.30%	
120%	99.66%	

Amount of Magnoflorine was found to be 0.02% in sample.

D. Linearity Palmatinee in Coronil tablet is shown in Fig. **(2.66)**.

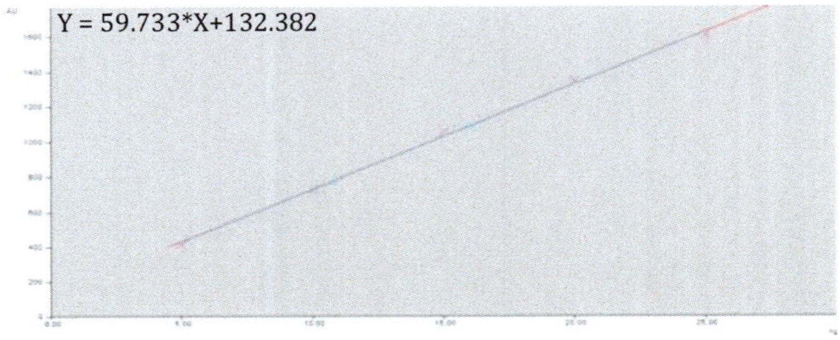

Fig. (2.66). Linearity of Palmatinee in Coronil tablet.

The correlation coefficient of Palmatine was determined by the regression equation is shown in Table **2.75**.

Table 2.75. Regression equation of Palmatine in Coronil tablet.

Parameter	**Palmatinee**
Linearity range (ng)	5 – 25
Regression equation	132.382 + 59.733*X
Correlation coefficient	0.999
RF	0.55

D.1: Detection of Palmatinee at 350 nm is shown in Fig. (**2.67**).

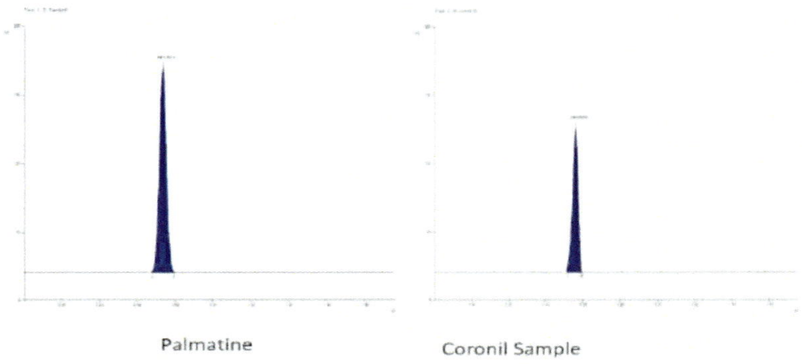

Fig. (2.67). HPTLC chromatogram of Palmatinee standard and Coronil tablet.

D.2: Limit of detection limit of quantification of Palmatine in Coronil tablet is shown in Table **2.76**

Table 2.76. LOD and LOQ of Coronil tablet.

LOD	0.03 ppm
LOQ	0.10 pm

D.3: Precision of HPTLC method for Palmatinee in Coronil is shown in Table **2.77**.

Table 2.77. Precision of Coronil tablet.

Precision	**% RSD**
Intra day	0.83%
Inter day	1.01%

D.4: Recovery of HPTLC method for Palmatinee in Coronil is shown in Table **2.78**.

Table 2.78. Recovery of Palmatinee Coronil tablet.

Recovery level	**% Recovery**	**Mean Recovery %**
80%	93.70%	96.91%
100%	97.20%	
120%	99.84%	

Result: Amount of Palmatinee was found to be 0.0034% in sample.

E: Linearity of Rosmarinic acid in Coronil is shown in Fig. **(2.68)**.

The correlation coefficient of linearity of Rosmarinic acid was determined by the regression equation is shown in Table **2.79**.

Table 2.79. Regression equation of Rosmarinic acid in Coronil tablet.

Parameter	**Rosmarinic acid**
Linearity range (ng)	100 – 350
Regression equation	13.836*X – 449.808
Correlation coefficient	0.999
RF	0.32

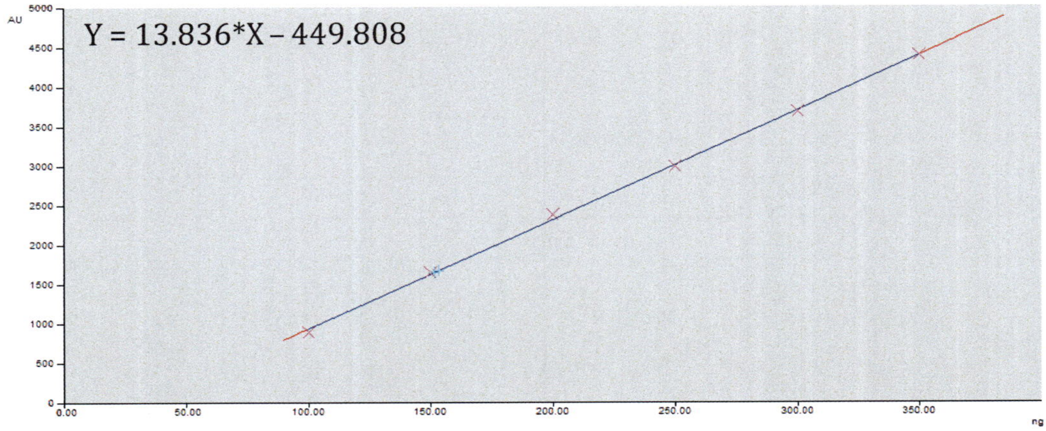

Fig. (2.68). Linearity of Rosmarinic acid in Coronil tablet.

E.1: Detection at 330 nm of Rosmarinic acid in Coronil table is shown in Fig. **(2.69)**.

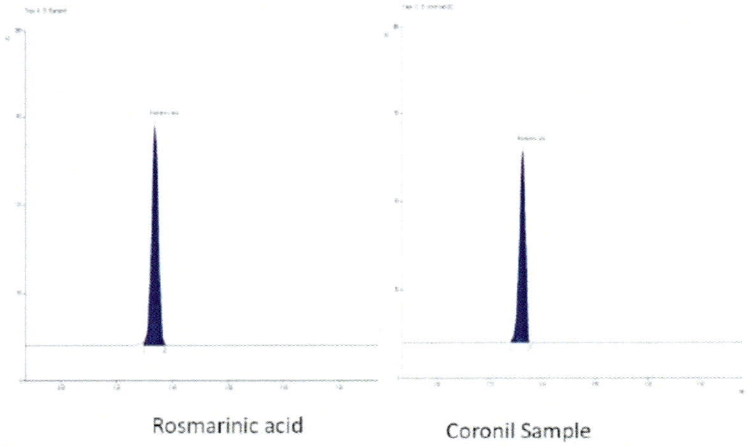

Fig. (2.69). HPTLC chromatogram of Rosmarinic standard and Coronil tablet.

E.2: Limit of Detection Limit of Quantification of Rosmarinic acid is shown in Table **2.80**.

Table 2.80. LOD and LOQ of Rosmarinic acid in Coronil tablet.

LOD	0.10 ppm
LOQ	1.31 ppm

E.3: Precision of Rosmarinic acid in Coronil tablet is shown in Table **2.81**.

Table 2.81. Precision of Rosmarinic acid in Coronil tablet.

Precision	% RSD
Intra day	0.95%
Inter day	0.52%

E.4: Recovery of Rosmarinic acid in Coronil tablet is shown in Table **2.82**.

Table 2.82. Recovery Rosmarinic acid in Coronil tablet.

Recovery level	% Recovery	Mean Recovery %
80%	95.34%	96.73%
100%	93.92%	
120%	100.75%	

Amount of Rosmarinic acid was found to be 0.017% in sample.

F: Analysis of Ursolic acid in Coronil tablet

F.1 Limit of detection limit of quantification of Ursolic acid in Coronil tablet is shown in Table **2.83**.

Table 2.83. LOD and LOQ of Ursolic acid in Coronil tablet.

LOD	0.51 ppm
LOQ	1.53 ppm

F.2: Precision of HPTLC method in detection of Ursolic acid in Coronil tablet is shown in Table **2.84**.

Table 2.84. Precision of Ursolic acid in Coronil tablet.

Precision	% RSD
Intra day	1.24%
Inter day	0.85%

F.3: Recovery of Ursolic acid in Coronil tablet is shown in Table **2.85**.

Table 2.85. Recovery of Ursolic acid in Coronil tablet.

Recovery Level	% Recovery	Mean Recovery %
80%	94.86%	95.64%
100%	92.59%	
120%	99.47%	

Result: The amount of Ursolic acid was found to be 0.07% in the sample.

Summary of HPTL Validation Report is shown in Table **2.86**.

Table 2.86. Summary report of Validation of Coronil tablet.

S. No.	Parameters	Acceptance Criteria	Result Obtained					
			Withaferin A	**Rosmarinic acid**	**Ursolic acid**	**Magnoflorine**	**Withanoside IV**	**Palmatinee**
1	System Suitability	% RSD of Retention time - NMT 2.0%	0.61%	0.27%	0.27%	0.58%	0.54%	1.42%
		% RSD of area – NMT 2.0%	0.99%	0.73%	1.04%	1.01%	0.80%	0.92%
2	Linearity	Correlation coefficient NLT 0.99	0.99	0.99	0.99	0.99	0.99	0.99
3	Precision							
3.1	System	%RSD of area – NMT 2%	0.99%	0.73%	1.04%	1.01%	0.87%	0.92%
3.2	Intermediate	%RSD of assay – NMT 2%	0.94%	0.52%	0.84%	1.05%	0.80%	1.00%
3.3	Method	%RSD of assay – NMT 2%	1.04%	0.95%	1.23%	0.97%	0.94%	0.83

Chemical Characterization of Divya Swasari Vati

UPLC/QToF MS Study of Divya Swasari Vati

Sample Preparation Method

10 ml methanol: water (80:20) was added to 100 mg of powdered sample and sonicated for 30 min. Then this solution was centrifuged for 5 min at 10000 rpm and filtered through a 0.22 µm nylon filter.

UPLC/QToF MS Condition

Analysis was performed on a Xevo G2-XS QToF of Waters with Acquity UPLC-I Class and Unifi software. Separation was carried out using the Nucleodur C18 Gravity column (100 x 2.0 mm, 1.8 µm). The column was maintained at 35°C throughout the analysis and sample temperature was kept at 20°C during the analysis. Detection was carried out by Xevo G2-XS QToF. The elution was carried out at a flow rate of 0.3 ml/min using gradient elution similar to Coronil with mobile phase 0.05% formic acid in water (mobile phase A) and 0.05% formic acid in acetonitrile (mobile phase B). 1 µl of test solution was injected during the analysis and recorded the chromatograph for 40 min. The representative UPLC chromatogram of Divya Swasari Vati in Positive and Negative modes is shown in Fig. **(2.70)**.

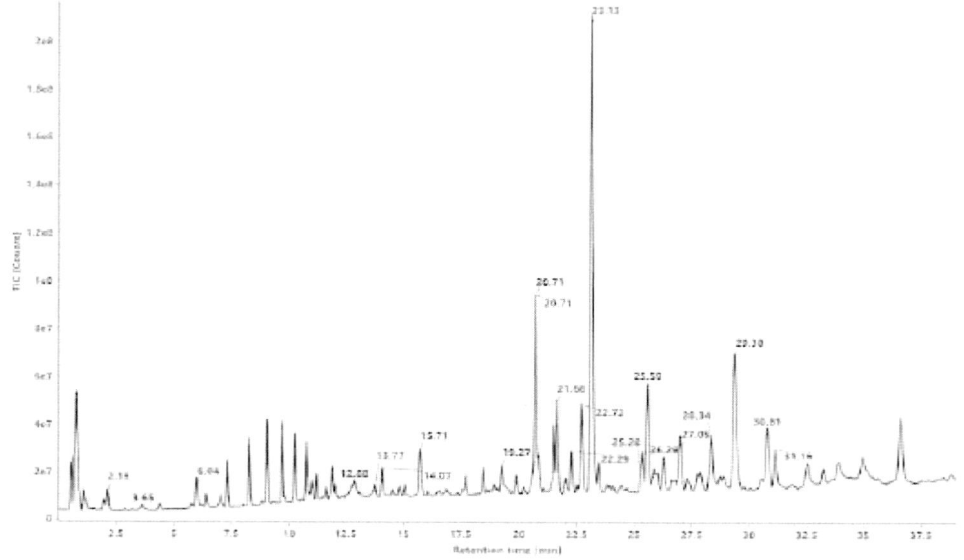

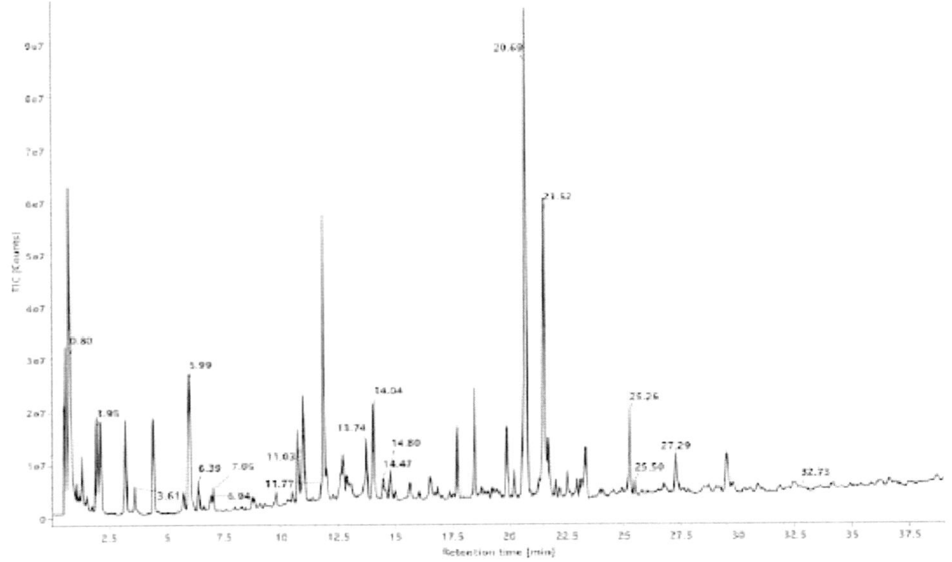

Fig. (2.70). Representative chromatograph of Divya Swasari vati in Positive and Negative mode using UPLC/QToF MS.

Conclusion: A total of 39 compounds were identified in Divya Swasari vati as shown in Table **2.87**.

HPLC-PDA Method Development for Standardization of Divya Swasari Vati

HPLC Condition

Method: The quantification of marker compounds was performed by HPLC system (Waters Corporation, USA) consisting of Binary pump (1525), Detector PDAD (2998) and Auto-sampler (2707). A reverse-phase column Sunfire C18 (5 µm, 4.6 x 250 mm) was used and the column temperature was maintained at 35.0°C. HPLC mobile phase A (0.1% orthophosphoric acid in water adjust pH 2.5 with diethylamine) and mobile phase B (0.1% orthophosphoric acid in a mixer of acetonitrile and water in the ratio of 88:12, adjust pH 2.5 with diethylamine) gradient composition as shown in Table **2.88** and **2.89** at a flow rate of 1.0 ml/min were used. 10 µl of standard solutions and test solution was injected during the analysis. Chromatograph at 278 nm wavelength for cinnamic acid, eugenol, 6-gingerol, piperine and chromatograph at 250 nm wavelength for glycyrrhizin, gallic acid and ellagic acid were recorded.

Table 2.87. UPLC/QToF MS Identified compounds of Divya Swasari Vati in positive and negative modes.

Positive Mode

S.No.	Component Name	Formula	RT (min)	Observed m/z	Neutral Mass (Da)	Response	Adducts
1	Gallic acid	$C_7H_6O_5$	2.13	171.0291	170.0215	53135	+H
2	Protocatechuic acid	$C_7H_6O_4$	3.65	155.034	154.0266	8791	+H
3	Methyl gallate	$C_8H_8O_5$	6.04	185.0447	184.0372	88168	+H
4	Ellagic acid	$C_{14}H_{6}O_{8}$	11.09	303.014	302.0063	13659	+H
5	Coumarin	$C_9H_6O_2$	12.88	147.0446	146.0368	431343	+H
6	Licurazide	$C_{26}H_{30}O_{13}$	13.77	551.1762	550.1686	193106	+H, +Na
7	Liquiritin apioside	$C_{26}H_{30}O_{13}$	14.07	551.1757	550.1686	344670	+H, +Na
8	Cinnamic acid	$C_9H_8O_2$	15.71	149.0603	148.0524	64974	+H
9	Eugenol	$C_{10}H_{12}O_{2}$	19.27	165.0894	164.0837	12221	+H
10	Piperanine	$C_{17}H_{21}NO_{3}$	19.4	288.1608	287.1521	156781	+H, +Na
11	Glycyrrhetic acid	$C_{30}H_{46}O_{4}$	20.71	471.3477	470.3396	489619	+H
12	Glycyrrhizin	$C_{42}H_{62}O_{16}$	20.71	823.4115	822.4038	2853912	+H, +Na
13	6-Gingerol	$C_{17}H_{26}O_{4}$	21.66	317.1738	294.1831	201999	+Na
14	Piperlonguminine	$C_{16}H_{19}NO_{3}$	22.29	274.1448	273.1365	1507842	+H, +Na
15	Feruperine	$C_{17}H_{21}NO_{3}$	22.72	288.1602	287.1521	3083079	+H, +Na
16	Piperine	$C_{17}H_{19}NO_{3}$	23.13	286.1449	285.1365	3444132	+H, +Na
17	Glabridin	$C_{20}H_{20}O_{4}$	25.28	325.1445	324.1362	520357	+H
18	Piperettine	$C_{19}H_{21}NO_{3}$	25.59	312.1605	311.1521	2570678	+H, +Na
19	Piperolein A	$C_{19}H_{25}NO_{3}$	26.29	316.1921	315.1834	1405243	+H, +Na
20	Retrofractamide A	$C_{20}H_{25}NO_{3}$	27.05	328.1919	327.1834	631777	+H, +Na
21	Dehydropipernonaline	$C_{21}H_{25}NO_{3}$	28.34	340.1915	339.1834	2587890	+H, +Na
22	Pipernonaline	$C_{21}H_{27}NO_{3}$	29.38	342.2072	341.1991	5437196	+H, +Na
23	Piperolein B	$C_{21}H_{29}NO_{3}$	30.81	344.223	343.2147	3424954	+H, +Na
24	Pipercide	$C_{22}H_{29}NO_{3}$	31.16	356.2231	355.2147	2030795	+H, +Na

Negative Mode

S. No.	Component name	Formula	RT (min)	Observed m/z	Neutral mass (Da)	Response	Adducts
1	Quinic acid	$C_{7}H_{12}O_{6}$	0.80	191.0555	192.0634	541598	-H, +HCOO
2	Galloylglucose	$C_{13}H_{16}O_{10}$	1.50	331.0665	332.0744	86204	-H

(Table 2.87) cont.....

Positive Mode							
S.No.	**Component Name**	**Formula**	**RT (min)**	**Observed m/z**	**Neutral Mass (Da)**	**Response**	**Adducts**
3	Gallic acid	$C_7H_6O_5$	1.95	169.0136	170.0215	629003	-H
4	Protocatechuic acid	$C_7H_6O_4$	3.61	153.0185	154.0266	177433	-H
5	Methyl gallate	$C_8H_8O_5$	5.99	183.0292	184.0372	1488232	-H
6	3,4-Di-O-galloylquinic acid	$C_{21}H_{20}O_{14}$	6.18	495.0775	496.0853	90807	-H
7	Chlorogenic acid	$C_{16}H_{18}O_9$	6.39	353.0874	354.0951	332141	-H
8	Digallic acid	$C_{14}H_{10}O_9$	6.94	321.0246	322.0325	129846	-H
9	Cryptochlorogenic acid	$C_{16}H_{18}O_9$	7.05	353.0873	354.0951	217928	-H
10	Ellagic acid	$C_{14}H_6O_8$	11.03	300.9986	302.0063	78625	-H
11	Quercetin-3-O-β-D-glucuronide	$C_{21}H_{18}O_{13}$	11.77	477.0677	478.0747	112047	-H
12	Licurazide	$C_{26}H_{30}O_{13}$	13.74	549.1616	550.1686	603182	-H, +HCOO
13	Liquiritin apioside	$C_{26}H_{30}O_{13}$	14.04	549.1614	550.1686	859570	-H, +HCOO
14	Liquiritin	$C_{21}H_{22}O_9$	14.47	417.1191	418.1264	140850	-H
15	N-feruloyltyramine	$C_{18}H_{19}NO_4$	14.80	312.1240	313.1314	115563	-H
16	Cinnamic acid	$C_9H_8O_2$	15.67	147.0446	148.0524	11414	-H
17	Glycyrrhizin	$C_{42}H_{62}O_{16}$	20.69	821.3994	822.4038	6320565	-H
18	Licoricesaponine K2	$C_{42}H_{62}O_{16}$	21.52	821.3991	822.4038	3647344	-H
19	Glabridin	$C_{20}H_{20}O_4$	25.26	323.1292	324.1362	1053337	-H, +HCOO
20	Sophoranodichromane B	$C_{25}H_{28}O_5$	25.50	407.1870	408.1937	203066	-H
21	Glabrol	$C_{25}H_{28}O_4$	27.29	391.1922	392.1988	633957	-H
22	Sophoranodichromane D	$C_{25}H_{28}O_5$	32.73	407.1865	408.1937	66126	-H

Table 2.88. HPLC mobile phase gradient composition for the study of Divya Swasari Vati for Cinnamic acid, Glycyrrhizin, Eugenol, 6-Gingerol and Piperine.

Time (min)	Flow (ml/min)	A %	B%	Curve
0	1.0	65	35	6
5	1.0	65	35	6
15	1.0	50	50	6
25	1.0	20	80	6
30	1.0	10	90	6
31	1.0	65	35	6
35	1.0	65	35	6

Table 2.89. HPLC mobile phase gradient composition for study of Divya Swasari Vati for Ellagic acid.

Time (min)	Flow (ml/min)	A %	B %	Curve
0	1.0	95	5	6
10	1.0	90	10	6
30	1.0	70	30	6
31	1.0	10	90	6
35	1.0	5	95	6
36	1.0	95	5	6
40	1.0	95	5	6

Gradient Program (HPLC): For Cinnamic acid, Glycyrrhizin, Eugenol, 6-gingerol and Piperine:

For Gallic acid and Ellagic Acid:

Sample Preparation Method: About 0.50 gm of Divya Swasari Vati sample was diluted with 10 ml of methanol and sonicated for 45 min. This solution was centrifuged at 10000 rpm for 5 min and filtered using a 0.45 µm nylon filter (Solution A). This solution A was used for the analysis of cinnamic acid and ellagic acid. 1.0 ml of solution A was diluted to 5 ml with methanol (Solution B) and diluted to 10 ml with the same solvent (Solution C). Solution B was used for the analysis of eugenol, glycyrrhizin, 6-gingerol, piperine and Solution C was used for the analysis of gallic acid.

Standard Preparation Method: Standards were purchased from Natural Remedies Pvt. Ltd., Bangalore and Sigma Aldrich, Bangalore. Standards were dissolved in methanol to prepare the appropriate concentration.

A typical HPLC chromatogram of standard and sample under different condition is shown in Fig. (**2.71**, 2.72 and 2.73).

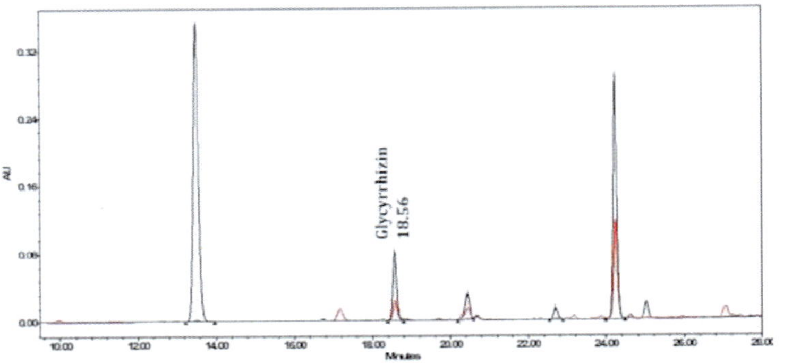

Fig. (2.71). Overlap chromatograph of standards mix (in black), glycyrrhizin (18.56 min) and Divya Swasari Vati (in red) at 250 nm.

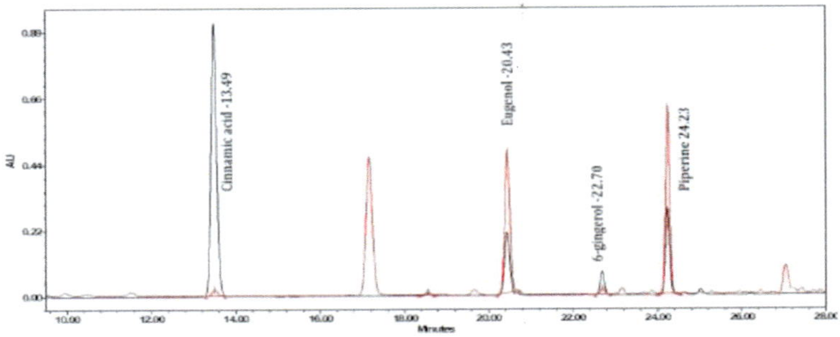

Fig. (2.72). Overlap chromatograph of standards mix (in black), cinnamic acid (13.49 min), eugenol (20.43 min), 6-gingerol (22.70 min), piperine (24.23 min) and Divya Swasari Vati (in red) at 278 nm.

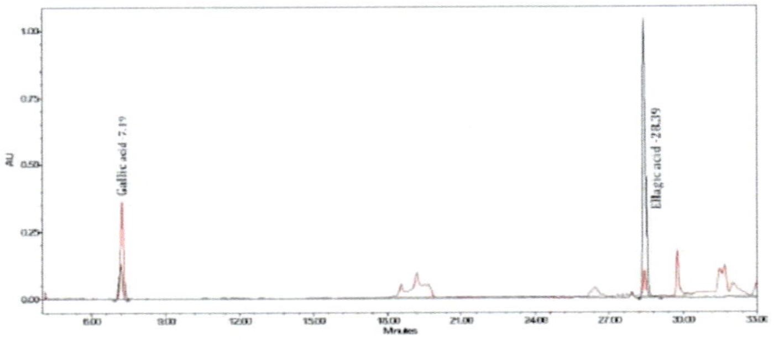

Fig. (2.73). Overlap chromatograph of standards mix (in black), gallic acid (1.19 min), ellagic acid (28.39 min) and Divya Swasari Vati (in red) at 250 nm.

HPLC-PDA Method Validation for Standardization of Divya Swasari Vati

Summary of Validation Report is shown in Table **2.90** and the result of marker compound are shown in Table **2.91** of Divya Swasari Vati.

Table 2.90. HPLC Validation summary report of Divya Swasari Vati.

S. No.	Parameter	Acceptance criteria	Results Obtained						
			Cinnamic Acid	**Glycy-rrhizin**	**Eugenol**	**6-Gingerol**	**Piperine**	**Gallic acid**	**Ellagic acid**
1	System Suitability	% RSD of Retention time - NMT 2.0%	0.10	0.18	0.21	0.16	0.12	0.05	0.22
		% RSD of area – NMT 2.0%	0.54	0.41	0.27	0.82	0.56	0.62	0.92
		USP trailing – NMT 2.0%	1.09	1.07	1.01	1.05	1.06	1.00	1.41
		Theoretical plates – NLT 2000	43405	138833	116934	221488	270171	12814	289710
2	Specificity	No interference at retention time of Standard	Complies						
3	Linearity	Correlation coefficient NLT 0.99	1.0000	0.9999	0.9997	1.0000	1.0000	0.9998	0.9999
4	Precision								
4.1	System	%RSD of area – NMT 2%	0.54	0.41	0.27	0.82	0.56	0.62	0.92
4.2	Intermediate	%RSD of assay – NMT 3%	1.25	0.78	0.56	1.54	0.63	0.93	1.25
4.3	Method	%RSD of assay – NMT 3%	1.06	0.85	0.52	0.91	0.38	1.14	1.06
5	Limit of detection	%RSD of area – NMT 33%	1.47	1.12	1.67	1.98	1.22	1.46	1.73

(Table 2.90) cont.....

S. No.	Parameter	Acceptance criteria	Results Obtained						
			Cinnamic Acid	Glycy-rrhizin	Eugenol	6-Gingerol	Piperine	Gallic acid	Ellagic acid
6	Limit of Quantification	%RSD of area – NMT 10%	0.54	0.41	0.27	0.82	0.56	0.62	0.92

Table 2.91. Results of marker compounds in Divya Swasari Vati.

S. No.	Name of Marker Compound	Result (µg/mg)
1	Gallic acid	0.964
2	Chlorogenic acid	0.689
3	Caffeic acid	0.006
4	Rutin	0.174
5	Cinnamic acid	0.025
6	Piperine	0.746
7	Glycyrrhizin	8.871

HPTLC Method Development for Standardization of Divya Swasari Vati Experiment Methods

Preparation of Sample Solution: 500 mg of sample was dissolved in 10 ml methanol: water (80: 20), sonicated for 20 minutes and then centrifuged to obtain a clear solution.

Preparation of Standard Solution: The stock solution was prepared by dissolving 10 mg of Gallic acid, Cinnamic acid & Piperine in 10 ml of methanol. The working solution was prepared from stock solution by dissolving 0.1ml of stock solution in 1ml of methanol.

Chromatographic Conditions

TLC plate: Silica gel 60 F254.

Mobile phase: Toluene: ethyl acetate: formic acid (9: 10: 1) ***Results:*** Results of Gallic acid in Divya Swasari Vati

Photo of developed TLC at 254 nm and chromatogram at 280 nm and 254 nm are shown in Fig. (**2.74**).

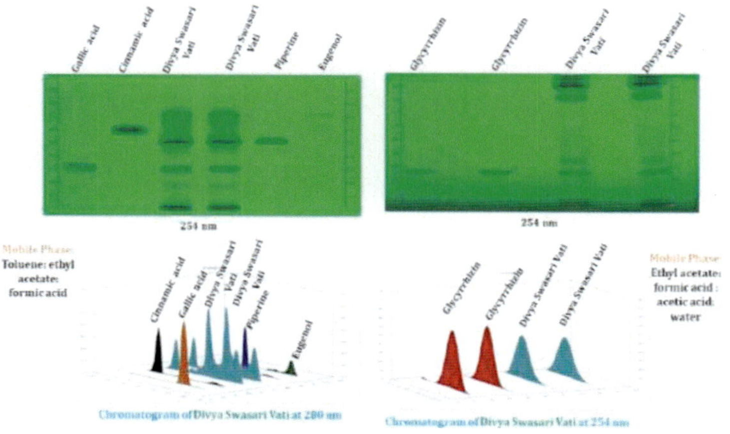

Fig. (2.74). HPTLC fingerprint of Divya Swasari Vati at 254 nm and chromatogram at 280 nm.

HPTLC Method Validation for Standardization of Divya Swasari Vati A.1:

Linearity of Gallic acid in Divya Swasari Vati is shown in Fig. **(2.75)**.

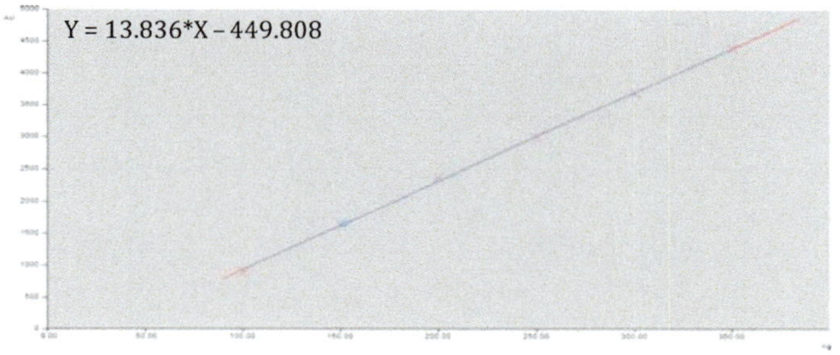

Fig. (2.75). HPTLC Linearity of Gallic acid in Divya Swasari Vati.

The correlation coefficient of linearity was determined by the regression equation is shown in Table **2.92**.

Table 2.92. Linearity of Gallic acid in Divya Swasari Vati.

Parameter	Gallic Acid
Linearity range (ng)	400 – 800
Regression equation	8.934*X + 865.273
Correlation coefficient	0.999
RF	0.31

A.2: Detection of Gallic acid in Divya Swasari Vati at 280 nm is shown in Fig. (**2.76**).

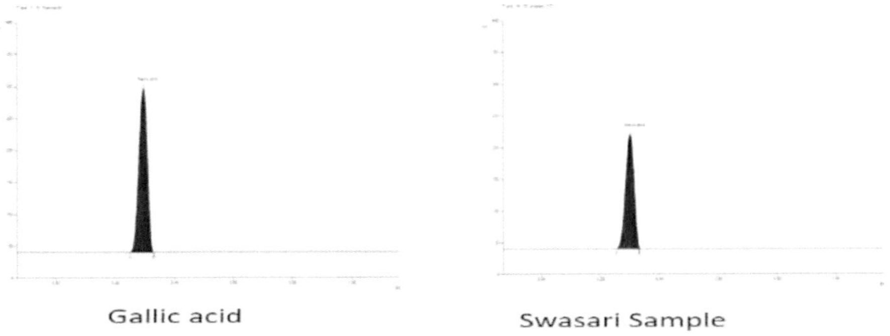

Fig. (2.76). HPTLC chromatogram of Gallic acid standard and Divya Swasari Vati.

A.3: Limit of detection and Limit of quantification of Gallic acid in Divya Swasari Vati is shown in Table **2.93**.

Table 2.93. LOD and LOQ of Gallic acid in Divya Swasari Vati.

LOD	0.18 ppm
LOQ	0.56 ppm

A.4: Precision of Gallic acid in Divya Swasari Vati is shown in Table **2.94**.

Table 2.94. Precision of Gallic acid in Divya Swasari Vati.

Concentration (ng)	**Intraday Precision**		**Interday Precision**	
	% RSD	**Mean (% RSD)**	**% RSD**	**Mean (% RSD)**
400	0.72	0.96	0.54	0.61
600	0.89		0.81	
800	1.27		0.46	

A.5: Recovery of Gallic acid in Divya Sawasari Vati is shown in Table **2.95**

Table 2.95. Recovery of Gallic acid in Divya Swasari Vati.

Recovery level	% Recovery	Mean Recovery %
80%	100.64%	95.97%
100%	95.06%	
120%	92.22%	

Result: amount of Gallic acid was found to be 0.324% in sample.

B:- Results of Cinnamic acid in Divya Swasari Vati

Photo of developed HPTLC of Divya Swasari Vati at 254 nm is shown in Fig. **(2.77)**.

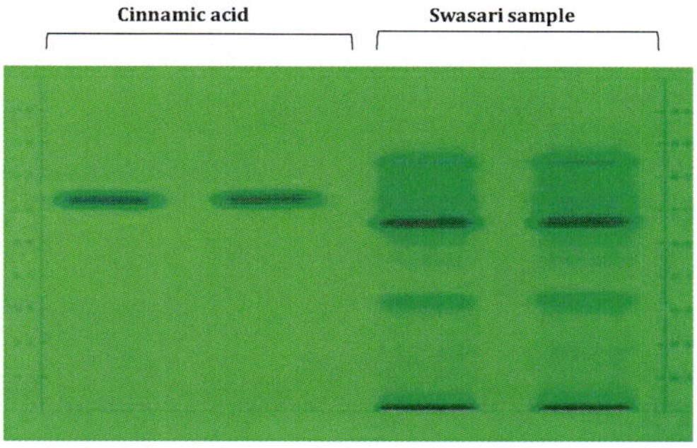

Fig. (2.77). HPTLC fingerprint of Cinnamic acid in Divya Swasari Vati.

B.1: Linearity of Cinnamic acid of Divya Swasari Vati is shown in Fig. **(2.78)**.

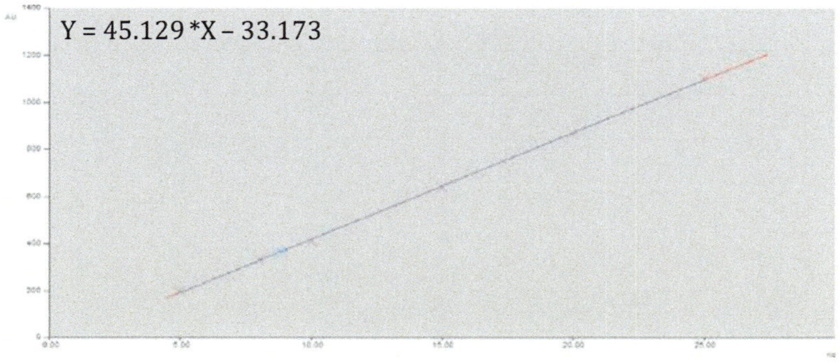

Fig. (2.78). HPTLC Linearity of Cinnamic acid in Divya Swasari Vati.

The correlation coefficient of linearity was determined by the regression equation for Cinnamic acid in Divya Swasari Vati is shown in Table **2.96**.

Table 2.96. Regression equation of Cinnamic acid in Divya Swasari Vati.

Parameters	Cinnamic Acid
Linearity range (ng)	5 – 25
Regression equation	45.129 *X – 33.173
Correlation coefficient	0.999
RF	0.64

B.2: Detection of Cinnamic acid at 280 nm in Divya Swasari Vati is shown in Fig. **(2.79)**.

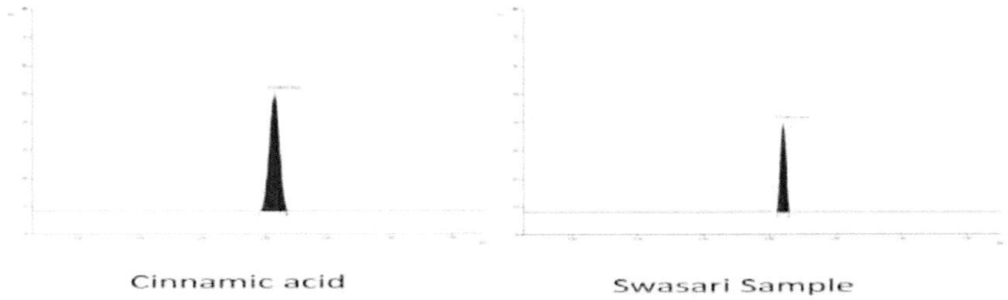

Fig. (2.79). HPTLC chromatogram of Cinnamic acid standard and Divya Swasari vati.

B.3 Limit of detection and limit of quantification of Cinnamic acid in Divya Swasari Vati is shown in Table **2.97**.

Table 2.97. LOD and LOQ of Cinnamic acid in Divya Swasari Vati.

LOD	0.003 ppm
LOQ	0.009 ppm

B.4: Precision of Cinnamic acid in Divya Swasari Vati is shown in Table **2.98**.

Table 2.98. Precision of Cinnamic acid in Divya Swasari Vati.

Concentration (ng)	Intraday Precision		Interday Precision	
	% RSD	Mean (% RSD)	% RSD	Mean (% RSD)
5	1.27	0.64	0.34	0.53
15	0.37		0.78	
25	0.28		0.46	

B5: Recovery of Cinnamic acid in Divya Swasari Vati is shown in Table **2.99**

Table 2.99. Recovery of Cinnamic acid in Divya Swasari Vati.

Recovery level	% Recovery	Mean Recovery %
80%	94.49%	92.66%
100%	90.39%	
120%	93.12%	

C: Results of Piperine in Divya Swasari Vati

Result: Amount of Cinnamic acid was found to be 0.002% in sample.

The HTLC fingerprint of Piperine at 254 nm in Divya Swasari Vati is shown in Fig. (**2.80**).

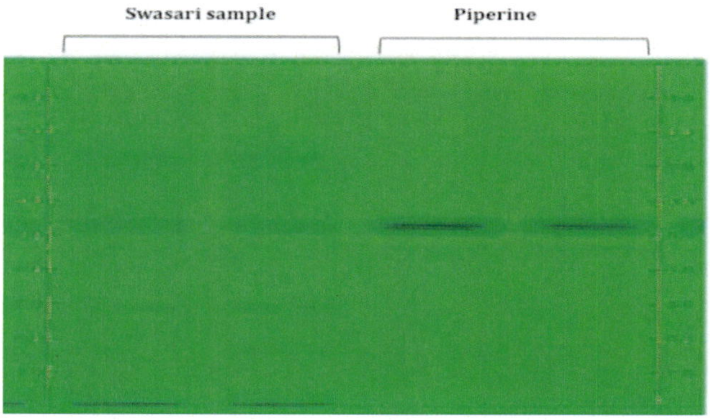

Fig. (2.80). HPTLC fingerprint of Piperine and Divya Swasari Vati.

C.1: Linearity of Piperine in Divya Swasari Vati is shown in Fig. (**2.81**).

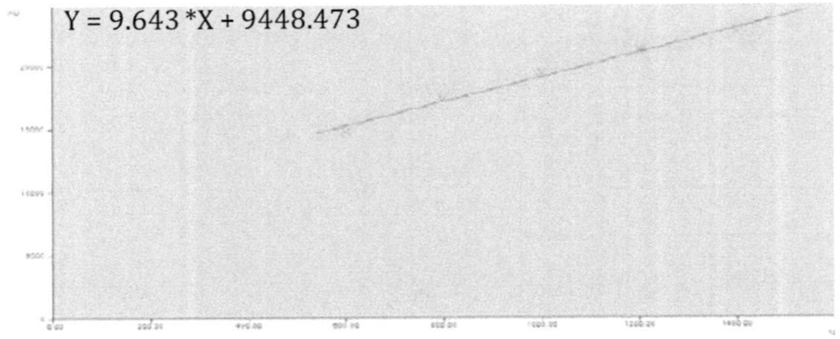

Fig. (2.81). Linearity of Piperine in Divya Swasari Vati.

The correlation coefficient of linearity was determined by the regression equation for Piperine in Divya Swasari Vati is shown in Table **2.100**.

Table 2.100. Regression equation of Piperine in Divya Swasari Vati.

Parameter	**Piperine**
Linearity range (ng)	600 – 1400
Regression equation	9.643 *X + 9448.473
Correlation coefficient	0.993
RF	0.54

C.2: Detection of Piperine at 434 nm in Divya Swasari Vati is shown in Fig. (**2.82**).

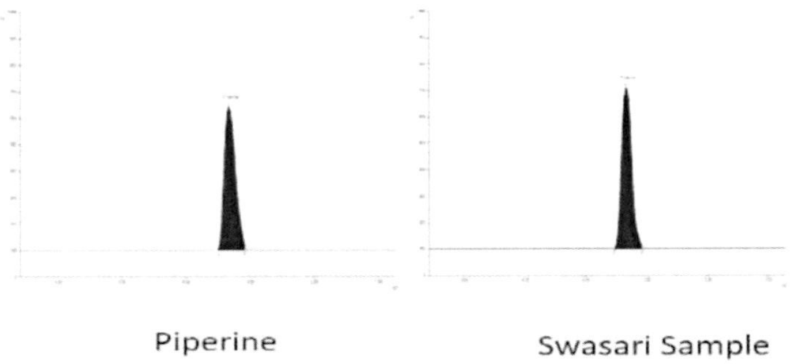

Fig. (2.82). HPTLC chromatogram of Piperine standard and Divya Swasari Vati.

C.3: Limit of detection and limit of quantification of Piperine in Divya Swasari Vati is shown in Table **2.101**.

Table 2.101. LOD and LOQ of Piperine in Divya Swasari Vati.

LOD	8.73 ppm
LOQ	26.45 ppm

C.4: Precision of Piperine in Divya Swasari Vati is shown in Table **2.102**.

Table 2.102. Precision of Piperine in Divya Swasari Vati.

Concentration (ng)	**Intraday precision**		**Interday precision**	
	% RSD	**Mean (% RSD)**	**% RSD**	**Mean (% RSD)**
600	1.35	1.11	0.08	0.37
1000	1.10		0.85	
1400	0.88		0.16	

C.5: Recovery of Piperine in Divya Swasari Vati is shown in Table **2.103**.

Table 2.103. Recovery of Piperine in Divya Swasari Vati.

Recovery level	**% Recovery**	**Mean Recovery %**
80%	97.65%	94.16%
100%	93.78%	
120%	91.06%	

Result: Amount of Piperine was found to be 0.501% in the sample.

CONCLUDING REMARKS

Taken together, a robust method of chemical profiling of the formulated Coronil and Divya Swasari Vati was established that employed a battery of techniques of analytical chemistry, such as HPTLC, HPLC and UPLC/QToF MS. A sequence of required chemical validations has emerged from the collections of studies mentioned in this chapter, which can be used as a guide for developing traditional formulations into modern medicines.

CHAPTER 3

Understanding the Mode of Action of the Medicine through *In-Vitro* Studies

Abstract: This chapter deals with the scientific authentication of the formulated Ayurvedic medicine. . Scientific research for mechanistic insights into the functionality is not a regulatory requirement for developing a herbal drug. Nevertheless, the outcomes from such scientific research works have been included in this chapter. Such scientific evidence on modes-of-actions of the herbal medicines helps in generating awareness among the end users, who could be from both scientific and non-scientific backgrounds. In this chapter, we have shared our scientific observations from the laboratory validations of the medicines, Coronil and Divya Swasari Vati,that have been developed. We have also discussed the modes of action of these medicines against the SARS-CoV-2 virus, as gathered from ***in-vitro*** experiments. Biochemical studies have shown that the medicines formulated by Patanjali Research Foundation Trust against the SARS-CoV-2 virus are capable of inhibiting the physical interactions between viral spike (S) protein and host ACE2 receptor protein. This interaction between S protein and ACE2 receptor is critical for COVID-19 infection. Our medicines were found to be effective in disrupting this interaction regardless of the initial mutation, like, D614G, that the SARS-CoV-2 virus has undergone to increase its infectivity. These medicines could also rescue the lung epithelial cells from S protein- and pseudovirus-induced cytokine storms. Pseudoviruses are non-pathogenic study viruses used for experimental purposes to understand the host entry mechanisms in viruses. In this case, the non-pathogenic viral genome was encased with SARS-CoV-2 S protein so that we can follow the S protein and ACE2 interactions. Besides, these pseudoviruses also had reporters inside them that helped us to monitor their entry into host cells. We found that cells, when treated with our medicines, showed lesser internalization of the viruses, suggesting that the medicines are preventing the virus entry. During COVID-19 pathogenesis, the pro-inflammatory cytokines put the immune response into an overdrive by inducing each other. We tried to mimic this *in-vivo* condition ***in-vitro*** by inducing inflammation in the lung epithelial cells with one pro-inflammatory cytokine and then checked the levels of others and how the treatment with our medicines altered this response. We observed that cells, when exposed to one pro- inflammatory cytokine showed an increase in the levels of others and interestingly when these cells were treated with Ayurvedic medicines, the cytokine levels reduced. Taken together, these *in-vitro* observations revealed that these Ayurvedic medicines disrupted physical interaction between viral S protein and host ACE2 receptor and attenuated the cytokine storm, implicating their potential in managing acute respiratory distress syndrome (ARDS), one of the prime causes of COVID-19 associated mortality.

Acharya Balkrishna

Keywords: SARS-CoV-2 pseudovirus, ACE2-S protein interaction, S^{D614G} protein, S^{W436R} protein, ELISA, RT-PCR.

3.1. EXPERIMENTAL VALIDATION OF COMPUTATIONAL OBSERVATION

ACE-2 is a single-pass type I membrane protein, with its enzymatically active domain exposed on the surface of cells in lungs and other tissues (Hamming *et al.*, 2004). The binding of the spike S protein of SARS-CoV-2 to the enzymatic domain of ACE-2 on the surface of cells results in endocytosis and translocation of both the virus and the enzyme into endosomes located within cells (Fig. **3.1 A**). This entry process also requires priming of the S protein by the host serine protease TMPRSS2, the inhibition of which is under current investigation as a potential therapeutic (Hoffmann, *et al.*, 2020).

Computational studies from our and other groups have shown that withanone can target ACE-2 and Receptor Binding Domain (RBD) of SARS-CoV-2 viral spike (S) protein interaction, SARS-CoV-2 main protease (M^{pro}) and TMPRSS2 (Kumar, Dhanjal, Bhargava, *et al.*, 2020; Kumar, Dhanjal, Kaul, *et al.*, 2020; Balkrishna, Pokhrel, *et al.*, 2021) (Fig. **3.1B**). However, experimental evidence has been lacking. Through an ELISA-based method, we have checked the effect of pure withanone on the interaction between human ACE-2 protein and RBD of SARS-CoV-2 viral spike (S) protein (Fig. **3.1 C**). In this method, overexpressed truncated S protein of SARS-CoV-2 expressing only the RBD was used while the human ACE-2 (hACE-2) used was full length. ELISA wells were coated with viral RBD to which biotinylated hACE-2 was added along with different concentrations of withanone. An inhibitor of ACE-2-RBD interaction provided with the kit was used as a positive control, while the reaction without any inhibitor was taken as a negative control. Inhibition of ACE-2-RBD interaction was calculated with respect to the negative control assuming the interaction to be 100%. The interaction was detected using HRP- conjugated streptavidin against biotinylated ACE-2 (Fig. **3.1 D**). We observed that withanone exhibited a dose-dependent inhibition of ACE-2-RBD interaction (IC_{50} = 0.33 ng/ml) (Fig. **3.1 E**). In the physiological context, this will translate into therapeutic efficacies of pure withanone. To validate this speculation, we treated the zebrafish model presenting COVID-19 pathologies with leaf extract from *W. somnifera* (Ashwagandha) enriched in withanone (WiNeWsE) (Fig. **3.1F**). WiNeWsE treatment relieved these fishes from pathological symptoms, like, behavioural fever (Balkrishna, Pokhrel, *et al.*, 2021).

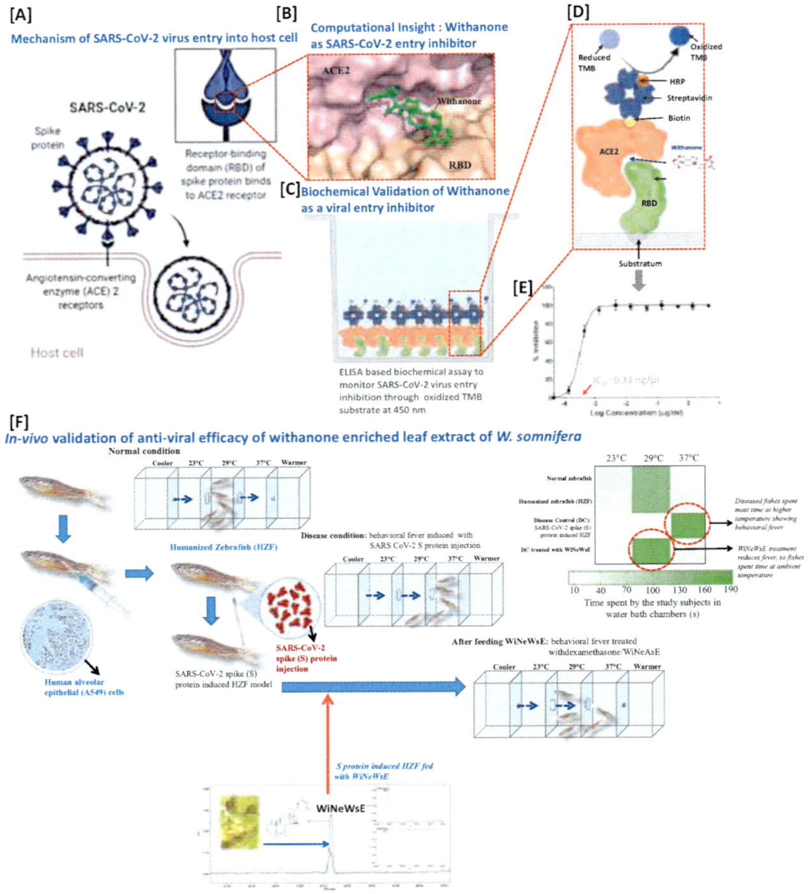

Fig. (3.1). Experimental validation of the viral entry inhibitory effect of withanone. **[A]** Schematic representation of the molecular mechanism of SARS-CoV-2 entry into the host cell. **[B]** withanone binds at the ACE-2-RBD interacting interface (demarcated with a red open box in the cartoon) as shown in a magnified view of the molecular docking visualization. **[C]** Pictorial depiction of the experimental procedure employed in evaluating the inhibitory effect of withanone on the biochemical interaction between host ACE-2 and viral RBD. **[D]** Biotinylated ACE-2 bound to RBD, immobilized to the substratum, is detectable through HRP-conjugated streptavidin due to oxidation of 3,3',5,5'-Tetramethylbenzidine (TMB). **[E]** Dose-response curve exhibiting the inhibitory effect of withanone on the interaction between human ACE-2 and RBD of SARS-CoV-2 S protein. IC_{50} is found to be 0.33 ng/ml. **[F]** *In-vivo* validation of the efficacy of *W. somnifera* leaf extract enriched with withanone (WiNeWsE) showing the induction of disease pathology in the zebrafish, subsequent treatment with WiNeWsE and concomitant amelioration of behavioural fever. Withanone enrichment in WiNeWsE was validated through HPLC *[Courtesy:*(Balkrishna, Pokhrel, *et al.*, 2021)*; Under CCBY License].*

We obtained a mechanistic insight into the functioning of withanone as a SARS-CoV-2 entry inhibitor with *in-vivo* validation demonstrating its efficacy in ameliorating COVID-19 like pathology. Taken together, this study laid the foundation for developing withanone and other virtually screened phytochemicals into treatment for COVID-19. In the initial phase, we developed *W. somnifera*, *T. cordifolia* and *O. sanctum* extracts into medicinal forms, chemically characterized them (as mentioned in detail in chapter 2) and followed their remedial efficacies through a retrospective observational clinical study (discussed in Chapter 6). Subsequently, for better patient compliance, we combined these medicines into the Coronil tablet and experimentally validated its anti-viral functionality.

3.2. CORONIL AS A POTENTIAL ANTIVIRAL AGENT AGAINST SARS-COV-2

Coronil is composed of aqueous extracts of Ashwagandha (*W. somnifera*), Giloy (*T. cordifolia*) and Tulsi (*O. sanctum*), all three of which have been predicted to be potential antiviral agents against SARS-CoV-2.

3.2.1. Insight into the Entry Inhibitory Mechanism of Coronil

From *in-silico* observations, Coronil is expected to inhibit physical interaction between ACE-2 and S protein. So, we tested Coronil for its inhibitory effect on ACE-2 and S protein interaction, as we did for withanone (Fig. **3.2**).

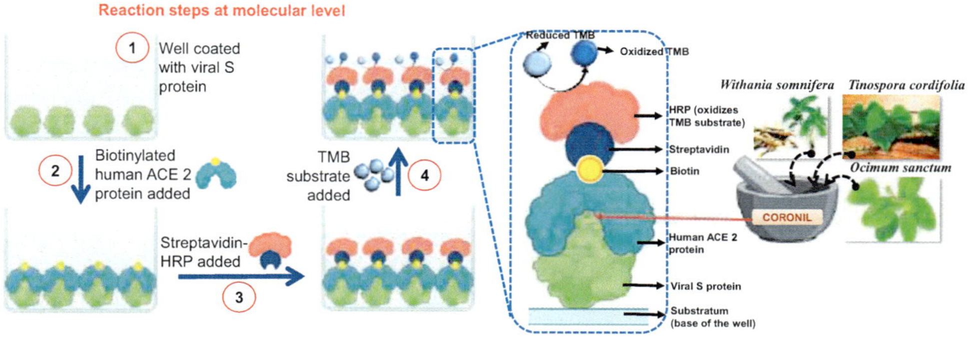

Fig. (3.2). Experimental design for validating the inhibition of SARS-CoV-2 entry into the host cell by Coronil. The method has an ELISA-based design wherein wells were coated with different mutations of viral spike (S) protein, namely, wild type (S^{WT}), D614G mutation (S^{D614G}) and W436R mutation (S^{W436R}). Biotinylated human ACE-2 protein was incubated in these wells, and subsequently, the interaction between these proteins was detected using streptavidin-conjugated horseradish peroxidase (HRP) and Tetramethylbenzidine (TMB) substrate by measuring the absorbance. Plausible alterations in the ACE-2-S protein interaction due to Coronil are also depicted. *[Courtesy:* (Balkrishna, Haldar, *et al.*, 2021)*; Under CCBY License]*

We observed that Coronil was capable of disrupting the physical interaction between ACE-2 and viral spike (S) protein. We included different variants of SARS-CoV-2 S proteins, namely, S^{WT}, S^{D614G} and S^{W436R}. S^{WT} is the variant that appeared at the beginning of the pandemic. S^{D614G} variant has aspartic acid 'D' at 614th position replaced by glycine 'G' and is identified to be responsible for enhanced infectivity by improving S protein incorporation into the virions during packaging (Korber *et al.*, 2020). Likewise, the variant S^{W436R} has an arginine 'R' at 436th position instead of the original tryptophan 'W'. While, the S^{D614G} variant is the one currently in circulation (Korber *et al.*, 2020), S^{W436R} is a predicted one, which is likely to offer an evolutionary advantage to the SARS-CoV-2 because of increased affinity for ACE-2 (J. Ou, *et al.*, 2020; Padhi and Tripathi, 2020). Coronil exerted a dose-dependent inhibitory effect on the interactions between ACE-2 and all variants of S proteins, thereby establishing the authenticity of this effect (Fig. **3.3**). The extent of inhibition varied for each mutant. Coronil inhibited ACE-2- S^{W436R} most efficiently showed a 20% inhibition at 0.55 µg/ml concentration only. For a similar magnitude of inhibition in cases of S^{WT} and S^{D614G} variants, 19.08 and 20.08 µg/ml of Coronil were required. Regardless of this variation in the observed effect of Coronil in the presence of different S proteins, the overall result shows that it could jeopardize the critical host-viral molecular interaction.

3.2.2. Coronil is an Entry Inhibitor of SARS-CoV-2 into the Host Cell

We designed a cell-based assay for evaluating the effect of impeding the ACE-2 and S protein interaction by Coronil. We used lung (pulmonary) epithelial cells, a type of cells that line the air sacs (scientifically called alveolus or alveoli) for this assay. SARS-CoV-2 exploits the ACE-2 receptors on the host cell with the S protein present on its envelope. Pathogenicity of this virus comes from its genome; therefore, a false/pseudotyped SARS-CoV-2 virus (VSVppSARS-CoV-2S) was prepared (Fig. **3.4**), which was non-pathogenic.

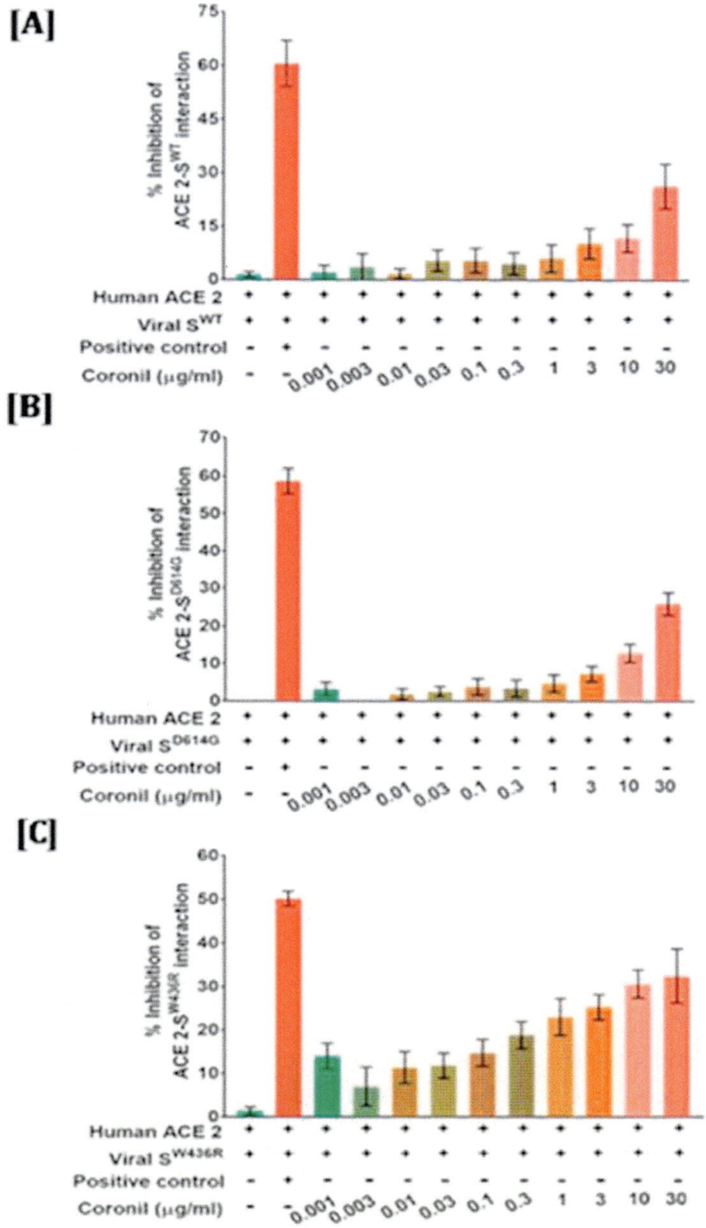

Fig. (3.3). Coronil inhibits interactions between human ACE-2 receptor and viral S proteins. **[A-C]** Graphs showing the dose-dependent effect of Coronil on the interactions between human ACE-2 receptor and different types of SARS-CoV-2 S proteins, namely, S^{WT} (A), S^{D614G} (B) and S^{W436R} (C) represented as percent (%) inhibition relative to the extent of ACE-2-S protein interactions observed in the reaction mix without any inhibitor. *[Courtesy:* (Balkrishna, Haldar, *et al.*, 2021)*; Under CCBY License].*

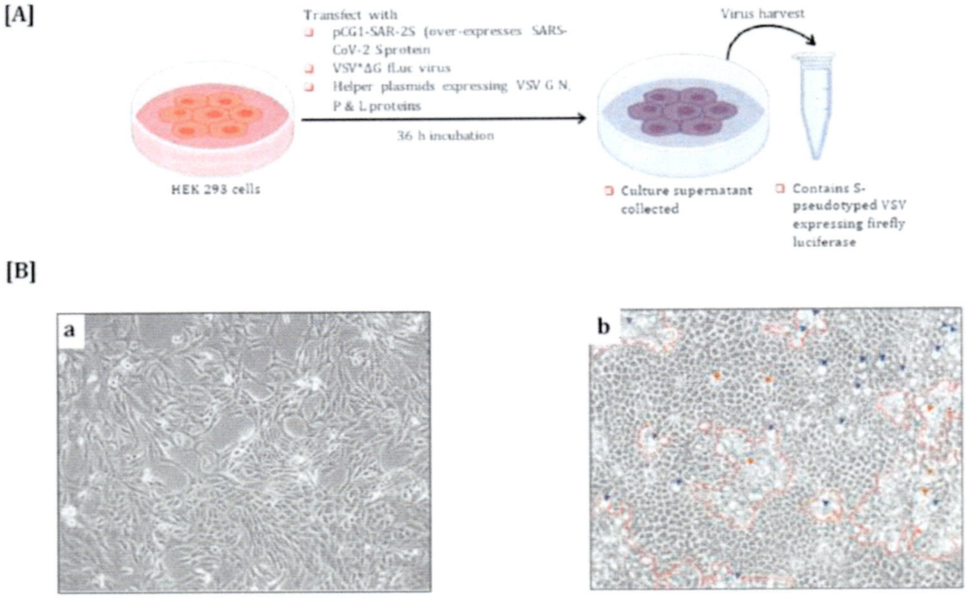

Fig. (3.4). Preparation of VSVppSARS-2S pseudovirus **[A]** Pictorial depiction of the steps involved in pseudotypic VSV with SARS-CoV-2 protein to obtain VSVppSARS-2S viruses. **[B]** Representative bright-field images of HEK293 cells before (a) and after (b) induced for pseudotyping. Manifestation of successful pseudotyping was observed as cytopathic effects in the form of cytopathic islands (demarcated with red dotted lines), plaques (blue arrowheads) and syncytia (red arrowheads) in (b). *[Courtesy:* (Balkrishna, Haldar, *et al.*, 2021)*; Under CCBY License].*

The genome of the vesicular stomatitis virus (VSV) was packaged with S protein of SARS- CoV-2 to form the VSVppSARS-2S pseudovirus. The genome of VSVppSARS-2S had a stably expressing firefly luciferase (*luc*) gene. Whenever VSVppSARS-2S will enter the host cell, the *luc* gene will get expressed to produce the luciferase enzyme, which can be detected by using D-luciferin as substrate. Luciferase acts upon D-luciferin to emit luminescence (light) which can be quantified to indirectly reflect the extent of viral entry into the host cell. We determined the cytosafety of Coronil in the lung cells we were using before treating them with it (Fig. **3.5**). Coronil did not show any toxicity in these cells confirming its safety as an exploratory therapeutic agent (Balkrishna, Solleti, Verma, *et al.*, 2020a).

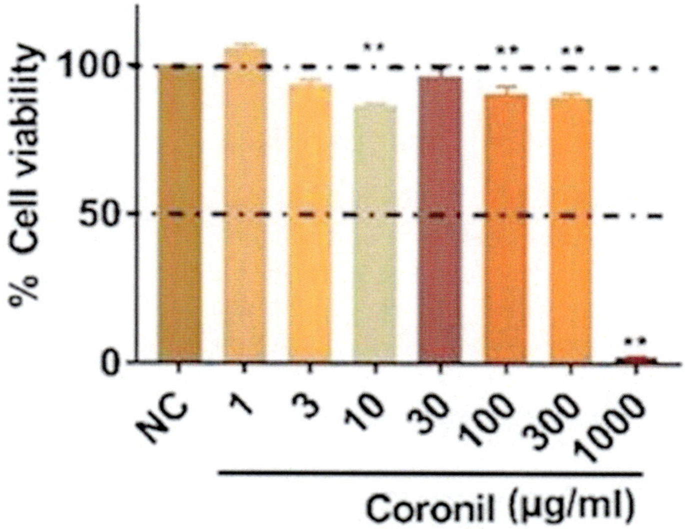

Fig. (3.5). Cell cytotoxicity assay of Coronil. Cytosafety of Coronil was ensured through Alamar blue staining of lung cells treated with different concentrations of Coronil. *[Courtesy:*(Balkrishna, Solleti, Verma, *et al.*, 2020a)*; Under CCBY License].*

We also observed that the treatment with Coronil significantly reduced the number of virus particles that could enter the cells as was evident from reduced fold change in luminescence, reflecting a proportional reduction in the entry of VSVppSARS-2S pseudoviruses (Fig. **3.6**) (Balkrishna, Haldar, *et al.*, 2021).

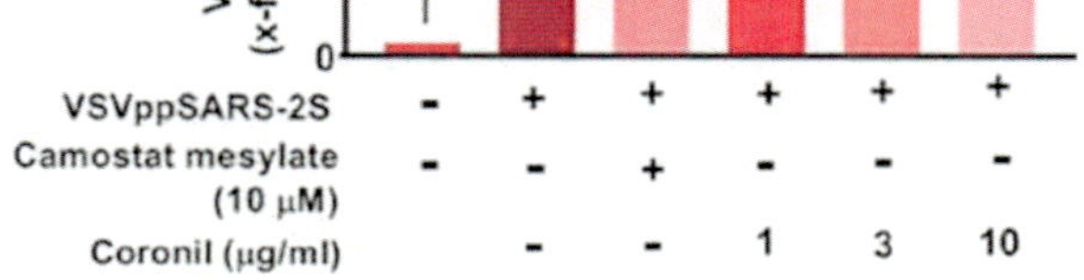

Fig. (3.6). Coronil inhibits VSVppSARS-2S pseudovirus entry into lung cells. The extent of VSVppSARS-2S pseudovirus entry into the lung cells was followed through the observed luciferase activity emanated from the firefly luciferase (*fLuc*) gene inserted into the genome of VSV. *[Courtesy:* (Balkrishna, Haldar, *et al.*, 2021)*; Under CCBY License]*

These observations clearly showed that Coronil inhibited ACE-2 – S protein interaction and prevented the entry of the virus into the host cells.

3.2.3. Coronil as an Anti-inflammatory Agent

Subsequent to SARS-CoV-2 entry into the human body, cytokine responses are mounted in which pro-inflammatory cytokines, interleukin-6 (IL-6), interleukin-1β (IL-1β) and tumour necrosis factor-α (TNF-α) is highly elevated. These cytokines affect each other's levels and are responsible for the complex cytokine response that follows SARS-CoV-2 infection in humans. It was mimicked *in-vitro* by treating the pulmonary epithelial cells with pro-inflammatory cytokine IL-1β and measuring the increase in IL-6 (Fig. **3.7 A**) and TNF-α (Fig. **3.7 B**). The dose-dependent effect of Coronil was checked in this setup. We observed that the levels of IL-6 and TNF-α in IL-1β treated cells were reduced in a dose-dependent manner upon treatment with Coronil. TNF-α is one of the master transcriptional regulators known to mediate cytokine response through a downstream effector, NF-κB, which is also a transcriptional regulator. So, we checked the effect of Coronil on TNF-α induced NF-κB-mediated response using a transactivation assay. For this purpose, we used a stable cell line HEK-Blue engineered to express secreted alkaline phosphatase (SEAP) enzyme from a promoter that is regulated by NF-κB/AP-1 (co-factor Activator protein-1). When TNF-α is added to these cells, cellular NF-κB expression is triggered which results in the switching on of SEAP expression. SEAP expression can be quantified through an enzymatic reaction. This quantification indirectly reflects the amount of TNF-α to which the cells have been exposed. Secreted TNF-α produced by Coronil treated pulmonary epithelial cells, which have been induced with inflammation, showed lower SEAP activity than the one from untreated cells (Fig. **3.7 C**). This indicated that Coronil helped in reducing the levels of TNF-α due to inflammation (Balkrishna, Solleti, Verma, *et al.*, 2020a).

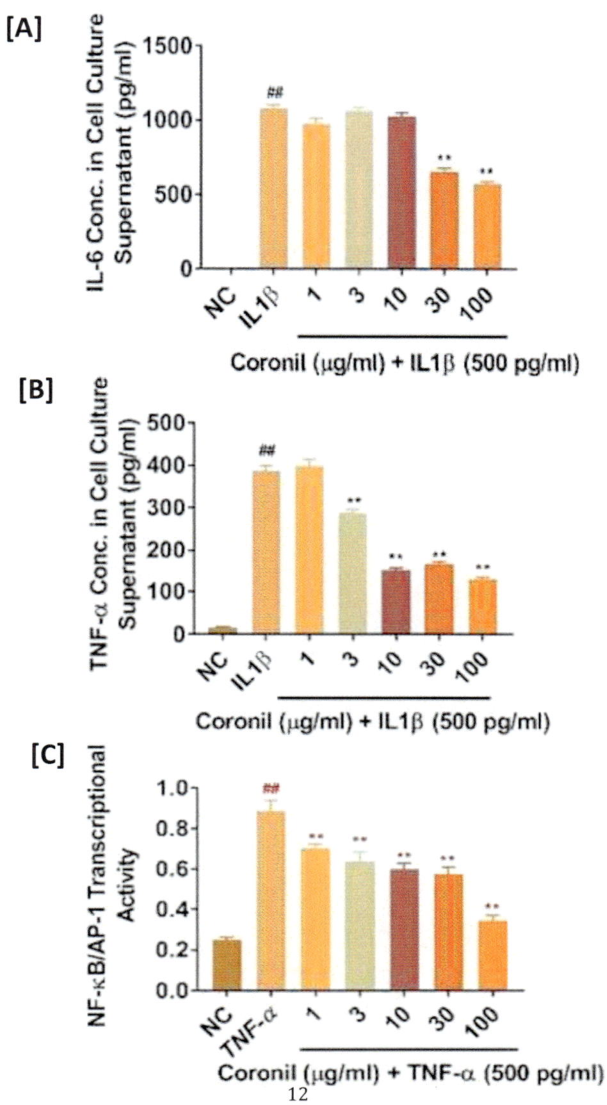

12

Fig. (3.7). Coronil decreases the pro-inflammatory responses *in vitro*. Lung cells were pre-treated with various concentrations of Coronil for 24 h followed by co-treatment with Coronil + IL-1β for 24 h and assayed for the secretion of cytokines **[A]** TNF-α and **[B]** IL-6 using ELISA. **[C]** HEK Blue TNF-α reporter SEAP assay was done for NF-κB/AP-1 transcriptional activity. HEK blue cells stably expressing the NF-κB/AP-1-SEAP reporter gene were pre-treated with various doses of Coronil followed by treatment with TNF-α and measuring SEAP activity after 24 h. *[Courtesy:* (Balkrishna, Solleti, Verma, *et al.*, 2020a)*; Under CCBY License].*

The above experimental set-up was an artificial stimulation of the cytokine storm that ensues SARS-CoV-2 infection. In order to check whether Coronil could manage the cytokine response evoked due to virus binding to the host cells, either S proteins or VSVppSARS-CoV-2S pseudoviruses were used to elicit such cytokine response in the lung cells. We observed that treating pulmonary epithelial cells with S proteins evoked a cytokine response akin to that found during COVID-19 infection. So, we checked whether Coronil could subdue this cytokine response. Lung cells were pre-treated with Coronil and then exposed to different variants of S protein. The levels of pro-inflammatory cytokines, TNF-α, IL-1β, and IL-6, were subsequently measured (Fig. **3.8**). We observed that treatment with Coronil prevented the surge in these cytokines, regardless of the variant of S protein involved. SD614G did not evoke a prominent cytokine response which corroborates with evidence that supports its reduced virulence (Fig. **3.9**) (Balkrishna, Haldar, *et al.*, 2021).

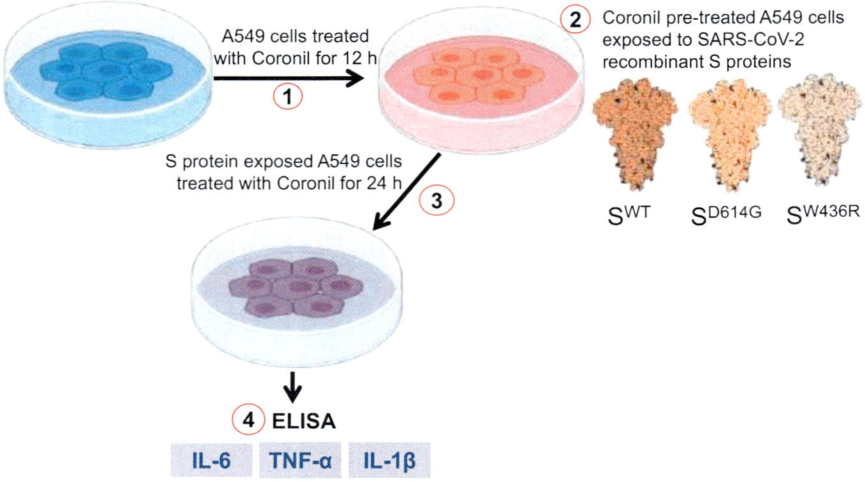

Fig. (3.8). Experimental set-up for studying S-protein induced pro-inflammatory responses. Pictorial representation of the experimental set-up. A549 cells were pre-treated with different concentrations of Coronil followed by incubation in different types of viral S proteins, S^{WT}, S^{D614G} or S^{W436R} to induce cytokine activation when co-treated with Coronil. *[Courtesy:* (Balkrishna, Haldar, *et al.*, 2021)*; Under CCBY License].*

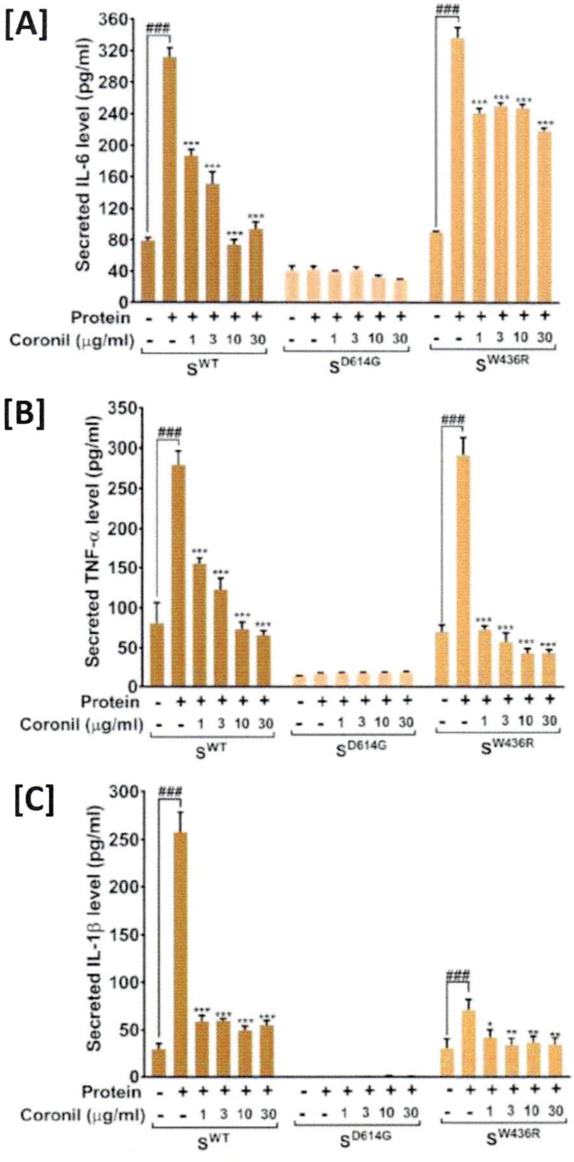

Fig. (3.9). Coronil inhibits viral S protein-induced cytokine response [A-C] Activation of pro-inflammatory cytokines, TNF-α (A), IL-1β (B) and IL-6 (C) in alveolar epithelial A549 cells treated with different SARS-CoV-2 S proteins and dose-dependent effect of Coronil treatment thereof was measured through ELISA. Observations are depicted as levels of secreted cytokines. *[Courtesy:* (Balkrishna, Haldar, *et al.*, 2021)*; Under CCBY License].*

Similarly, we induced cytokine storm in the lung cells pre-treated with Coronil, by incubating them with different concentrations of Coronil to check whether it could rescue the cells from VSVppSARS-CoV-2S pseudovirus induced cytokine surge (Fig. **3.10**).

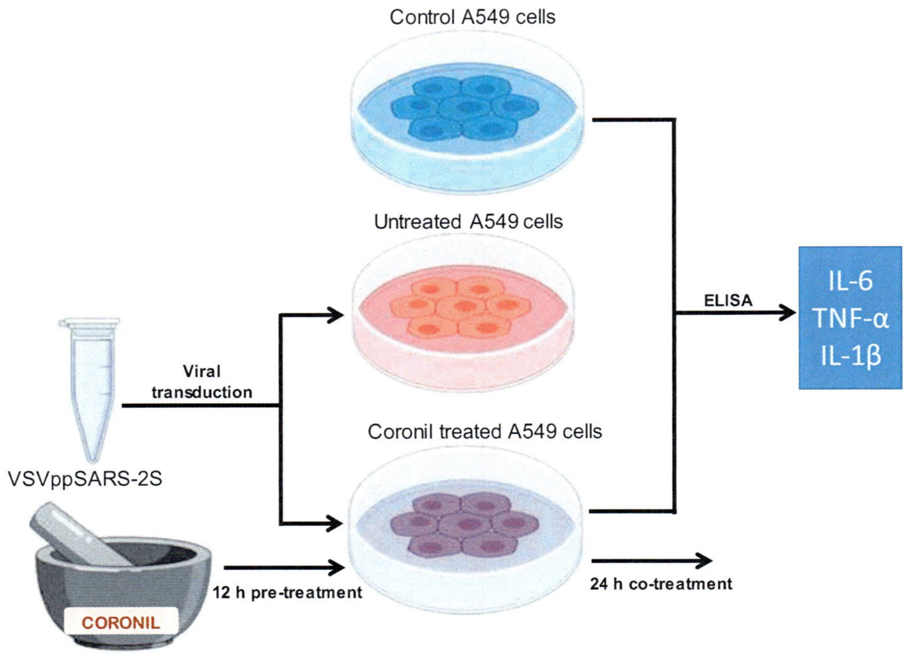

Fig. (3.10). Experimental set-up for studying pseudovirus-induced pro-inflammatory responses. Pictorial representation of the experimental set-up. A 549 cells were pre-treated with different concentrations of Coronil followed by transduction with VSVppSARS-2S pseudovirus, to induce cytokine storm. The Coronil treatment was maintained during viral transduction. *[Courtesy:* (Balkrishna, Haldar, *et al.*, 2021)*; Under CCBY License].*

We observed that treatment with Coronil reduced the cytokine levels in the infected cells (Fig. **3.11**) (Balkrishna, Haldar, *et al.*, 2021). These observations meant that Coronil is not only capable of potentially preventing viral entry into the host cell but also probably, effective against the 'cytokine storm' believed to be the sole reason behind severe COVID-19 prognosis.

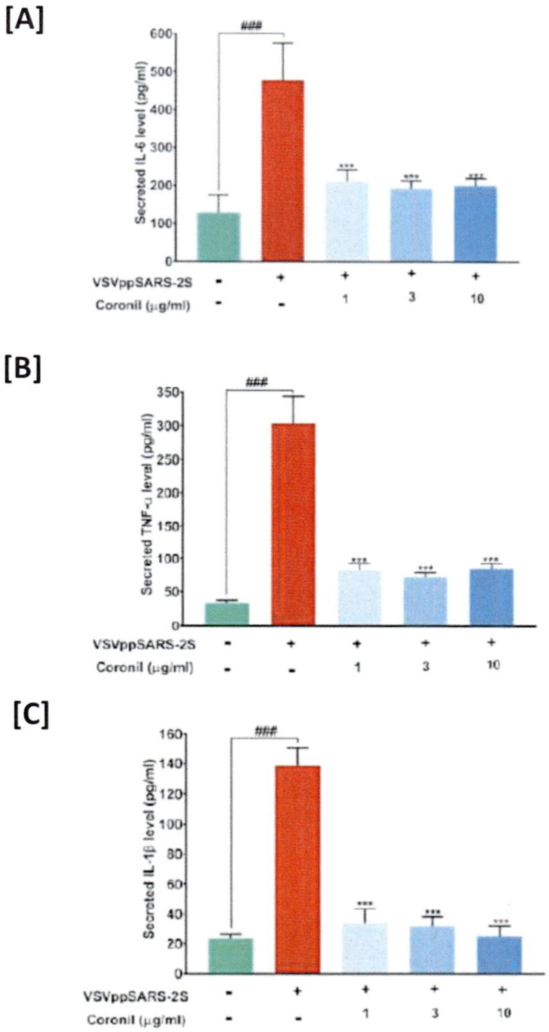

Fig. 3.11. Coronil reduced pseudovirus elicited cytokine response *in vitro***[A-C]** Measured levels of secreted IL-6 (A), TNF-α (B) and IL-1β (C) show the evoked cytokine responses and their reduction upon Coronil treatment. *[Courtesy:* (Balkrishna, Haldar, *et al.*, 2021)*; Under CCBY License].*

All these studies not only provided experimental validation for Coronil as a potential antiviral agent against SARS-CoV-2 but also helped us in gaining insight into the molecular mechanism employed by Coronil in acting against the SARS-CoV-2 virus. Sharing observations obtained from such research activities are likely to help in earning scientific credibility among the educated population and consequently, increase the commercial visibility of Coronil.

3.3. POTENTIALS OF SWASARI AGAINST SARS-COV-2

We intended to come up with a prophylactic and therapeutic remedy for COVID-19. While Coronil appeared, from our research, to be both prophylactic and therapeutic, we tested another age-old, known Ayurvedic formulation, Swasari Vati for its effectiveness in reducing lung inflammation in the context of COVID-19 infection.

3.3.1. Scientific Rationale of Using Swasari against SARS-CoV-2

For systemic symptomatic treatment of COVID-19, poly-herbo-mineral formulation, Tablet Swasari Ras has been generated for providing relief in lung congestion and to reduce mucus accumulation in the lungs. We have several thousand patients' clinical data in Patanjali Electronic Medical Record (PEMR) system.

Tablet Swasari Ras is a poly herbo-mineral formulation; its constituents are mentioned in classical ancient Ayurveda, for the treatment of disorders related to the respiratory tract such as cough, bronchitis, asthma, rhinitis and excessive mucous formation. This formulation has been used in clinical settings at several chikitsalayas across India, on several thousand patients as per Patanjali Electronic Medical Records (PEMR). Scientists at Patanjali Research Institute have also validated Swasari Ras in preclinical studies (Balkrishna, Solleti, Singh, *et al.*, 2020a). Swasari Ras consists of Mulethi, Lavanga, Dalchini, Karkatashringi, Rudanti, Ardraka, Maricha, Pippali and Akarkara. Swasari Ras contains several bioactive plant metabolites that are responsible for producing anti-inflammatory activity in respiratory diseases and alleviates the vitiated Tridosa (Vata-Kapha and Pitta). Swasari Vati also contains calcium mineral components such as, Kapardak bhasma, Abhraka bhasma, Godanti bhasma and Mukta shukti bhasma. These mineral components are free from any metallic sources and have been traditionally known for efficacy in the treatment of cough, asthma, inflammation and other lung disorders.

Tablet Swasari Ras is a unique combination of various plant parts, namely, fruit of *Glycyrrhiza glabra* (Liquorice/Mulethi), buds of *Syzygium aromaticum* (Cloves/ Lavanga), bark of *Cinnamomum zeylanicum* (Cinnamon/Dalchini), galls of *Pistacia integerrima* (Zebrawood/ Karkatashringi), fruit of *Cressa cretica* (Salt Cresse/Rudanti), rhizome of *Zingiber officinale* (Ardraka/Ginger), fruit of *Piper nigrum* (Maricha/Black pepper), fruit of *Piper longum* (Long pepper/Pippali), root of *Anacyclus pyrethrum* (Spanish chamomile/Akarkara).

Glycyrrhiza glabra (Mulethi), decreases the mucus production in the lungs (Nishimoto *et al.*, 2010), interferes with replication and/or cytopathogenic effect induced by many respiratory viruses such as SARS coronavirus (Cinatl *et al.*, 2003), respiratory syncytial virus (RSV), HIV (Harada, 2005) involving clustering of fusion-activated proteins and fluidization of the plasma membrane and viral envelope. Glycyrrhizin exerts an antioxidative response against H5N1 Influenza A virus (Wolkerstorfer *et al.*, 2009) and inhibits virus replication and pro-inflammatory gene expression (Michaelis *et al.*, 2010, 2011). Further, it inhibits the expression of Th2 cytokines, IL-4 and IL-5 levels and eosinophilia by decreasing the IgE- stimulating cytokines, airway hyperresponsiveness (Ram *et al.*, 2006) the incidence of which is increasing globally. The existing therapy is inadequate and has many adverse effects. It needs a better therapeutic molecule preferably of natural origin, which has negligible or no adverse effects. In view of this, we evaluated Glycyrrhizin (GRZ), in bacterial lipopolysaccharide (LPS) induced TNF-α and IL-1β levels in lungs (Xie *et al.*, 2012) asthma and chronic obstructive pulmonary disease (COPD) and oxidative stress in lungs (Hassan Khattab, *et al.*, 2018). It contains glycyrrhizin as a major bioactive ingredient, along with glycyrrhetinic acid, flavonoids, isoflavonoids, and chalcones as active compounds. Its roots have been traditionally used for cough, colds, asthma, and COPD (Ram, *et al.*, 2011).

The barks of *Cinnamomum zeylanicum* (Dalchini) is one of the oldest herbal medicine possessing an array of pharmacological metabolites including trans-cinnamaldehyde, eugenol, and linalool, which represent 82.5% of the total composition. It exerts anti-inflammatory, analgesic, antipyretic, immunomodulatory, anti- complementary properties (Chericoni, *et al.*, 2005). Cinnamon has antioxidant properties (Jayaprakasha, Mohan Rao and Sakariah, 2003) and suppresses IL-1β, IL-6 and TNF-α in LPS-activated macrophages in MAPK dependent pathway (Kim, Na and Lee, 2018) and bleomycin-induced idiopathic pulmonary fibrosis (Yan *et al.*, 2018) but its effect on Idiopathic Pulmonary Fibrosis (IPF) is unknown. The present study was performed to investigate the anti-fibrotic effect and mode of action of cinnamaldehyde on IPF.

Idiopathic pulmonary fibrosis (IPF) was induced by intra-tracheal administration of bleomycin in mice. Submicron emulsion of cinnamaldehyde was given by intraperitoneal injection once every day for 7 or 21 continuous days after bleomycin administration. Lung histological and injury indices were analyzed along with the protein expression levels of inflammation and oxidative stress, as well as EMT marker alpha-smooth muscle actin (α-SMA). Type-A procyanidine polyphenols of Cinnamon improve lung function, decreases inflammatory cell infiltration in lung tissue and goblet cell hyperplasia and mucus hypersecretion (Kandhare, *et al.*, 2013). Further, cinnamon bark oil is a potent fungus toxicant against respiratory tract mycoses (Singh, *et al.*, 1995).

Traditionally, the essential oil of *Pistacia integerrima* (Karkatashringi) is used for the treatment of various respiratory diseases like chronic bronchitis, and other ailments of the respiratory tract. It abolishes bronchoconstriction (Adusumalli, Madan Ranjit and Sankaranarayan Harish, 2013; Shirole, Shirole and Saraf, 2015) by inhibiting Phosphodiesterase-1 and regulating smooth muscle cell activity (Rauf *et al.*, 2015). In the lungs, it exerts anti-inflammatory effects by reducing the levels of TNF-α, IL-4, IL-5, IL-1β, and IL-6. It also inhibits acute lung injury (Rana, Shahzad and Shabbir, 2016) besides, combatting intranasal challenges (Xie *et al.*, 2012). Ethyl gallate present in *P. integerrima* attenuates acute lung injury through Nrf2 signalling (Mehla, *et al.*, 2013).

Cressa cretica (Rudanti), has been used for cough and other respiratory problems due to its bronchodilatory and mast cell stabilizing activity (Priyashree, Jha and Pattanayak, 2010) and antitussive activity (Sunita, Jha and Pattanayak, 2009). Its aerial parts contain noctacosanol-1, β-sitosterol, 6-hydroxy-3,4-dimethyl coumarin, 6-methoxy-7,8-methylenedioxy coumarin, β-sitosterolglucoside, quercetin, kaempferol and rutin that modulate the antioxidant environment within the cells. The rhizome of *Zingiber officinale* (Ardaka) has been used in the treatment of cold and bronchitis (Ram *et al.*, 2011). It has antiviral activity against the respiratory syncytial virus (Chang *et al.*, 2013), n-gingerol present in ginger prevents Th2-mediated immune responses and airway inflammation and 6-gingerol was sufficient to suppress eosinophilia (Ahui *et al.*, 2008). The compound also inhibits the production of TNF-α, IL-1β, and IL-12 (Tripathi, *et al.*, 2007).

Piper nigrum (Maricha) and *Piper longum* (Pippali) are used for treating various bronchial diseases, tuberculosis, due to their anti-oxidant, anti-inflammatory, anti-bacterial effect (Huang, *et al.*, 2010; Vinay *et al.*, 2012). Piperine is a major component of *Piper nigrum* and *P. longum*. *P. longum* is a rich source of alkaloids and amides; pipericide, piperine, piperlonguminine, piplartine, and aristolactams (Chatterjee and Dutta, 1967). *P. nigrum* inhibits allergic inflammation by inhibiting Th2/Th17 responses and mast cell activation and regulating the balance of cytokines production from Th1, Th2, Th17, and Treg cells. *P. nigrum* also inhibited GATA3, IL-4, IL-6, IL-1β, RORγt, IL-17A, TNF-α expression and increased the secretions of IL-10, INF-γ (Bui *et al.*, 2017). Piperine also reduced histologic damage and myeloperoxidase (MPO) activity in the pancreas (Bae *et al.*, 2011). *Piper longum* exhibited endothelial barrier protective effects and leukocytes migration *in vivo*, suppressed IL-6 and TNF- α levels by acting upon NF-*k*B and ERK1/2 pathways (Lee *et al.*, 2013). Fruits of *P. longum* inhibited the release of Th-2-mediated cytokines, eosinophil infiltration in the lungs (Kim and Lee, 2009).

Syzygium aromaticum (Lavanga) has anti-inflammatory (Zhang, *et al.*, 2013) properties and it inhibits eosinophilia, by modulating cytokine levels in an NF-κB pathway-dependent manner (Pan and Dong, 2015) in lungs. Further, it has free radical scavenging (Barboza, da Silva Maia Bezerra Filho, Silva, Jand Venes R Medeiros, *et al.*, 2018) and antioxidant properties (Abd El Motteleb, Selim and Mohamed, 2014). It is efficacious against herpes simplex virus type 1 (HSV-1) (Nolkemper *et al.*, 2006) and the influenza A virus (Reichling *et al.*, 2009). Eugenol is a phenylpropanoid phenolic compound constituting 45–90% of the essential oil of *S. aromaticum* (Zhang *et al.*, 2013).

The roots of *Anacyclus pyrethrum* (Akarkara) exerts immune-modulatory and immune-stimulating activities (Wu *et al.*, 2007) along with anti-inflammatory and antioxidant properties (Sujith, Darwin and Suba, 2011). It is a rich source of N-isobutyldienediynamide and polysaccharides along with saponins, sesamin, inulin, gum and traces of essential oil (Sujith, Darwin and Suba, 2011).

Swasari Ras contains Abhraka bhasma, Mukta shukti bhasma, Kapardak bhasma, and Godanti bhasma. These bhasmas are unique incinerated Ayurvedic mineral preparations, treated with herbal juice or decoction (Pal, Sahu and Haldar, 2014; Jantan *et al.*, 2019) and are rich in calcium. Abhraka bhasma is calcined mica ash that has anti-inflammatory properties and provides relief from chronic and incessant cough and respiratory illnesses. Prepared from the shell of Pearl oyster, Mukta shukti bhasma has been traditionally used for its anti-inflammatory properties (Vadnere, Pathan and Singhai, 2013) and lung diseases. Kapardak bhasma is prepared from the shell of sea animal *Cypraea moneta* (Pal, Sahu and Haldar, 2014) and has reported anti-asthmatic properties. Godanti bhasma is a combination of calcium-rich gypsum and aloe vera juice. It has an anti-inflammatory function and antipyretic activity (Dubey, *et al.*, 2012).

The presence of these poly-herbs and bhasma combination in Tablet Swasari Ras with proven lung protective properties would serve as a superior formulation for symptomatic treatment of respiratory illnesses observed in COVID-19 patients (Fig. **3.12**).

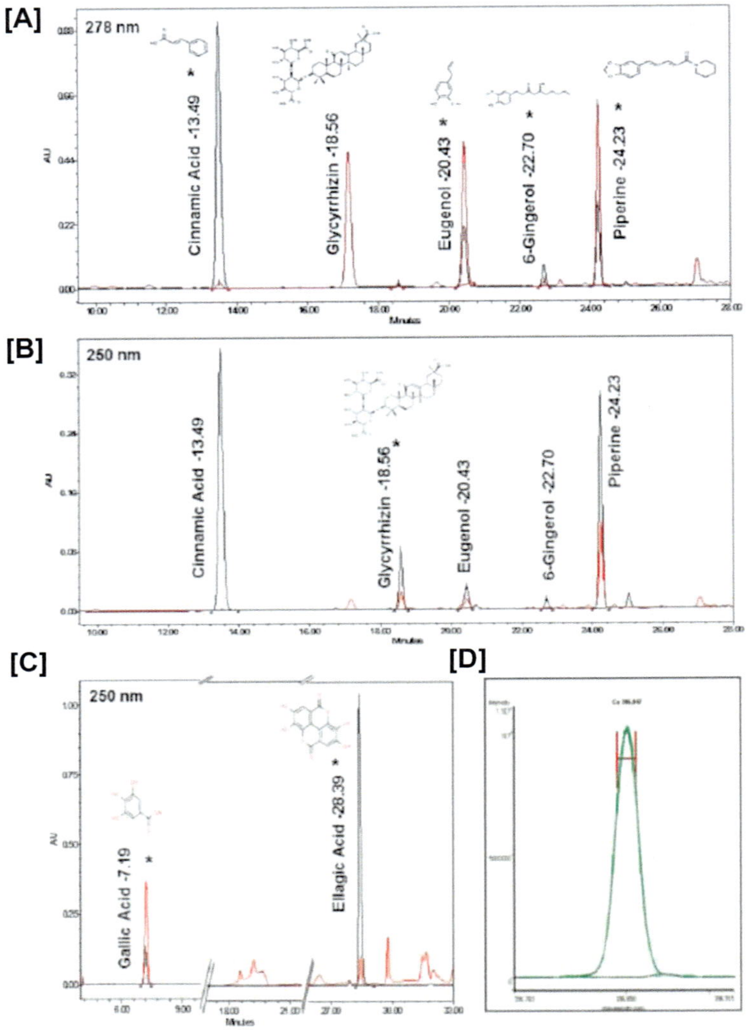

Fig. (3.12). Phytochemical profiling of Swasari HPLC (A-C) identified the presence of various bioactive secondary metabolites with proven biological activity namely, Cinnamic acid, Eugenol, 6-Gingerol, Piperine, Glycyrrhizin, Gallic acid and Ellagic acid in Swasari Vati. Further, ICP- OES analysis (D) identified the presence of calcium minerals in it. *[Courtesy:* (Balkrishna, Solleti, Singh, *et al.*, 2020b)*; Under CCBY License].*

We have also validated Swasari Ras in our pre-clinical models of lung diseases. Treatment of Swasari Ras reduced excessive mucus production and airway remodelling; decreased pro-inflammatory cytokines in the inflamed lungs; and kept a healthy oxidation state of the lungs.

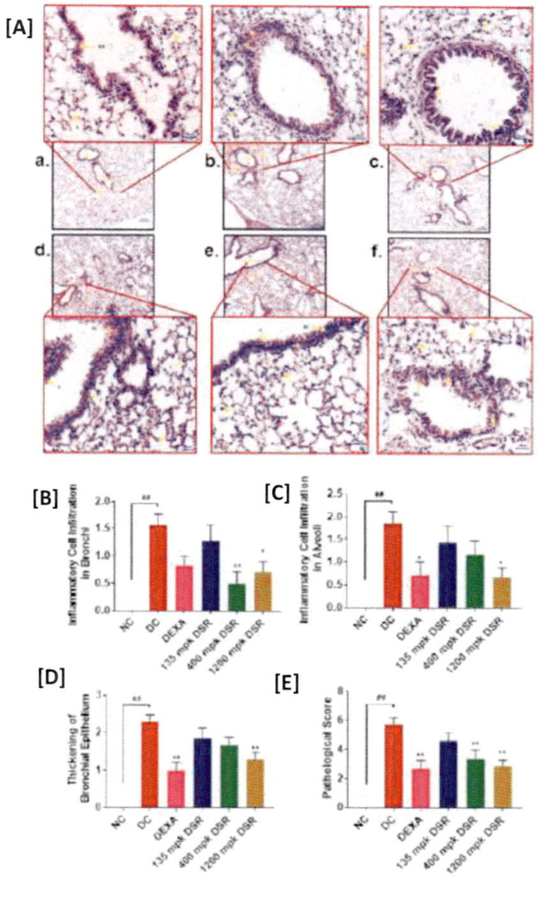

Fig. (3.13). Swasari ameliorated etiologies of lung airway inflammation **[A]** Swasari decreases lung airway inflammation and asthma-related histopathological changes. Ovalbumin allergen-induced pathological features **[B]** are reduced upon oral Swasari Ras treatment in a dose-dependent manner **[D-F]**, similar to Dexamethasone, DEXA **[C]**.*[Courtesy:* (Balkrishna, Solleti, Singh, *et al.*, 2020b)*; Under CCBY License].*

3.3.2. Swasari against SARS-CoV-2 Specific Inflammation

An improvised version of Swasari, named Divya Swasari Vati (DSV) was evaluated for its effectiveness in reducing lung inflammation in the context of COVID-19 infection. Lung epithelial cells were used, like, those used while testing Coronil. These cells were exposed to the variants of viral spike (S) protein, used during experimentation with Coronil, such as S^{WT}, S^{D614G} and S^{W436R} to induce the surge in the levels of pro-inflammatory cytokines, namely, TNF-α, IL-1β and IL-6. Cells pre-treated with DSV experienced a lesser surge in the levels of these cytokines, indicating that DSV efficiently attenuated S protein-induced cytokine responses, like, Coronil. Cytosafety of DSV was first established on these cells before conducting the actual experiment. DSV was found to be safe at over the range of its effective dose (Fig. **3.14**) (Balkrishna, Verma, *et al.*, 2020).

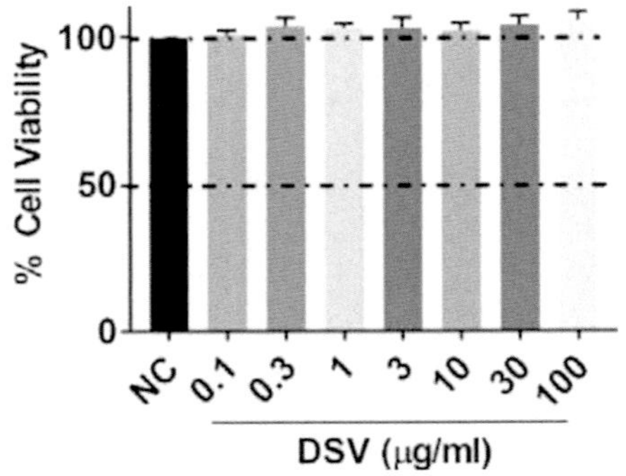

Fig. (3.14). Cell cytotoxicity assay of DSV. Cytosafety of DSV was ensured through Alamar blue staining of lung cells treated with different concentrations of DSV. *[Courtesy:* (Balkrishna, Verma, *et al.*, 2020)*; Under CCBY License].*

The myriad interplay of pro-inflammatory cytokines leading to 'cytokine storm' was also studied under a simplified *in vitro* set-up (using HEK-Blue cells and SEAP assay), wherein, one cytokine (for example, IL-1β) was induced to evoke the activation of other cytokines, like, TNF-α and IL-6, and see how well DSV could subside this complex surge of cytokines. We noted that DSV was quite potent in handling this simulated cytokine surge (Fig. **3.15**) (Balkrishna, Verma, *et al.*, 2020).

DSV exhibited anti-inflammatory responses of a magnitude similar to those observed for Coronil. So, we checked the efficacy of DSV in managing the cytokine response elicited by different variants of viral spike (S) protein, namely, S^{WT}, S^{D614G} and SW^{436R}. Lung cells were pre-treated with different concentrations of DSV and then exposed to the S proteins, while, continuing the DSV treatment. We observed that SD614G did not elicit a significant cytokine response which falls in line with the finding that this variant of S protein is less virulent, and virulence is manifested by a cytokine storm. Otherwise, like Coronil, DSV was capable of efficiently managing the cytokine surge induced by the other two S proteins (Fig. **3.16**).

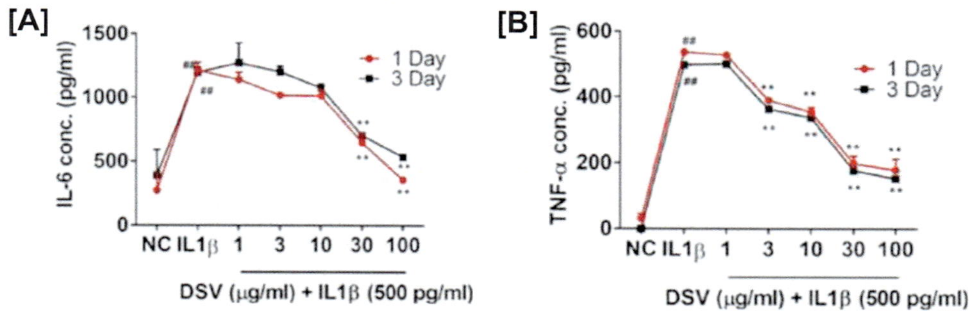

Fig. (3.15). Effect of DSV on cytokine cross-talk *in vitro*.**[A, B]** Cells were pre-treated with different concentrations of DSV for either 1 day or 3 days before the addition of IL-1β and DSV in the desired concentration. Cell supernatant was used in ELISA for the estimation of IL-6 (A) and TNF-α (B) expressions 24 hours post-stimulation. *[Courtesy:* (Balkrishna, Verma, *et al.*, 2020)*; Under CCBY License].*

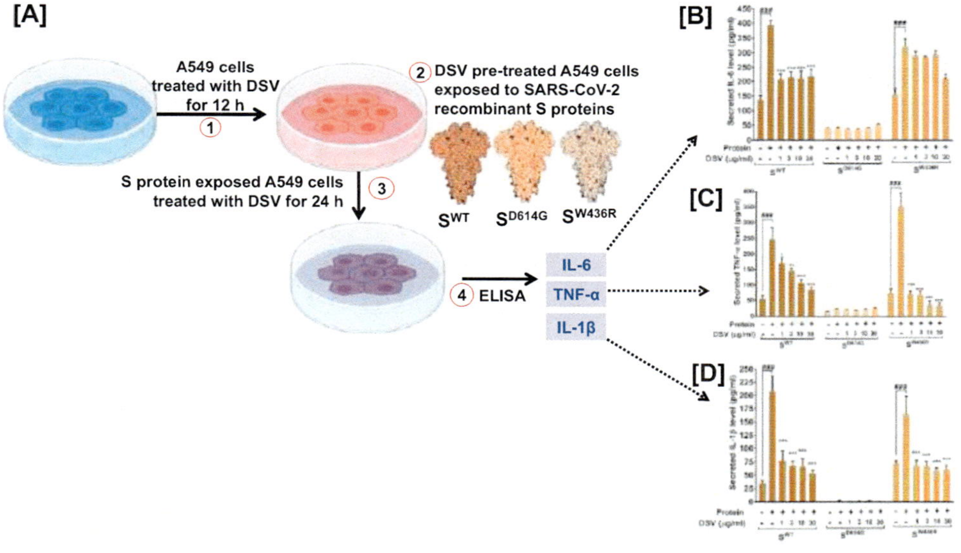

Fig. (3.16). DSV attenuates cytokine activation by viral S protein **[A]** Pictorial representation of the experimental set-up. A 549 cells were treated with different types of viral S proteins, S^{WT}, S^{D614G} or S^{W436R} to induce cytokine activation and subsequently treated with different concentrations of DSV. **[B-D]** Effect of DSV treatment on cytokine activation by S proteins was evaluated through ELISA and represented as levels of IL-6 (B), TNF-α (C) and IL-1β (D) secreted into the medium by A549 cells.

Observing similar responses for DSV as we found for Coronil, we evaluated the effect of DSV on VSVppSARS-2S pseudovirus-induced cytokine response. The experimental set-up was identical to that of Coronil, except for Coronil, DSV was used for treating the cells. We noted that upon DSV treatment the levels of TNF-α, IL-1β, and IL-6 were reduced as we observed for Coronil. This reflected that DSV also attenuated the VSVppSARS-2S pseudovirus-induced cytokine response (Fig. **3.17**).

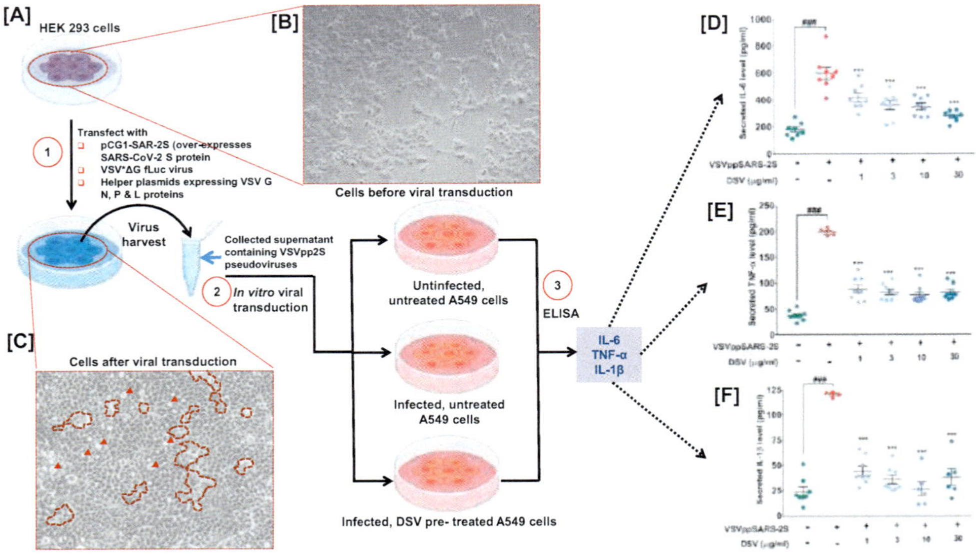

Fig. (3.17). Viral pseudotyping, transduction and effect of DSV on elicited cytokine response.**[A]** Schematic diagram depicting the steps (shown as numbers within red circles) involved in the entire experiment beginning with pseudotyping of VSV with SARS-CoV-2 S protein to obtain VSVpp2S viruses using HEK293 cells, followed by their infection of alveolar epithelial A 549 cells and subsequent determination of the effect of DSV treatment on the levels of secreted pro-inflammatory cytokines, TNF-α, IL-1β and IL-6. **[B]** Image of non-transduced HEK293 cells shown for comparison with the transduced ones showing cytopathic effects. **[C]** Pseudotyping was monitored through the appearance of plaques (red arrowheads) and cytopathic islands (demarcated with broken orange lines). **[D-F]** Levels of IL-6 (D), TNF-α (E) and IL-1β (F) secreted into the medium by VSVpp2S transduced A549 cells were determined through ELISA and represented as scatter plots.

With such observations, similar to Coronil, we went ahead and checked the effect of DSV on the physical interaction between ACE-2 and spike (S) protein of SARS-CoV-2 using an experimental set-up like the one used for Coronil. We observed that DSV, like Coronil, was effective as an inhibitor against ACE-2 and S protein, regardless of its variant in question, although, the IC_{20} values of 23.33, 7.78 and 2.28 μg/ml, for S^{WT}, S^{D614G} and S^{W436R}, respectively, suggested that, DSV was also more efficient in preventing the interaction between ACE-2 and S^{W436R} variant of viral S protein (Fig. **3.18**).

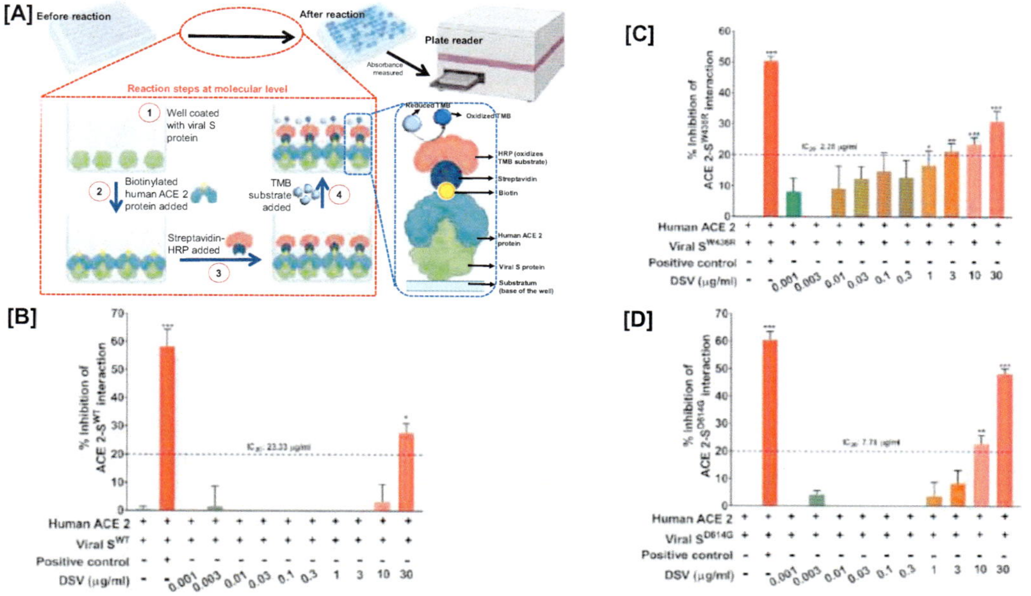

Fig. (3.18). DSV inhibits the interaction between human ACE-2 receptor protein and SARS-**CoV-2 S protein .[A]** Diagrammatic representation of the experimental principle employed for the study. Biotinylated ACE-2 allowed to bind to immobilized viral S proteins detected through streptavidin-conjugated horse-radish peroxidase (HRP) using TMB substrate. **[B-D]** Inhibitory effect of DSV treatment on the interactions between human ACE-2 and different variants of viral S proteins, S^{WT} (B), S^{D614G}(C) and S^{W436R} (D). A known inhibitor supplied with the kit was included as a positive control. Reaction without inhibitor or DSV was assumed to be 100% and inhibition of interaction was calculated relative to the absorbance obtained from this reaction.

These studies provided insight into the mode of actions of the two Ayurvedic medicines formulated against COVID-19. In doing so, these studies helped in establishing scientific proof in favour of the potency of Ayurveda in treating COVID-19. This evidence not only offered mechanistic insights into the functioning of these Ayurvedic medicines as potent anti-COVID-19 therapeutics (Fig. **3.19**), but also served as the *in vitro* studies mandatory for taking any drug forward for pre-clinical and clinical studies.

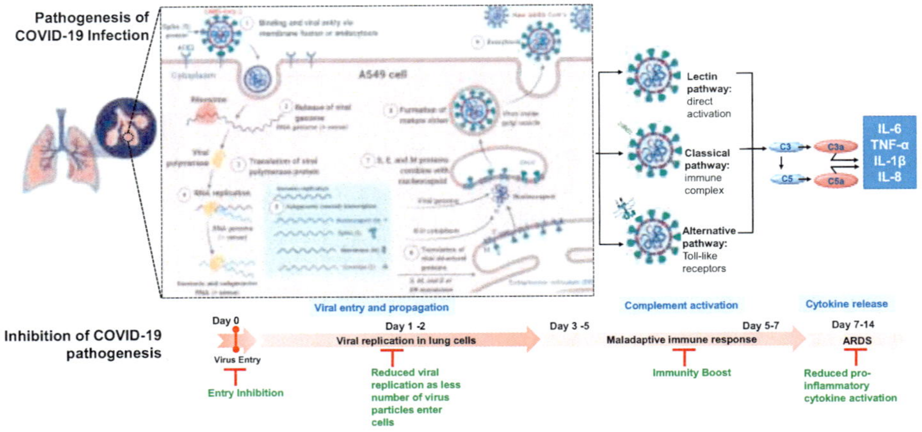

Fig. (3.19). Deciphered mode of action of Coronil and DSV as antiviral agents against SARS-CoV-2. Experimental evidence reveal that Coronil and DSV are likely to act at almost all the steps of SARS- CoV-2 pathogenesis thereby providing multi-step protection from the infection. This is in addition to the immense immune-boosting capabilities of both medicines. *[Courtesy:* (Balkrishna, Haldar, *et al.*, 2021)*; Under CCBY License]*

CONCLUDING REMARKS

In a nutshell, employing different cell biological techniques, the mode-of-actions of Coronil and Divya Swasari Vati have been deciphered. The observations show that these drugs can inhibit entry of SARS-CoV-2 pseudoviruses into human lung alveolar epithelial cells and can also ameliorate the detrimental cytokine responses generated by SARS-CoV-2 spike protein-mediated infection.

CHAPTER 4

Use of *In Vivo* Models in Preclinical Drug Discovery and Development

Abstract: This chapter deals with the *in vivo* preclinical studies involving the COVID-19 zebrafish model conducted on the Ayurvedic medicines mentioned in the last chapter to further validate their efficacy against COVID-19. Animal models are needed in order to understand the disease's progress and associated symptoms. While it is possible to understand the disease characteristics based on historical evidence and previous research on similar disease-causing organisms, newer species of disease-causing agents have been recently discovered. These newer organisms without any previous history, pose the biggest challenge in drug discovery and development. In these cases, the use of relevant animal models of disease becomes important in order to understand the disease progression as well as the interaction of the body with the disease-causing agent. In the current SARS-CoV-2 infections, the virus is potentially lethal in humans. In such cases, the danger of using humans to test new drugs becomes ethically unacceptable unless the drug has been tested in animal models against the virus. The use of higher primates, like monkeys, or small animals like dogs and rodents, which are generally accepted pre-clinical models of drug discovery, has a myriad of ethical concerns. Despite this, several different models of SARS-CoV-2 infection are currently in use, ranging from non-human primates, such as rhesus macaques (Rhesus monkey), and rodent models, such as transgenic mice and hamsters. While it is difficult to incorporate all the different pathological features of the disease in a single model, it is important to choose the correct model animal in order to answer the primary question that the investigator seeks. For example, rodents lack the coagulopathy component, which is often seen in severe SARS-CoV-2 infections. By the same token, the narrow spectrum of viral infectivity and the inability to the cross-species barrier by the virus is an important consideration while studying the disease pathology. This was seen in a rhesus monkey model where no overt clinical signs were detected even though prolonged viral shedding was detected in the upper respiratory tract of animals. With these issues in mind, we developed a humanized zebrafish model to test the efficacy of Coronil and Divya Swasari Vati in decreasing the pathogenic characteristics associated with SARS-CoV-2 spike protein expression. Zebrafish has proven to be a solid model system for investigating human viral pathophysiology, and various human viruses, including chikungunya and influenza, can colonize zebrafish, making it an appealing and alternative model system. Zebrafish have well-defined innate and adaptive immune systems that are strikingly comparable to those of humans. Unlike mouse models, zebrafish have swim bladders as buoyancy organs, and human cells could be transplanted into swim bladders to create xeno-transplanted humanized models for respiratory disorders, such as SARS-CoV-2 infection. The implantation of human lung cells into the zebrafish's air bladder increases the model's relevance and

Acharya Balkrishna

gives human-equivalent methods of inquiry. Different groups have successfully employed this strategy to replicate lung cancer in zebrafish as well as COPD and Pseudomonas aeruginosa pathogenesis. Results obtained from treating the humanized zebrafish model injected with the S protein of SARS-CoV-2 with either Coronil or Divya Swasari Vati are shared in this chapter, along with a proposed mode of action for both of these Ayurvedic formulations.

Keywords: Behavioural fever, Cytokine response, Humanized zebrafish, *In vivo* studies, Preclinical, SARS-CoV-2 S protein-induced inflammation.

4.1. RATIONALE FOR THE USE OF *IN VIVO* MODELS

Animal models are needed in order to understand the disease's progress and associated symptoms. While it is possible to understand the disease characteristics based on historical evidence and previous research on similar disease-causing organisms, newer species of disease-causing agents have been recently discovered. These newer organisms without any previous history pose the biggest challenge in drug discovery and development.

It becomes important for researchers to use relevant models of disease or induce disease in small animals to replicate the disease progression and to understand the interaction of the body with the disease-causing agent. Once such a model has been developed and successfully used, the process of drug discovery can start.

The introduction of unknown chemical agents to humans is fraught with danger, and therefore, it is ill-advised to test drugs directly in humans. Even if a particular drug was previously cleared for human use, it is important to understand the interactions between the drug and the new disease it is being tested against. This has many reasons, the most important being the potential transformation of the drug by the pathogen into a newer metabolite which could cause untold damage to the human body. For this reason, animal testing forms an integral part of drug discovery and development.

In the current SARS-CoV-2 infections, the virus is potentially lethal in humans. In such cases, the dangers of using humans to test new drugs become ethically unacceptable unless the drug has been tested in animal models against the virus. In the case of newer pathogens for which medications are not available, patient management to prevent mortality takes the center stage rather than outright eradication of the pathogen. Symptomatic treatment for the changes seen as a result of the viral infection is important so that the body's immune system is not over-burdened and can fight back on its own, or with a little help from various drugs that give symptomatic relief. Therefore, the immediate use of untested drugs in patients with active infections becomes a double-edged sword, wherein the drug may pose an unnecessary burden on the patient while having minimal to no effect on disease eradication.

4.2. WHY ZEBRAFISH?

The use of higher primates like monkeys, or small animals like dogs and rodents, which are generally accepted preclinical models of drug discovery has a myriad of ethical concerns. Despite this, several different models of SARS-CoV-2 infection are currently in use, ranging from non-human primates such as rhesus macaques (Rhesus monkey), and rodent models such as transgenic mice and hamsters. While it is difficult to incorporate all the different pathological features of the disease in a single model, it is important to choose the correct model animal in order to answer the primary endpoint that the investigator desires. For example, rodents lack the coagulopathy component, which is often seen in severe SARS-CoV-2 infections. By the same token, the narrow spectrum of viral infectivity and the inability to cross the species barrier by the virus is an important consideration while studying the disease pathology. This was seen in a rhesus monkey model where no overt clinical signs were detected even though prolonged viral shedding was detected in the upper respiratory tract of animals.

Keeping these concerns in mind, we employed a humanized zebrafish model to see if Coronil and Divya Swasari Vati may help reduce the pathogenic characteristics associated with SARS-CoV-2 spike protein expression. For researching the human viral disease, zebrafish has proven to be a reliable model system. It is a small and adaptable organism that is very easy to manipulate, and the signalling pathways, interactions with chemical modifiers, and host-virus communications on mucosal tissues may all be studied in great detail. Zebrafish have well-defined innate and adaptive immune systems that are strikingly comparable to those of humans. Furthermore, the interaction of viral glycoproteins with olfactory sensory neurons in the fish nasal area is well understood. The loss of olfactory sensibility is one of the early clinical indications of established SARS-CoV-2 infection, hence such an interaction model is required.

Several human viruses, including chikungunya and influenza, can invade zebrafish, making it an appealing and novel model system. Unlike mouse models, zebrafish have swim bladders that serve as buoyancy organs, and human cells could be implanted in them to create xenotransplanted humanized models for respiratory disorders like SARS-CoV-2 infection. The transplantation of human lung cells into the swim bladder of the zebrafish enhances the relevance of the model and provides a human equivalent means of investigation. This approach has been successfully used for modelling lung cancer in zebrafish and in modelling COPD and *Pseudomonas aeruginosa* pathogenesis by different groups.

In our study, human lung epithelial cells (A549) were injected into the swim bladder and allowed to colonize for a period of 7 days. Following that, the SARS-CoV-2 recombinant spike protein was injected at the location of A549 introduction and allowed to establish the illness phenotype. Once the illness phenotype was determined, the fish were fed human-relevant doses of the reference medication Dexamethasone (0.08 g/kg/day) and the test formulation Coronil and Divya Swasari Vati. In one set of experiments, the fish were dosed for 3 days and terminated on the 4th day, and in the other, the dosing was for 6 days and terminated on the 7th day (Fig. **4.1**).

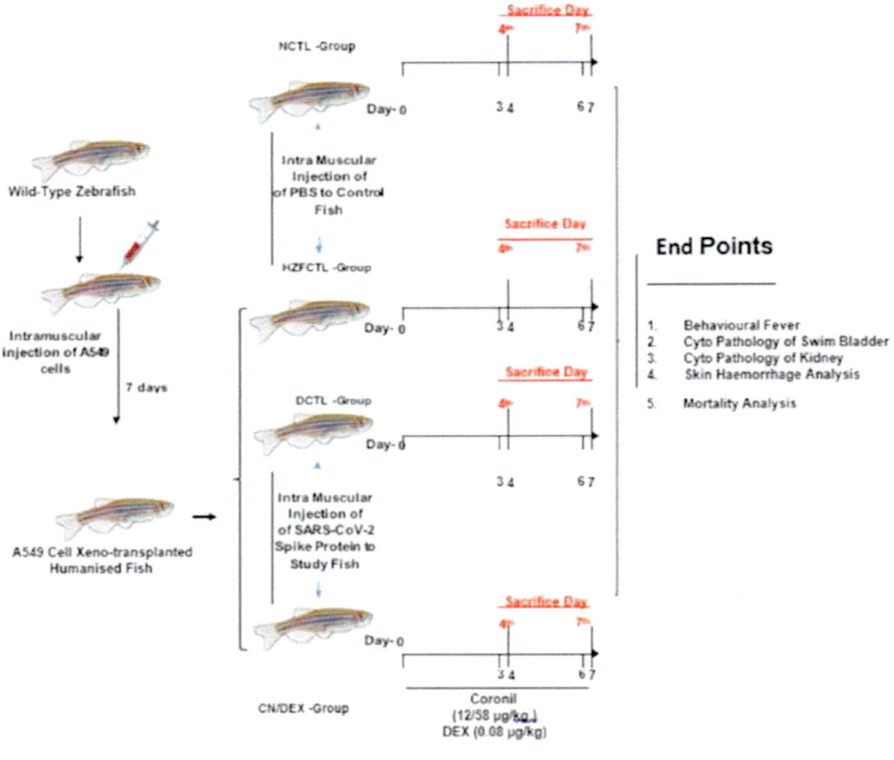

Fig. (4.1). Schematic representation of the study design for testing the efficacy of Coronil and Divya Swasari Vati in reducing the disease phenotype induced by SARS-CoV-2 spike protein in a humanized zebrafish model. ***[Courtesy:*** **(Balkrishna, Solleti, Verma,** ***et al.*****, 2020b)*****; Under CCBY License]***.

4.3. ESTABLISHMENT OF XENOTRANSPLANTED HUMANIZED ZEBRAFISH MODEL

In our study, human alveolar epithelial cells, A549 cells, were injected into the anterior lobe of the swim bladder of zebrafish. The swim bladder is a two-lobed, gas-filled organ that is used for buoyancy in zebrafish. It is connected to the esophagus and air enters the bladder when a fish gulps air.

After 7 days, the swim bladders were dissected out of a few experimental fish and studied for morphological and cytological changes (Fig. **4.2**). There were no morphological changes in the swim bladder suggesting that there were no unintended consequences of transplanting human cells into the swim bladder.

When the cytological smears were examined, human lung cells were easily identified as darkly staining cells, thus confirming the establishment of a human lung epithelial cell within the swim bladder without any serious side effects. These groups of fish were now designated as humanized zebrafish (HZFCTL).

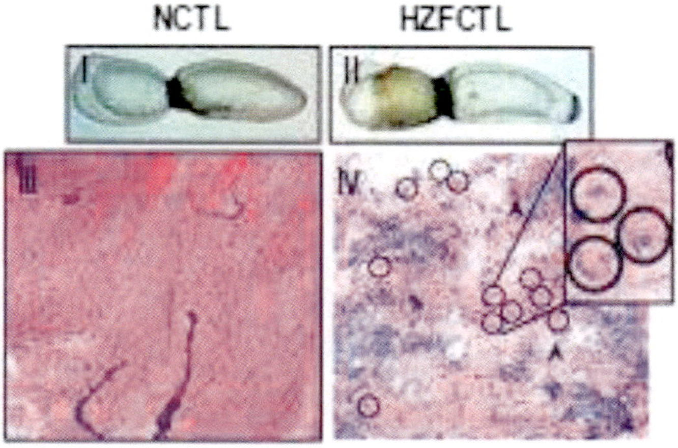

Fig. (4.2). Cytology staining to identify colonization of human lung cells (A549) in swim bladder. Representative images of swim bladders from **(i)** Normal control (NCTL) and **(ii)** Humanized zebrafish Control (HZFCTL) after a 7-day transplant showing normal morphological traits. Cyto-smears of **(iii)** NCTL and **(iv)** HZFCTL showed normal cytological features along with transplanted cells (zoom-in represents xeno-transplanted cells). Black arrows indicate cells of zebrafish origin and black circles represent cells of human origin. AL-anterior lobe, PL-posterior lobe. Scale bars, 1000 μm at 1X magnification. *[Courtesy:* (Balkrishna, Solleti, Verma, *et al.*, 2020b)*; Under CCBY License]*.

4.4. INDUCTION OF DISEASE PHENOTYPE IN HUMANIZED ZEBRAFISH MODEL USING SARS-COV- 2 SPIKE PROTEIN

The spike protein of the SARS-CoV-2 virus is needed for the interaction with and entry of the virus into the host cells. Though the virus can survive in the environment and on surfaces, it requires a host cell for its multiplication. The spike protein interacts with a protein called Angiotensin-Converting Enzyme 2 (ACE-2) present on the host cell surface and through this interaction and subsequent events, the viral RNA enters the host cell (Dosch, Mahajan and Collins, 2009). Once inside the host cell, the RNA undergoes replication by subverting the normal cellular processes to form multiple copies of the virus that eventually bud out of the cell to start a new cycle of infection.

Though the primary target for SARS-CoV-2 is the airway epithelium, the ACE-2 receptor required for entry of the virus into human cells is present on a multitude of cell types. These include the oral and nasal mucosa, lung, stomach, small intestine, colon, spleen, liver, kidney, and brain. The potential for infection in all of these organs is one of the reasons for systemic infection seen in the most severe cases.

Studies have shown that the use of recombinant spike protein in cell culture models and animal models can stimulate the changes in cytokine profile that is generally seen in a natural infection. Moreover, the spike protein is the first target of neutralizing antibodies produced in a recovering patient during the course of an infection. Multiple studies with either computer-generated docking models or with inhibitory agents that block the interaction of the spike protein confirmed the importance of this protein in the disease process.

In our investigation, the addition of purified recombinant spike protein to the humanized zebrafish model increased the infiltration of pro-inflammatory cells into the air bladder, such as macrophages and granulocytes. (Fig. **4.3**) (Balkrishna, Solleti, Verma, *et al.*, 2020a).

Semi-quantitative PCR was used to examine changes in the expression of IL-6, IL-10, and TNF- genes in zebrafish after spike protein production. When compared to both the normal control (NCTL) and the xeno-transplanted fish (HZFCTL), the expression of all three cytokines was considerably higher (p0.0001) in fish administered the SARS-CoV-2 spike protein (DCNTL) (Fig. **4.4**). The presence of these cytokines can generate further inflammation and, in the case of severe infections, a "cytokine storm" can lead to systemic shock.

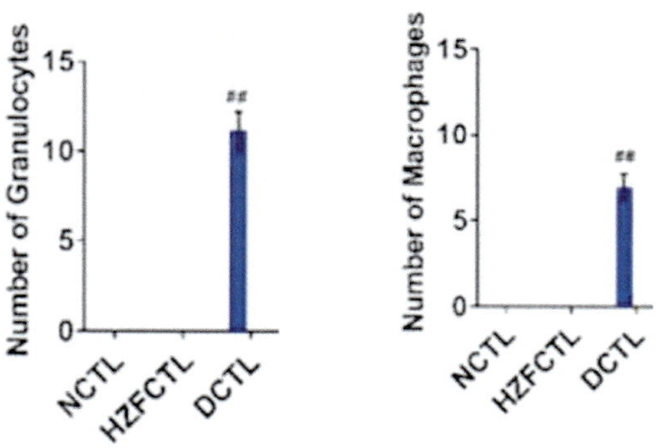

Fig. (4.3). Introduction of SARS-CoV-2 spike protein, increases the infiltration of pro-inflammatory cytokines in the swim bladder. Quantitative enumeration of granulocytes and macrophages using swim bladder cyto-smear. n=24 for each test group. ## represents statistical significance compared to HZFCTL (p <0.001). *[Courtesy:* (Balkrishna, Solleti, Verma, *et al.*,)*; Under CCBY License].*

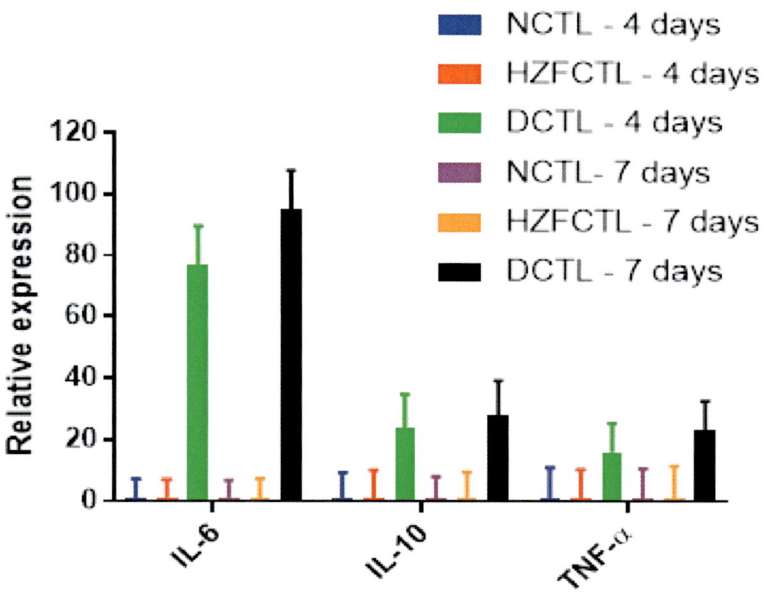

Fig. (4.4). Pro-inflammatory cytokines are induced post-SARS-CoV-2 infection. Quantitative enumeration of gene expression levels of different pro- inflammatory cytokines in humanized zebrafish upon spike protein challenge. n= 24 for each test group. ## represents statistical significance compared to HZFCTL (p<0.001).

In humans, SARS-CoV-2 is accompanied by a high fever (in approximately 90% of cases). Unlike humans, zebrafish are ectothermic, preferring water temperatures ranging from 26 to 29 degrees Celsius, and they migrate to areas of a water body that reflect their body temperature (Avdesh *et al.*, 2012). The duration spent by individual fish in interconnected chambers with water at varying temperatures (23 °C, 29 °C, and 37 °C) is quantified as behavioural fever. As expected, both NCTL and HZFCTL fish spent more time at 29 °C on the fourth and seventh days, and less time at 37 °C (Table **4.1**). Spike protein challenge caused behavioural fever in DCTL, and the fish spent more time at 37 °C and less time at 29 °C on the fourth and seventh days.

Table 4.1. Time (in seconds) spent by experimental fish in various temperature chambers.

Study Groups	Time (in seconds) Spent in Temperature Gradient Chamber					
	4th day			7th day		
	23 °C	29 °C	37 °C	23 °C	29 °C	37 °C
NCTL	35.58 ± 3.0	129.63 ± 1.4	14.92 ± 2.7	24.13 ± 0.7	130.00 ± 0.8	25.88 ± 0.7
HZFCTL	37.79 ± 1.5	134.00 ± 1.5	8.21 ± 2.0	25.88 ± 1.3	135.75 ± 1.5	18.38 ± 1.3
DCTL	15.96 ± 1.6	7.04 ± 1.3	157.08 ± 1.6	2.38 ± 1.1	4.75 ± 1.3	172.88 ± 1.3

Data expressed as mean ± S.D. values (n = 24).

The presence of pro-inflammatory cells inside the swim bladder increased expression of pro-inflammatory cytokines, and the increased behavioural fever suggests that the use of SARS-CoV-2 spike protein in a humanized zebrafish model is a good model to study the effects of different ayurvedic medicinal formulations in rescuing the disease phenotype.

4.5. *IN VIVO* MODEL FOR DEMONSTRATION OF EFFECTIVENESS OF CORONIL IN REDUCING SARS-COV-2 SPIKE PROTEIN-INDUCED DISEASE PHENOTYPE

The anti-inflammatory and anti-viral capabilities of Coronil's herbal components and constituent phyto-compounds are well recognized. *T. cordifolia* has been utilized for thousands of years for its therapeutic benefits and contains alkaloids, glycosides, steroids, and polysaccharides (Panchabhai, Kulkarni and Rege, 2008). *W. somnifera* has been shown to improve physical and mental health as well as rejuvenate the body (Ernst, 2010). It possesses well-described anti-inflammatory, antibacterial, analgesic, anti-stress, neuroprotective, cardioprotective, and immunomodulatory properties (Vyas, Bhandari, and Patidar, 2011) and includes bioactive components such as steroidal saponin, alkaloids, and steroidal lactones (Ernst, 2010). The leaves of *O. sanctum* have been used to treat rheumatism, bronchitis, and pyrexia, as well as to boost cellular and humoral immunity (Pattanayak, *et al.*, 2010).

In this section of the investigation, a SARS-CoV-2 spike protein challenge resulted in the induction of behavioural fever, and Coronil therapy reduced this behavioural fever just somewhat. Furthermore, Coronil-mediated suppression of swim bladder collapse supports a role for Coronil in oedema rescue. In the case of SARS-CoV-2 infection, the innate immune response in the lungs recruit macrophages and monocytes, releases cytokines, and initiates adaptive T and B cell immunological responses to resolve the infection. A defective immune response, on the other hand, can result in severe lung and even systemic pathology in some situations (Tay *et al.*, 2020). In the study, a spike protein challenge promoted the accumulation of macrophages and granulocytes in DCTL fish. More importantly, the fact that CN therapy reduced inflammatory cell accumulation while increasing lymphocytic accumulation suggests that adaptive immune response may have played a role in pathology rescue.

Changes in the survival of the fish were also observed and recorded every day. The disease control fish showed 8.7% mortality after 2 days and 13.8% mortality after 5-days, while the normal control and the humanized zebrafish did not have any mortality (Fig. **4.5**).

Fig. (4.5). Survival of the different study groups of zebrafish was analyzed and plotted as a Kaplan-Meier survival curve. ***[Courtesy:* (Balkrishna, Solleti, Verma, *et al.*, 2020b)*; Under CCBY License].***

4.5.1. Coronil Attenuates SARS-CoV-2 Spike Protein-Induced Inflammation in Swim Bladder

The zebrafish swim bladder is a gas-filled chamber that is two-lobed, an anterior and a posterior lobe, connected by a wide ductus communicans. Both the lobes function in synchrony to maintain buoyancy in the fish. A thin mesothelial layer comprising of epithelial cells and smooth muscle cells form a gas-filled chamber and the whole structure is encased in a Tunica Externa.

The presence of human lung epithelial cells in the swim bladder ensures that any changes in the cells are easily captured for analysis. Moreover, the correlation with human disease becomes easier. Introduction of the SARS-CoV-2 spike protein-induced inflammatory changes in the swim bladder and was seen by increased oedema in the anterior lobe by the 4th day time point (Fig. **4.6**). Continued induction further deteriorated the condition of the swim bladder seen by the collapse of the anterior lobe by the 7th day.

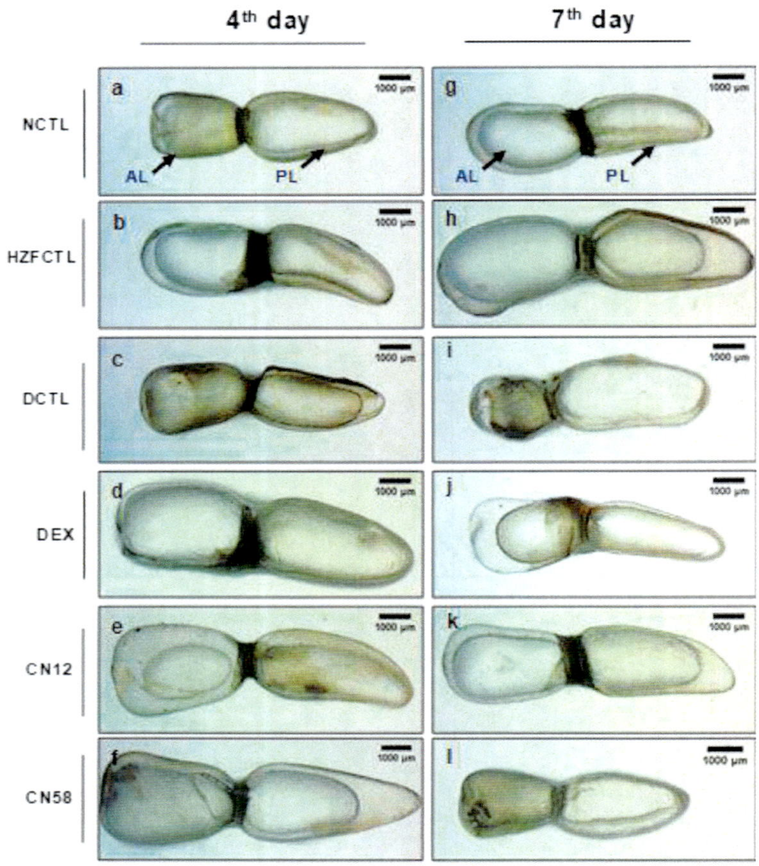

Fig. (4.6). Coronil reduces SARS-CoV-2 induced swim bladder structural abnormality and oedema. The left panel (A to F) shows results obtained at the 4th day time point, while the right panel (G to L) shows the 7th day time point. (A and G) Normal control (NCTL) (B and H), Humanized zebrafish control (HZFCTL), (C and I) SARS- CoV-2 spike protein-induced disease control (DCTL), (D and J) Dexamethasone (DEX) treatment groups, (E and K) Treatment with12 μg/kg body weight (CN12), and (F and L) Treatment with 58 μg/kg (CN58) AL-anterior lobe, PL- posterior lobe. The circle inside the swim bladder indicates a watermark at the contact between the glass slide and the swim bladder during image acquisition. Scale bar, 1000 μm at 1X magnification. *[Courtesy:* (Balkrishna, Solleti, Verma, *et al.*, 2020b)*; Under CCBY License].*

In the study, Dexamethasone was used as a reference control as it was proven to have a role in reducing inflammation in a clinical setting. Treatment with Dexamethasone in the 4th day group reduced oedema seen in the disease control group as seen by slight inflation of the swim bladder with an intact tunica externa and gas gland. Prolonged treatment with Dexamethasone was unable to mitigate the severity of the spike protein induction. The swim bladder had an enlarged anterior lobe while the posterior lobe was much narrower. The ductus communicans was also seen to be narrower when compared to the normal control possibly due to the increased pressure inside the lobes of the swim bladder at the 7th day time point. These observations suggest that Dexamethasone is perhaps unable to combat the severe changes due to the prolonged presence of the spike protein.

When human equivalent doses of Coronil, 12 μg/kg body weight (CN12) and 58 μg/kg (CN58), were used in the treatment group, the swim bladder inflammation was mitigated on the 4th day. Both the lobes were comparable in size, shape and colour with that of the swim bladder in the normal control or the humanized zebrafish control groups. Similar results were also seen at the 7th day time point suggesting that the human equivalent doses were able to reverse the inflammation seen with the spike protein.

Cytology smears prepared from whole swim bladders were stained with Hematoxylin-Eosin to determine the cellular changes due to the introduction of spike protein as well as for identification of immune cell infiltration. The normal swim bladder is composed of squamous and columnar epithelial cells (labelled as E and shown by black arrowhead), smooth muscle cells (labelled as S and shown by black arrowhead), and collagen (Fig. **4.7a**, 4th day and 4.7g, 7th day). These different cell types were seen in the cytology of both the normal control and the humanized zebrafish control (Fig. **4.7b**, 4th day and 4.7h, 7th day) groups. The absence of any degraded cells or cellular debris indicated that there was no change in the swim bladder due to the introduction of human lung epithelial cells.

The various immune cells were identified based on their nuclear morphology and the colour of the cytoplasm with Eosin stain. Granulocytes are composed of four different cell types, neutrophils (segmented nucleus with 2 to 3 lobes), basophils (peripheral and eccentrically placed, an unsegmented nucleus with lightly staining basophilic cytoplasm), eosinophils (peripheral and eccentrically placed, an unsegmented nucleus with darkly staining acidophilic cytoplasm), and mast cells (centrally located nucleus in an oval or irregularly shaped cell). Macrophages were identified by their large centrally located nucleus with visible cytoplasm. Lymphocytes have a centrally located spherical nucleus with very little cytoplasm.

At the 4th day time point, the disease control group showed nuclear and cellular debris and oedema in cytological staining. As depicted in the representative image (Fig. **4.7c**), there was an increased presence of granulocytes (green arrowhead) and macrophages (brown arrowhead). Compared to the disease control, the group treated with Dexamethasone showed the presence of lymphocytes (yellow arrowhead) in the cytology smears (Fig. **4.7d**) at the 4th day time point. Low dose (Fig. **4.7e**) and high dose Coronil treatment (Fig. **4.7f**) showed increased infiltration of lymphocytes while granulocytes and macrophages were also detected.

Interestingly, the 7th day disease control group did not show any immune cell infiltrates (Fig. **4.7i**). However, the cytological smear showed the presence of oedema and cellular debris. Treatment with Dexamethasone resulted in a reduction in the number of macrophages and granulocytes but an increase in the number of lymphocytes (Fig. **4.7j**). Both the doses of Coronil treatment, showed a reduction in the number of granulocytes and macrophages while the number of lymphocytes was higher than that of the disease control group (Fig. **4.7k**, CN12 and **4.7l** CN58).

As seen in this result, reduction in the number of inflammatory cells along with a reduction in the cellular debris with only mild to moderate cellular degradation, indicate the rescue of disease phenotype induced by the spike protein in the presence of Coronil.

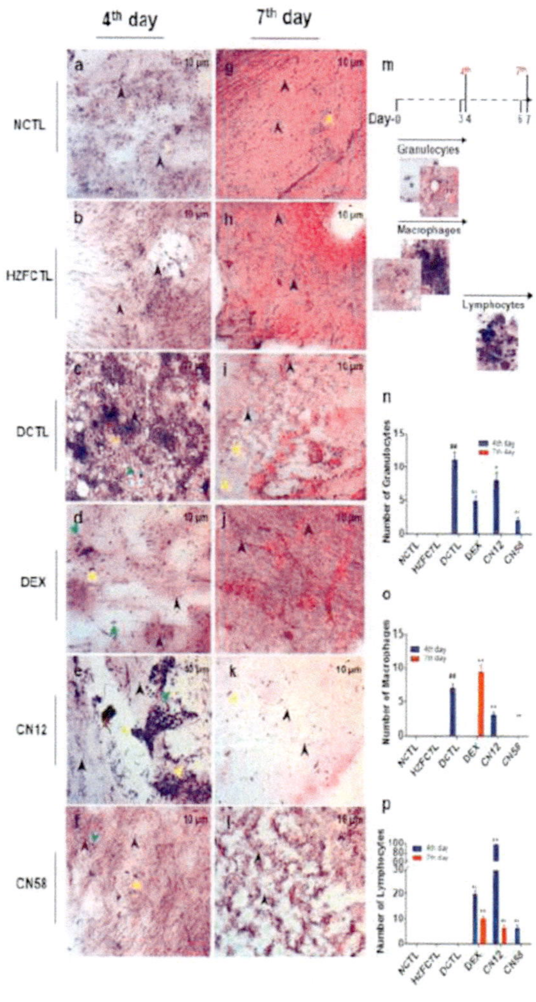

Fig. (4.7). Coronil rescues from SARS-CoV-2 spike protein-induced inflammation in swim bladder cytosmears after Hematoxylin-Eosin staining. **(a)** Normal control at 4th day and **(g)** at 7th day, **(b)** Humanized zebrafish control at 4th day and **(h)** at 7thday, **(c)** Disease control at 4th day and **(i)** at 7th day, **(d)** Dexamethasone treatment at 4th day and **(j)** at 7th day, **(e)** Coronil (12 µg/kg) at 4th day, **(f)** Coronil (58 µg/kg) at 4th day; **(k)** Coronil (12 µg/kg) at 7thday, and **(l)** Coronil (58 µg/kg) at 7th day. Scale bars, 10 µm at 200X magnification. Black arrowheads denote normal cells, green for granulocytes, brown for macrophages, and yellow arrowhead denotes lymphocytes. *[Courtesy:* (Balkrishna, Solleti, Verma, *et al.*, 2020b)*; Under CCBY License]*

Quantitation of the number of immune cells infiltrates in the disease control group showed a significantly higher ($p < 0.001$) number of granulocytes (Fig. **4.8**) at both the time points. Macrophages which are phagocytic cells were not detected in the disease control group at both the time points (Fig. **4.8b**). Lymphocytes which are part of the adaptive immunity were absent in the group that was challenged with the spike protein of SARS-CoV-2 suggesting that the adaptive immunity may not be triggered due to the lack of a favourable cytokine milieu.

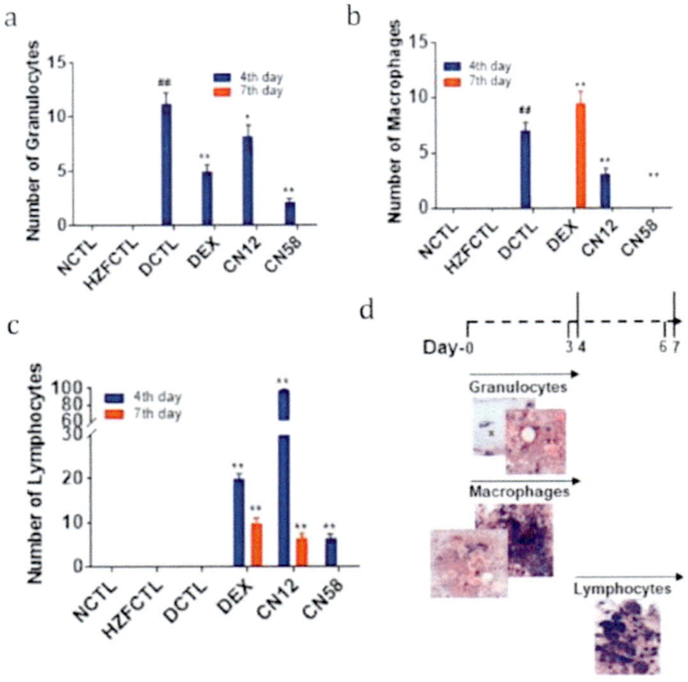

Fig. (4.8). Quantitative estimation of immune cell infiltration in the swim bladder assessed by cytology. **(a)** Number of Granulocytes, **(b)** Number of Macrophages, **(c)** Number of Lymphocyte infiltrates. (d) schematic showing the time point for the identification of the different immune cell types that infiltrate the swim bladder as seen by cytology. Data are represented as mean ± S.D. for a sample number of 24. (##) represents P <0.001 compared to the normal control and (**) represents p<0.001 compared to the disease control group. *[Courtesy:* (Balkrishna, Solleti, Verma, *et al.*, 2020b)*; Under CCBY License].*

Treatment with Dexamethasone significantly reduced the number of Granulocytes at the 4th day time point and was completely absent on the 7th day. In contrast, macrophages were absent on the 4th day while there was an increase by the 7th day. There was a significant increase in the number of lymphocytes compared to the disease control group at both the time points but the number was slightly lower on the 7th day compared to the 4th day.

Coronil treatment showed a dose-dependent reversal of the cytological disease markers at both the time points tested for. The number of Granulocytes and macrophages were significantly lower than the disease control, in a dose-dependent manner (Figs. **4.8a** and **4.8b**). Macrophages were totally absent in the 58 µg/kg treatment group by the 7th day. Lymphocytes were significantly higher on the 4th day compared to the 7th day suggesting that 3-day treatment was enough to reverse most of the disease phenotype caused by the presence of the spike protein. Interestingly, the number of lymphocytes was higher in the group treated with 12 µg/kg compared to the group that was treated with 58 µg/kg (Fig. **4.8c**). This data suggests that the initial response to the presence of the spike protein is an increase in the number of pro-inflammatory cells and by the 4th day, the number of these cells is reduced accompanied by a significantly higher infiltration of lymphocytes in response to the treatment with either Dexamethasone or Coronil (Fig. **4.8d**).

In SARS-CoV-2 infection, granulocyte and monocyte abnormalities, lymphopenia and aberrant cytokine secretion have been observed (Yang, *et al.*, 2020). In the early stages of respiratory viral infections including corona virus, the airways are infiltrated by polymorpho-nuclear neutrophils (PMN) (Tsui *et al.*, 2003; Haick, *et al.*, 2014) and their presence has been correlated with severe disease pathology or clinical symptoms (Nagata, *et al.*, 2008). The presence of PMN activates the innate and adaptive immunity and through this exert antiviral activity (Tsui, *et al.*, 2003; Mantovani *et al.*, 2011). However, the involvement of PMNs in coronaviral infections is not completely known (Haick, *et al.*, 2014).

SARS-CoV-2 spike protein becomes heavily glycosylated after infection. This conceals the virus's immunogenic epitopes from the host humoral immune system and aids in the evasion of the host immune system (Walls, *et al.*, 2019). We could not find any lymphocytes and macrophages in DCTL after the fourth day time point, which could be due to the masking of glycoprotein by the zebrafish host system. Our results confirm past studies on SARS-CoV that indicated the presence of granulocytes during the early stage of infection. The observed decrease in SARS-CoV-2 spike protein caused granulocyte and macrophage infiltration following Coronil treatment shows that the numerous phyto-compounds discovered in Coronil play an anti-inflammatory role.

Lymphopenia is common in SARS-CoV-2 infection (Zhao *et al.*, 2020), and absolute lymphocyte count has also been recommended as a diagnostic for coronavirus infection severity. The presence of a low number of lymphocytes (immune dysfunction) during the early stages of infection may suggest a serious disease (Wagner, *et al.*, 2020; Zhao, *et al.*, 2020). Lymphocytes emerged only in the treatment groups in the current investigation, indicating that the adaptive immune system was activated in the presence of Coronil. The presence of lymphocytes may have played an important role in scavenging the spike protein.

4.5.2. Coronil Inhibits SARS-CoV-2 Spike Protein-Induced Renal Cell Necrosis

The SARS-CoV-2 infection causes renal dysfunction, severe acute tubular necrosis, and inflammatory cell infiltration in addition to pneumonia (Batlle *et al.*, 2020; Benedetti *et al.*, 2020). We searched for alterations in kidney structure and the presence of degenerative and necrotic cells to measure systemic injury. The normal control (Fig. **4.9a**) and the HZFCTL (Fig. **4.9b**) demonstrated normal morphological features at the 4th and 7th day time points (Fig. 4.9g and correspondingly). The kidney had a well-defined design with adequate internal tubule packing. In the disease control, a spike protein challenge resulted in the loss of a few tubular segments and vascular degeneration which is indicative of renal necrosis on the 4th day (Fig. **4.9c**) as well as the 7th day (Fig. **4.9i**).

Dexamethasone treatment restored normal renal architecture on the fourth day (Fig. **4.9d**). The 7th day kidney, however, revealed modest structural abnormalities (Fig. **4.9j**), indicating that Dexamethasone was unable to reverse the inflammatory damage caused by the SARS-CoV-2 spike protein for a longer period of time. Surprisingly, Coronil therapy restored the damage induced by the spike protein at both concentrations examined on the fourth day (Fig. **4.9e**; 12 g/kg and (Fig. **4.9f**; 58 g/kg). On the seventh day, morphological alterations in the kidneys dissected out of the Coronil treatment groups yielded similar results (Figures Fig. **4.9k** and **4.9l**, respectively). In this study, Coronil mediated recovery of SARS-CoV-2 spike protein injected in zebrafish kidneys suggests the role of Coronil in protecting against systemic damage.

To further analyze the renal damage caused by the spike protein and recovery mediated by Coronil, cytological smears were stained by Hematoxylin-Eosin. The cytological smears from the NCTL at the 4th day (Fig. **4.10a**) and 7th day (Fig. **4.10g**), and HZFCTL at both 4th (Fig. **4.10b**) and 7th day (Fig. **4.10h**) time points exhibited well arborized tubular network of mesonephros with evenly scattered glomerulocytes without any observable signs of necrosis and degeneration. Spike protein challenge in disease control induced disorganized cellular arrangement and erythrocyte aggregation in a time-dependent manner (**Fig. 4.10c** on 4th day and **4.10i** on 7th day).

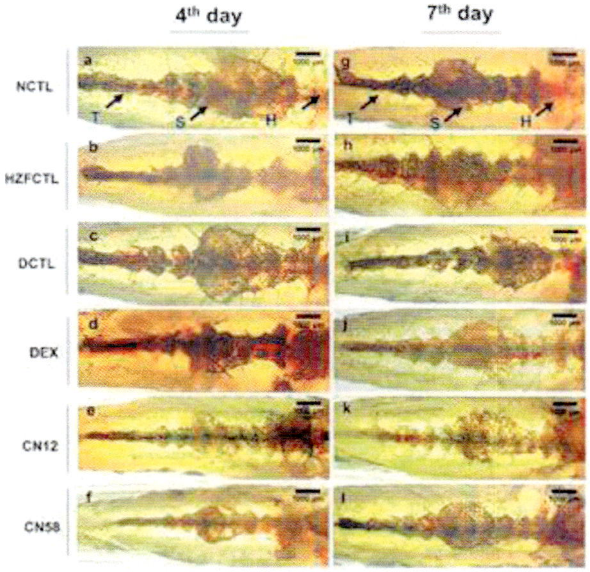

Fig. (4.9). Gross anatomy of the kidney to test the effect of SARS-CoV-2 spike protein and Coronil on renal architecture. **(a)** Normal control at 4th day, **(b)** HZFCTL at 4thday, **(g)** NCTL at 7thday, **(h)** HZFCTL at 7thday. **(c)** Disease control with loss of tubular segmentation and vascular degeneration at 4th day. **(i)** DCTL at the 7th day **(d, j)** Dexamethasone treatment at the 4th and 7th day respectively. **(e, f)** 4th day time point with 12 µg/kg and 58 µg/kg Coronil. **(k)** CN12 on the 7th day and **(l)** CN58 on the 7th day. H—Head; S—Saddle; T—Tail of kidney. Scale bars, 1000 µm at 1X magnification. *[Courtesy:* (Balkrishna, Solleti, Verma, *et al.*, 2020b)*; Under CCBY License].*

Dexamethasone treatment significantly reduced the disorganized architecture that was seen with the disease control group while also reducing the number of degenerative and necrotic cells in the cytology smears on the 4th day (Fig. **4.10d**) and on the 7th day (Fig. **4.10j**). More importantly, treatment with Coronil rescued spike protein-induced renal cell degradation as seen by recovery of the disorganized internal structures in the kidney. There was a gradual improvement in the kidney structure as seen by cytology on 4th day (Fig. **4.10e**, Coronil 12 µg/kg and 4.10f, 58 µg/kg) and on the 7th day (Fig. **4.10k**, Coronil 12 µg/kg and 4.10l, 58 µg/kg).

Quantitative estimation of the degenerative and necrotic cells present in the kidney was done on the cytology smears. An average number was arrived at by counting the number of degraded cells in 3 fields from each fish. The normal control and the HZF groups did not have any detectable degenerative or necrotic cells as expected. In contrast, the disease control group had a significantly higher ($p < 0.001$) number of both degenerative cells (Fig. **4.11a**) and necrotic cells (Fig. **4.11b**) on the 4th day. The percentage of both these cell types was even higher by the 7th day indicating unchecked tissue damage due to the presence of the spike protein. Treatment with Dexamethasone significantly reduced the percentage of both the degenerative and necrotic cells when compared to the disease control. The numbers of cells were higher on the 7th day compared to the 4th day, but this number was still lower than that of the disease control. This suggested that Dexamethasone was not able to completely reverse the necrotic damage seen in the kidney. Longer treatment with Coronil was able to reduce the number of degenerative cells in a dose-dependent fashion but was unable to completely reverse the necrotic cell damage at both the doses studied.

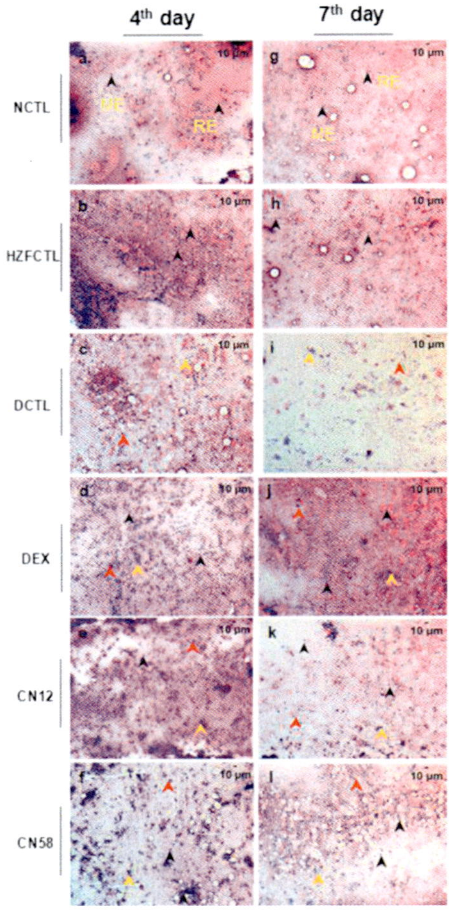

Fig. (4.10). Coronil rescues renal cell damage due to SARS-CoV-2 spike protein as seen in Hematoxylin-Eosin-stained cytology smears. 4th day representative images **(a)** Normal control, **(b)** HZFCNTL, **(c)** Disease control, **(d)** Dexamethasone, **(e)** 12 µg/kg Coronil and **(f)** 58 µg/kg Coronil. 7th day representative images **(g)** Normal control, **(h)** HZFCNTL, **(i)** Disease control, **(j)** Dexamethasone, **(k)** 12 µg/kg Coronil and **(l)** 58 µg/kg Coronil. Black arrow—normal cell, Red arrow—necrotic cell and Yellow arrow—degenerating cell. RE represents Renal Epithelium and ME Mesonephros. Scale bars, 10 µm at 200 X magnification. *[Courtesy:* (Balkrishna, Solleti, Verma, *et al.*, 2020b)*; Under CCBY License].*

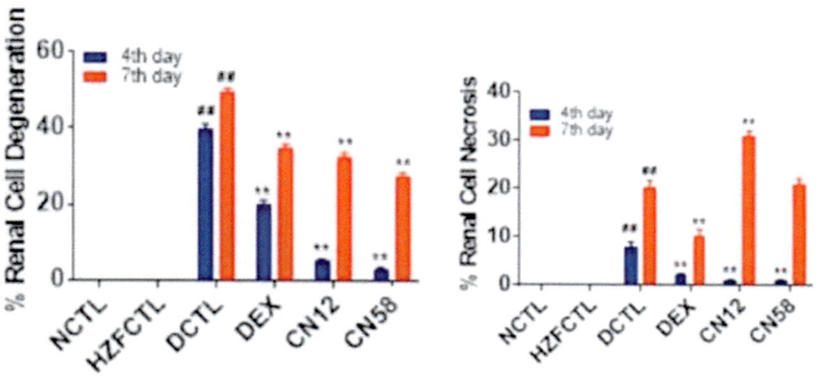

Fig. (4.11). Coronil rescues from SARS-CoV-2 spike protein-induced renal cell damage. Cytosmears of whole kidney necropsies were made and stained with H&E. The average degenerative and necrotic nuclei per 3 fields were quantified to study renal pathological features at both the 4th and 7th day time points. **(a)** quantitative estimation of percentage degenerative cells presents in the cytology smears. **(b)** percentage of necrotic cells estimated in the renal cytology smears. n = 24 for each test group. ## represents statistical significance compared to HZFCTL and ** represents significance compared to DCTL ($p < 0.001$). *[Courtesy:* (Balkrishna, Solleti, Verma, *et al.*, 2020b)*; Under CCBY License].*

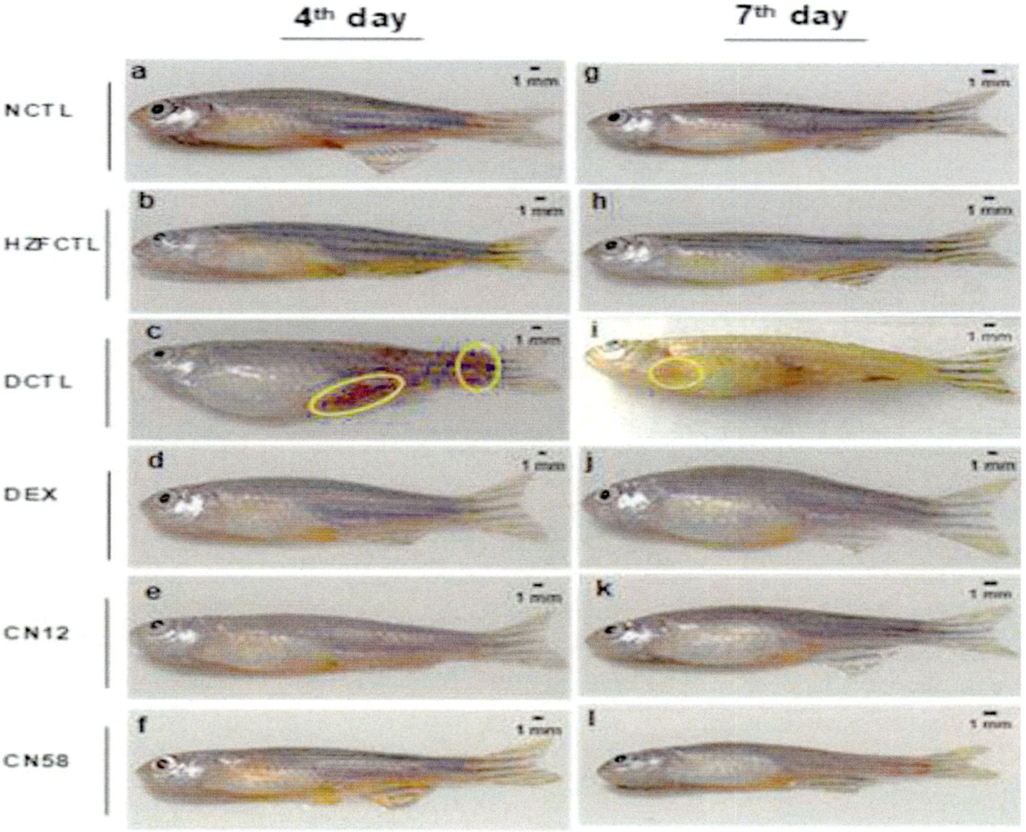

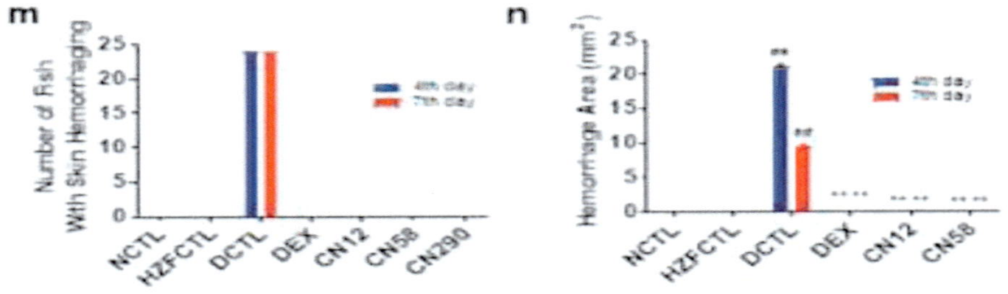

Fig. (4.12). Representative images of fish from different control and treatment groups showing the reversal of skin haemorrhage with Coronil treatment. The fish were euthanized at the end of the study and whole animal imaging was used to detect the presence of hemorrhagic spots on the skin. Images a to f show 4th day time point while g to l show 7th day **(a, g)** Normal control, **(b, h)** HZF, **(c, i)** disease control, **(d, j)** Dexamethasone treatment groups, **(e, k)** 12 μg/kg Coronil, and **(f, l)** 58 μg/kg Coronil treatment groups. *[Courtesy:* (Balkrishna, Solleti, Verma, *et al.*, 2020b)*; Under CCBY License].*

4.5.3. Coronil Attenuates SARS-CoV-2 Spike Protein-Induced Hemorrhage

SARS-CoV-2 is also known to cause vascular leakage due to the disruption of endothelial cell junctions and this can be seen as hemorrhagic spots on the skin of zebrafish. The normal (Fig. **12a**, 4th day; 4.12g, 7th day) and HZF (Fig. **12b**, 4th day; 4.12h, 7thday) control groups did not show any hemorrhagic spots on the skin and all the fish in the groups were free of skin haemorrhage. In contrast, all the disease control fish showed signs of skin haemorrhage near one or more fins, pelvic, anal, dorsal and caudal fin regions (Fig. **12c**, 4th day, 4.12i, 7th day). The representative figure for the 4th day time point shows hemorrhagic spots near the pelvic and caudal fins while it was detected near the gills on the 7th day. Fish that were treated for dexamethasone for 3 days (Fig. **4.12d**, 4th day time point) and for 6 days (Fig. **12j**, 7th day time point), did not show the presence of a skin haemorrhage in any of the fish. The group treated with 12 μg/kg Coronil (Fig. **12e**., 4th day; 4.12k, 7th day) and with 58 μg/kg Coronil (Fig. **4.12f** 4th day; 4.12l 7th day) showed statistically significant recovery from the spike protein-induced skin haemorrhage. None of the fish in these groups had hemorrhagic spots on the skin similar to the control and HZF groups.

The area of the skin haemorrhage was measured in each fish using the Image J software. Each fish was photographed at high resolution and the area of haemorrhage was demarcated using the free selection tool in the software. Only the fish that were in the disease control fish showed the presence of skin haemorrhage and was absent in all the other groups. The results were presented as a graph in Fig. (**4.13a**). The area was measured using the area measurement tool for each fish in mm^2. The disease control fish showed a significantly higher area of skin haemorrhage compared to the normal and HZF groups at the 4th day time point (Fig. **4.13b**). The area of skin haemorrhage was lower in the 7th day disease control group compared to the 4th day but was still significantly higher than the normal and HZF control groups as well as the Dexamethasone and Coronil treatment groups.

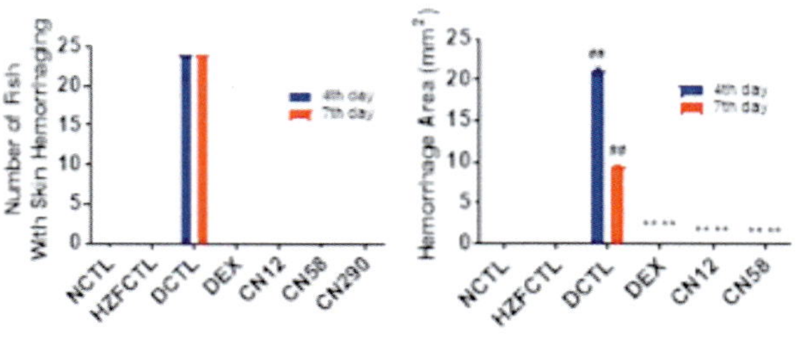

Fig. (4.13). Skin haemorrhage seen in the fish as a result of induction with the spike protein of SARS-CoV-2 virus. Number of fish that showed the presence of skin haemorrhage, **(b)** quantitative estimation of the average area of skin haemorrhage seen on individual fish. Data represented as mean ± S.D. of n=24, ## represents statistical significance compared to HZFCTL and ** represents significance compared to DCTL ($p < 0.001$). *[Courtesy:* (Balkrishna, Solleti, Verma, *et al.*, 2020b)*; Under CCBY License].*

4.5.4. Coronil Dampens the Gene Expression Levels of Pro-inflammatory Cytokines

Semi-quantitative gene expression in tissue samples was used to measure the amounts of the cytokines IL-6, IL-10, and TNF-. Total RNA was extracted from all zebrafish groups, and cDNA was produced using the reverse transcription. At 4 and 7 days, the disease control fish had a significant rise (p 0.0001) in the expression levels of all three cytokine genes. At 4 days, there was a somewhat significant (p 0.05) reduction in IL-6 expression levels with 12 g/kg Coronil, and this reduction was very significant with 58 g/kg Coronil (Fig. **4.14a**). There was a decrease in IL-10 gene expression levels, although it was not statistically significant. On the fourth day, an identical pattern was found with TNF-α.

When the gene expression levels were estimated on the seventh day, there was a significantly substantial reduction in IL-6 levels with both concentrations of Coronil (Fig. **4.14b**). Both IL-10 and TNF- levels were lowered at both Coronil concentrations, however, only at 58 g/kg Coronil was it statistically significant. These findings point to a putative mode of action for Coronil in the rescue of SARS-CoV-2 pathology *via* a decrease in the gene expression levels of pro-inflammatory cytokines IL-6, IL-10, and TNF-α. This reduction in the pro-inflammatory milieu can result in a number of downstream alterations that can contribute to additional symptom relief.

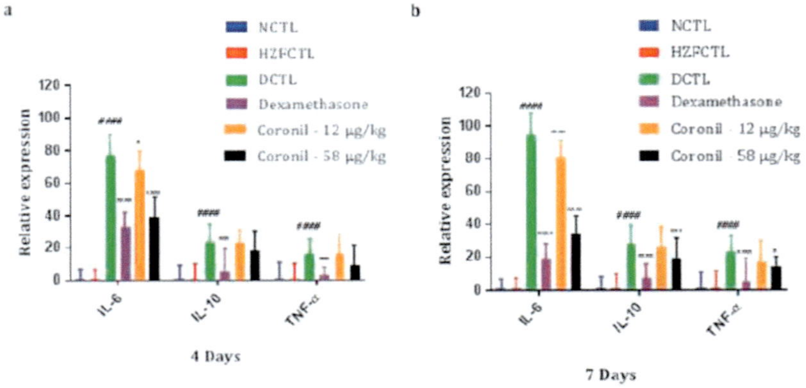

Fig. (4.14). Gene expression levels of pro-inflammatory cytokines IL-6, IL-10, and TNF-α as estimated by semiquantitative RT-PCR. Data points are represented as mean ± SD of n = 24. Data were analyzed by two-way ANOVA followed by Tukey's multiple comparisons test. #### p <0.0001 compared to normal control. **** p <0.0001 compared to DCTL, *** p <0.001 compared to DCTL and * p <0.05 compared to disease control. *[Courtesy:* (Balkrishna, Solleti, Verma, *et al.*, 2020b)*; Under CCBY License].*

A subset of patients with severe SARS-CoV-2 infection develops "cytokine storm syndrome," which is characterized by hyper-cytokinemia and multi-organ failure (Coperchini, *et al.*, 2020). SARS-CoV-2 infection of the respiratory tract results in the release of pro-inflammatory cytokines such as IL-1, IL-6, and TNF- (Conti, *et al.*, 2020; Coperchini *et al.*, 2020; Huang *et al.*, 2020). The ACE2 receptor is highly expressed in alveolar epithelial type II cells (pulmonary pneumocytes), indicating that these cells play an important role.

The roles of nuclear factor-kappa B (NF-κB) and activator protein-1 (AP-1) in lung inflammation and cytokine release are well established (Moon, 2020). Coronil's inhibitory action on the NF-B/AP-1 pathway suggests that it may play a role in limiting the infection's powerful cytokine output. The activation of NF-B is mediated by ROS and PPAR, and PPAR is well recognized. NF-κB activation is mediated by ROS and PPARα, and PPARα is known to regulate immunity to the presence of DNA in the cytoplasm (Tao, *et al.*, 2019). Several different naturally available ingredients have been shown to ameliorate the NF-κB activation seen in a host of metabolic disorders through the PPARα pathway (Hernandez-Baltazar, Zavala-Flores and Villanueva-Olivo, 2017; Illesca, *et al.*, 2019). SARS-CoV-2 is a cytopathic virus that infects airway epithelial cells and induces pyroptosis and vascular leakage (Tay, *et al.*, 2020). Toll-like receptor (TLR) identification of SARS-CoV-2 results in the generation of IL-1, which mediates lung inflammation, fever, and fibrosis (Conti, *et al.*, 2020). IL-6 is produced by a variety of cells and is crucial in regulating acute-phase inflammatory responses (Brocker *et al.*, 2010), and it is stimulated by both IL-1 and TNF-α (Hunter and Jones, 2015). IL-1β also induces the expression of TNF-α, which is an important cytokine for systemic inflammation and acute-phase reaction. TNF-α and IL-6 both stimulate immune cells to cause inflammation (Lee, *et al.*, 2018). TNF-α is a critical cytokine in viral infections as well as several chronic inflammatory and autoimmune illnesses. TNF-α has been found to facilitate SARS-CoV-2 interaction with ACE2 and subsequent virus entry into host cells in the context of SARS-CoV-2 infection (Haga, *et al.*, 2008). Both TNF-α and IL-6 signal the immune cells to induce inflammation (Lee, *et al.*, 2018).

4.5.5. Coronil Reduces SARS-CoV-2 Spike Protein-induced Behavioural Fever

Both the normal control and HZF groups showed no evidence of behavioural fever because they spent more time at 29 °C on the fourth and seventh days and less time at 37 °C (Table **4.2**). Spike protein challenge in disease control caused behavioural fever, and the fish spent more time at 37 °C and less time at 29 °C on the fourth and seventh days. Interestingly, Coronil treatment considerably relieved behavioural fever on the seventh day in a dose-dependent manner, as evidenced by a slight increase in time spent at 29 °C compared to disease control (Fig. **4.15**). This demonstrates Coronil's protective effect on fever reduction, a hallmark of an immunomodulatory action.

Table 4.2. Time (in seconds) spent by experimental fish in various temperature chambers.

Study Groups	4th Day			7th Day		
	23 °C	29 °C	37 °C	23 °C	29 °C	37 °C
NCTL	35.58 ± 3.0	129.63 ± 1.4	14.92 ± 2.7	24.13 ± 0.7	130.00 ± 0.8	25.88 ± 0.7
HZFCTL	37.79± 1.5	134.00 ± 1.5	8.21 ± 2.0	25.88 ± 1.3	135.75 ± 1.5	18.38 ± 1.3
DCTL	15.96 ± 1.6	7.04 ± 1.3	157.08 ± 1.6	2.38 ± 1.1	4.75 ± 1.3	172.88 ± 1.3
DEX	21.13 ± 2.3	30.46 ± 2.3	128.29 ± 1.9	45.54 ± 1.6	57.54 ± 2.0	76.92 ± 2.1
CN12	0	19.08 ± 2.1	160.92 ± 2.1	0	5.04 ± 1.7	174.96 ± 1.7
CN58	0	19.92 ± 2.1	160.08 ± 2.1	17.54 ± 1.7	21.50 ± 1.8	140.96 ± 2.0

Data expressed as mean ± S.D. values (n = 24).

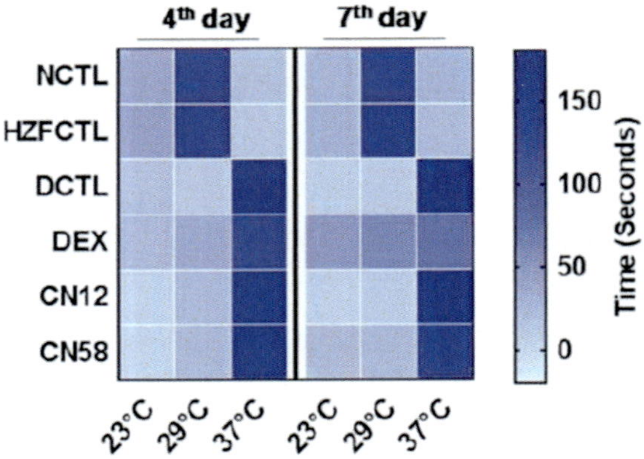

Fig. (4.15). Coronil reduces SARS-CoV-2 spike protein-induced behavioural fever. On the 4th and 7th day time points, zebrafish from various groups spent time (in seconds) at the assigned temperatures (low temperature 23°C, normal temperature 29°C, and behavioural fever 37°C). The colour intensity shows the amount of time spent in each temperature chamber. Coronil treatment reduced SARS-CoV-2 spike protein-induced behavioural fever in a dose-dependent manner upon Coronil treatment at the seventh day time point. *[Courtesy:* (Balkrishna, Solleti, Verma, *et al.*, 2020b)*; Under CCBY License].*

We effectively constructed a model for SARS-CoV-2 spike protein driven disease phenotype in zebrafish and verified the disease rescue characteristics of an Indian tri-herbal drug, Coronil, at human similar doses in this work. Various cellular and molecular endpoints were used to determine the anti-inflammatory capabilities. Coronil, when used as a supplemental therapy during SARS-CoV-2 infection, may improve disease pathology by functioning as an immunomodulator. The current preclinical study's findings warrant further clinical trials of Coronil in human subjects infected with SARS-CoV-2.

4.6. *IN VIVO* MODEL FOR DETERMINING THE EFFECTIVENESS OF DIVYA SWASARI VATI IN REDUCING SARS-COV-2 SPIKE PROTEIN-INDUCED DISEASE PHENOTYPE

We employed the herbal formulation Divya Swasari Vati (DSV) as a viable therapy option in a SARS-CoV-2 infection in this investigation. The formulation is a concoction of numerous herbs and bhasmas (ash obtained from cremated mineral components treated with herbal concoctions) and has been given in the ayurvedic medical system for chronic cough, common cold, asthma, phlegm accumulation in the chest and other lungs related problems. Since ancient times, the many diverse components of Divya Swasari Vati pharmaceutical formulation have been utilized as home treatments for the common cold, asthma, and persistent cough in India.

We studied the impact of disease phenotype induction with a recombinant spike protein from SARS-CoV-2 on the overall morphology and cytology of the zebrafish air bladder using a humanized zebrafish (Wild-type *Danio rerio*) model. The kidney was examined for systemic effects of SARS-CoV-2 spike protein induction as necrotic damage. Changes to the pro-inflammatory cytokine gene expression were determined semi-quantitatively in the zebrafish and were replicated *in vitro* using A549 cells.

As determined by HPLC, Divya Swasari Vati contains a mixture of different phyto- compounds such as Gallic acid, Ellagic acid, Cinnamic acid, Eugenol, 6-Gingerol, Piperine, and Glycyrrhizin. Glycyrrhizin has previously been demonstrated to be the most effective at preventing the reproduction of SARS-associated virus while causing the fewest adverse side effects (Cinatl, *et al.*, 2003; Chen, *et al.*, 2020). *Pistacia. integerrima* essential oils have been shown to have an anti-asthmatic effect due to their ability to reduce TNF- activity (Balkrishna, Verma, *et al.*, 2020). TNF-α levels in plasma were shown to be greater in severe cases of SARS-CoV-2 virus infection in patients (Qin, *et al.*, 2020). The ariel sections of the *Cressa cretica* plant contain bioactive substances like Coumarin derivatives, which have anti-inflammatory and anti-oxidant properties (Sunita, Jha and Pattanayak, 2009). Extracts of the whole plant are known to have a bronchodilatory activity and the combination of airway dilation and anti-inflammatory qualities may play a critical role in reducing the severity of the symptoms associated with the SARS-CoV-2 infections, and a major cause of mortality, by improving lung function.

Clove (*Syzygium aromaticum*) and Cinnamon (*Cinnamomum zylancium*) are good sources of Eugenol which is a known anti-inflammatory agent and a free radical scavenger (Chericoni, *et al.*, 2005; Barboza, da Silva Maia Bezerra Filho, Silva, Jand Venes R. Medeiros, *et al.*, 2018). Cinnamon has been demonstrated to inhibit the activity of IL-1, IL-6, and TNF- in LPS-activated macrophages (Kim, Na and Lee, 2018). Another phyto-constituent found in Divya Swasari Vati pharmaceutical formulation, methyl gallate, was proven to inhibit neutrophil recruitment and macrophage activation in an experimental model of arthritis inflammation (Correa, *et al.*, 2016). In our study, the wide variety of anti-inflammatory phyto-constituents present in DSV was seen in a drastic reduction in the infiltration of pro-inflammatory cells into the swim bladder containing transplanted lung cells.

Ginger, *Zingiber officinale*, either dried or fresh, has been used for generations as a home medicine against common colds, asthma, and bronchitis, and it is often used to defend against most infections when combined with black pepper. SARS-CoV-2 infection is caused by a loss of vascular integrity, and black pepper reduced leukocyte migration in vivo in an LPS-induced rat model by enhancing endothelial barrier integrity (Lee, *et al.*, 2018).

Ayurveda is unique in its use of different 'Bhasma' (ash formed from various animal exoskeletons or minerals after treating with herbal concoctions). Bhasmas are an easily absorbable source of trace elements, and their benefits are improved by their inclusion in herbal decoctions and subsequent cremation. They keep the body alkaline by neutralizing toxic acids (Pal, Sahu and Haldar, 2014). Divya Swasari Vati is made up of seven different bhasmas, the majority of which have anti-inflammatory properties (Mishra, *et al.*, 2014; Sahoo *et al.*, 2019; Balkrishna, Verma, *et al.*, 2020). Several of the symptoms of SARS-CoV-2 infection revolve around inflammation and strong cytokine responses. The various herbal and mineral components of Divya Swasari Vati act as anti-inflammatory agents and may be useful in symptomatic alleviation.

4.6.1. SARS-CoV-2 Spike Protein-Induced Edema in the Swim Bladder which is Reversed by Administration of Divya Swasari Vati

The xeno-transplantation of A549 cells into the swim bladder had no negative effects on the organ's morphology and was structurally identical to that of a normal fish. The tunica externa, as well as the smooth muscle mesothelium lining, were discovered to be intact (Fig. **16**). On the 4th day, the swim bladder of the disease control fish was structurally swollen in the anterior lobe, indicating oedema. Dexamethasone (0.08 g/kg body weight) treatment resulted in modest inflation of the swim bladder with intact tunica externa in the fish. This points to a partial reversal of the illness phenotype rather than a complete reversal. Swim bladders from fish treated with Divya Swasari Vati for three days after a spike protein injection were strikingly identical to those of normal control fish at all three doses (6 g/kg body weight, 28 g/kg, and 142 g/kg body weight).

The presence of the spike protein for a longer period of time, as seen on the 7th day, had a more dramatic effect on the swim bladder isolated from the disease control group. Because of the presence of edematous gas, the anterior lobe of the bladder was discovered to be structurally collapsed. The Dexamethasone group also had a structural abnormality with a larger anterior lobe and a narrower posterior lobe, indicating that the medicine did not have an effect for a longer period of time. Among the DSV-treated fish, the group treated with 6 g/kg body weight showed structural collapse but a minor reduction in anterior lobe expansion, indicating that the dosage was insufficient. The 28 g/body weight group had an enlarged and deformed anterior lobe, indicating oedema. The high dosage group, with 142 g/kg body weight, recovered normal swim bladder properties in terms of size, shape, and colour, similar to the control group.

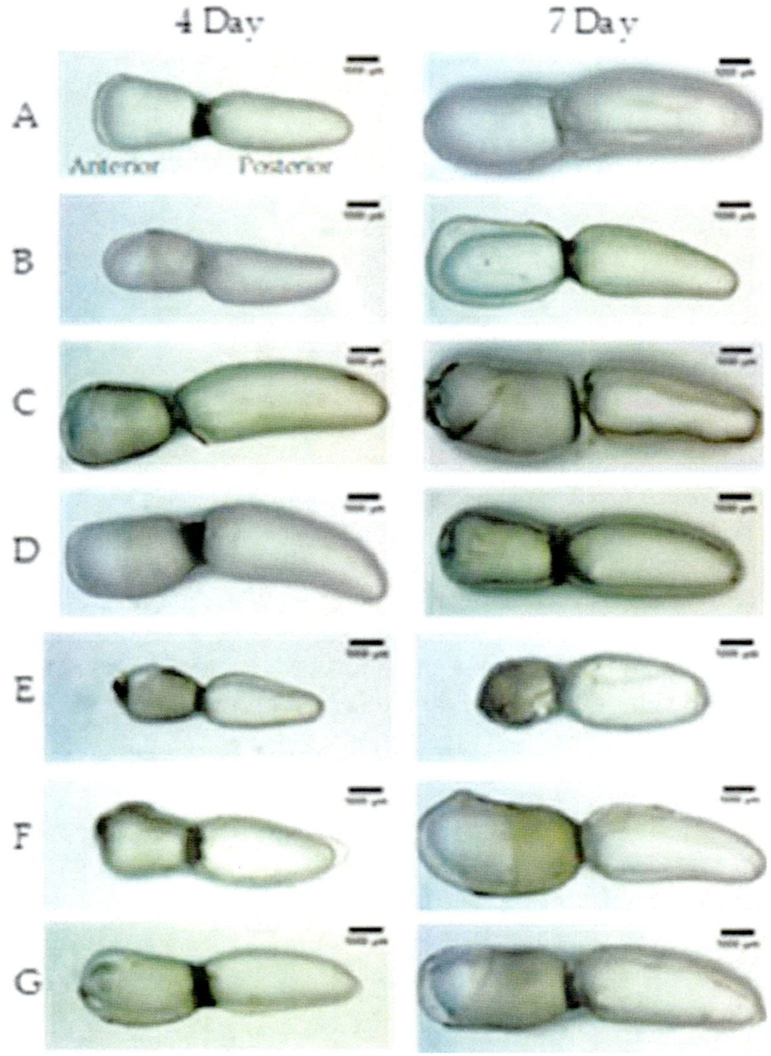

Fig. (4.16). Divya Swasari Vati reduced swim bladder oedema. Lateral view of swim bladder with the dorsal region on top and the cranial facing region to the left. The anterior and posterior lobes are labelled. Images were taken at 10X magnification. **(A).** Normal Control **(B).** Humanized Zebrafish with xeno-transplanted A549 cells (HZF) **(C).** Diseased fish with SARS-CoV-2 spike protein (Disease control) **(D).** Dexamethasone (0.08 μg/kg) treatment **(E).** Divya Swasari Vati treatment (6 μg/kg) **(F).** Divya Swasari Vati treatment (28 μg/kg) **(G).** Divya Swasari Vati treatment (142 μg/kg). *[Courtesy:* (Balkrishna, Solleti, Verma, *et al.*, 2020b)*; Under CCBY License].*

4.6.2. Restoration of Cytological Profile and Reversal of Pro-inflammatory Cell Infiltration in Swim Bladder after Treatment with Divya Swasari Vati

The swim bladder is made of several different layers consisting of columnar epithelium (identified by oval nuclei), squamous epithelium (spherical nuclei), smooth muscle (elongated nuclei), and collagen that shows up as eosinophilic staining in Hematoxylin-Eosin stained cytology slides. Both the normal control and the HZF groups exhibited the typical staining seen in healthy fish (Fig. **4.17**). Cellular debris and oedema were found in the cytology slides of disease control fish, most likely as a result of the pro-inflammatory response induced by spike protein production. This was determined by the presence of basophilic debris in the smears, as well as the presence of granulocytes and macrophages, both of which were absent in the normal control and HZF groups.

Treatment with Dexamethasone showed a slight reduction in the pro-inflammatory environment as seen by less amount of cellular debris, and importantly the infiltration of lymphocytes. Granulocytes were also detected suggesting that there was an incomplete rescue from the disease phenotype. Fish treated with Divya Swasari Vati at 6 g/kg and 28 g/kg body weight revealed considerable granulocyte infiltration and an increased lymphocyte count, with normal epithelial and myocyte cell cytology. Treatment with 142 g/kg demonstrated a considerable recovery of disease morphology with a reduction in pro-inflammatory granulocytes. The cytology from the 4-day time point group shows a significantly greater higher ($p < 0.0001$, compared to the DCTL) lymphocyte count and less cellular debris (Table **4.3**).

Table 4.3. Quantification of the immune cell infiltration in the air bladder cytology.

-	4th Day			7th Day		
-	Granulocyte	Macrophage	Lymphocyte	Granulocyte	Macrophage	Lymphocyte
NCTL	0	11 ± 5.2	7 ± 3.5	0	0	0
HZFCTL	0	5* ± 2.9	0*	20* ± 5.0	0	0
DCTL	11 ± 5.2	7.1* ± 4.6	0*	31$^{*\pm}$ 6.6	0	0
Dexamethasone	5* ± 2.9	5.3* ± 3.1	0*	53.9* ± 5.7	9* ± 5.4	10* ± 6.2
DSV-6 µg/kg	7.1* ± 4.6	3.4* ± 3	0*	113.2* ± 5.5	0	23.7* ± 5.0
DSV-28 µg/kg	5.3* ± 3.1	0	0	0	0	19.2* ± 6.8
DSV-142 µg/kg	3.4* ± 3	0	0	0	0	16* ± 6.3

On a Hematoxylin and Eosin-stained air bladder from each fish, lymphocytes, macrophages, and granulocytes were counted. The results are given as mean S.D. Statistical analysis was performed using ANOVA and significance as denoted by (*) represents $p < 0.0001$ when compared with the disease control group.

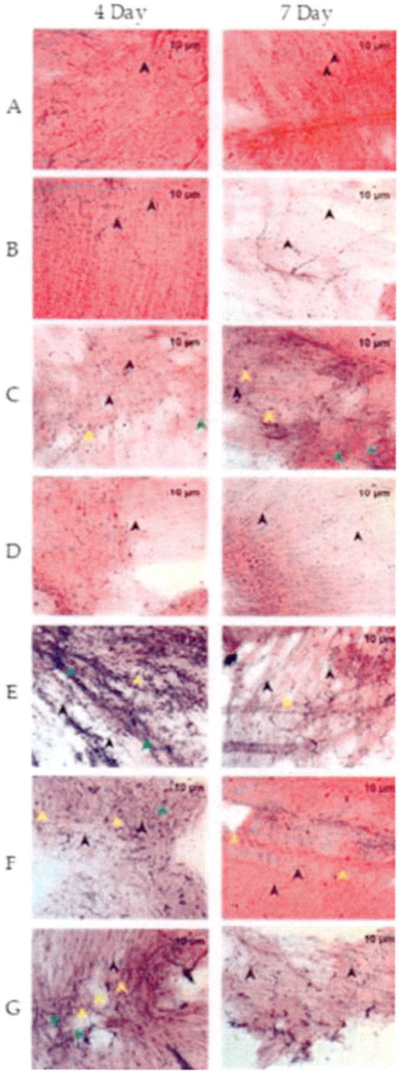

Fig. (4.17). At 20X objective magnification, cytological analysis of the entire swim bladder was performed after staining with Hematoxylin and Eosin. **(A)** Normal Control **(B)** Humanized Zebrafish with xeno-transplanted A549 cells (HZF) **(C)**. Disease control with SARS-CoV-2 spike protein **(D)**. Dexamethasone (0.08 µg/kg) treatment **(E)**. Divya Swasari Vati treatment (6 µg/kg) **(F)**. Divya Swasari Vati treatment (28 µg/kg) **(G)**. Divya Swasari Vati treatment (142 µg/kg). Black arrowheads depict the nuclei of normal cells, E- Epithelial cells, and S- Smooth muscle cells. Green arrowheads show granulocytes and brown arrowheads show macrophages. *[Courtesy:* (Balkrishna, Solleti, Verma, *et al.*, 2020b)*; Under CCBY License].*

In comparison to a 4-day induction with the SARS-CoV-2 spike protein, a 7-day induction exhibited no infiltration of granulocytes, macrophages, or lymphocytes beyond the typical distribution of epithelial and myocytes. However, the presence of basophilic nuclear debris and attenuated eosinophilic stain revealed the vestiges of a heightened inflammatory response. The Dexamethasone treated group did not show the presence of infiltrating granulocytes but had a significantly higher ($p<0.0001$) number of macrophages and lymphocytes (Table **4.3**). Cytological staining also identified prominent cellular debris. At 7 days, the Divya Swasari Vati-treated group revealed a gradual dose-dependent rescue of disease indicators detected by cytology, as well as a significantly increased infiltration of lymphocytes but no evidence of macrophages or granulocytes. In contrast to a 4-day induction with the SARS-CoV-2 spike protein, a 7-day induction showed no infiltration of granulocytes, macrophages, or lymphocytes beyond the normal distribution of epithelial and myocytes. The presence of basophilic nuclear debris and attenuated eosinophilic stain, on the other hand, suggested the remnants of a heightened inflammatory response.

4.6.3. Divya Swasari Vati Treatment Reversed the SARS-CoV-2 Spike Protein-Induced Cytokine Gene Expression *In vivo*

Semi-quantitative RT-PCR was used to determine the levels of expression of the cytokines IL-6, IL-10, and TNF-α. Total RNA was extracted from all zebrafish groups, and cDNA was reverse transcribed. After 4 and 7 days of the study period, the illness control fish showed a significant ($p<0.0001$) rise in the expression levels of all three cytokine genes (Fig. **18**). Dexamethasone treatment for 3 and 6 days significantly reduced expression ($p<0.0001$). At the 4-day time point, a low dose of Divya Swasari Vati at 6 g/kg showed no significant reduction in IL-6 levels. All of the other treatments resulted in a highly significant ($p<0.0001$) decrease in IL-6 gene expression levels. Only the high dose of Divya Swasari Vati (142 g/ kg) significantly reduced IL-10 levels on the 4-day and 7-day time points. TNF- was down-regulated at substantial levels ($p<0.0001$) only with 142 g/kg on 7th day, however, this reduction was only marginally significant ($p<0.01$) at 4-day.

We can conclude that Divya Swasari Vati plays an important role in the reduction of the 'Cytokine Storm' and promotes a healing immune response to the presence of the SARS-CoV-2 spike protein based on the cytological identification of inflammation and the reduction in the gene expression levels of the pro-inflammatory cytokines when treated with DSV.

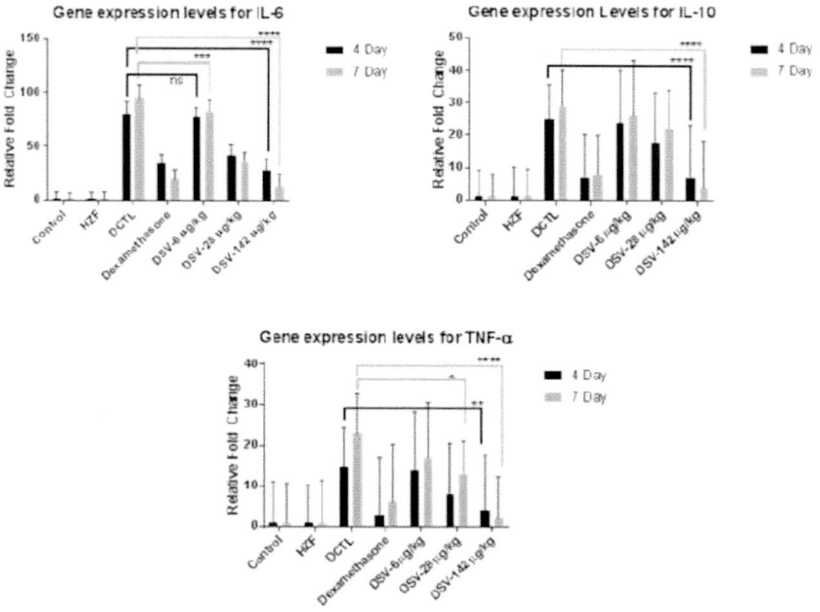

Fig. (4.18). Gene expression levels of IL-6, IL-10, and TNF-α *in vivo*. **(A)** IL-10 showed a highly significant reduction with 142 µg/kg of DSV treatment and with Dexamethasone, while the other concentrations were not significant at p<0.001. **(B).** The reduction in IL-10 was highly significant with DSV therapy at 142 g/kg and with Dexamethasone, but not at the other dosages. **(C).** Dexamethasone showed a significant (p <0.005) reduction of TNF-α levels at 4 days and p<0.0001 at 7 days. Divya Swasari Vati showed similar effects as the Dexamethasone group with 142 µg/kg dosage and only a slight reduction (p<0.05) with 28 µg/kg dosage after 7 days, rest of the treatments were not significant. (*) denotes p<0.05, (**) denotes p <0.05, (***) denotes p <0.001, (****) denotes p<0.0001. *[Courtesy:* (Balkrishna, Solleti, Verma, *et al.*, 2020b)*; Under CCBY License].*

4.6.4. SARS-CoV-2 Spike Protein-Induced Tubular Degeneration and Necrosis of the Kidney was Rescued Divya Swasari Vati Treatment

Multiorgan failure due to systemic shock is known to occur in about 11% of patients with untreated SARS-CoV-2 infection (Chen, *et al.*, 2020). We discovered renal tissue damage as a result of SARS-CoV-2 spike protein-induced organ failure in our investigation.

The kidney in zebrafish is made up of three physically separate regions: the head, the saddle (trunk), and the tail, which extends from the anterior to the posterior of the body. It is connected to the parenchymal liver and is positioned in the dorsal wall of the body cavity. Morphologically, control fish kidneys had well-defined and packed mesonephric nephrons in the head kidney. The glomerular tufts can be seen, and they are followed by the proximal and distal tubules. The melanocyte pigmentation was visible in the mesonephros and the pigmentation was distributed evenly suggesting normal anatomy (Fig. **4.19**). Post transplantation of the A549 cells, the HZF group of fish did not show any discernable changes in the kidney. Induction of the illness phenotype with the SARS-CoV-2 spike protein, on the other hand, revealed the existence of necrosis at 4-day analysis, as evidenced by tubule segment loss and vascular degeneration.

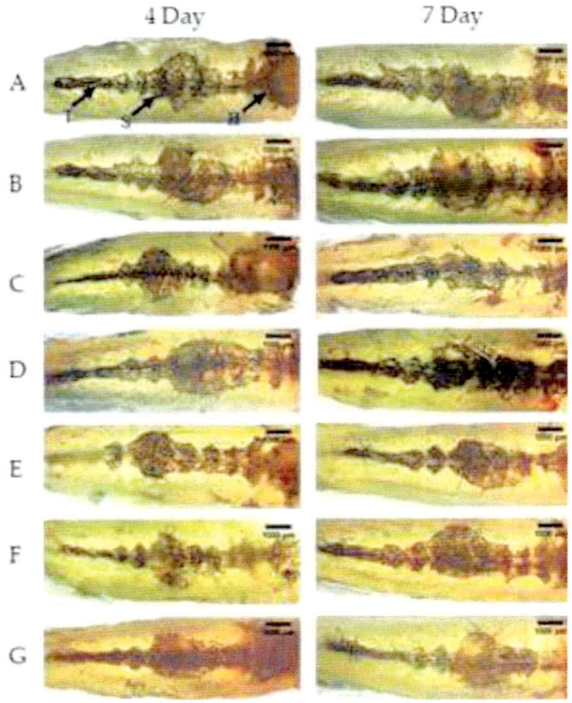

Fig. (4.19). Divya Swasari Vati rescued tissue damage in the kidney. At 10X magnification, a structural study of the kidney is performed. Head (H), Trunk or Saddle (S), and Tail (T) are the three parts of the kidney that span from the anterior to the posterior of the body. **(A).** Normal Control **(B).** Humanized Zebrafish with xeno-transplanted A549 cells (HZFCTL) **(C).** Diseased fish with SARS-CoV-2 spike protein (DCTL) **(D).** Dexamethasone (0.08 µg/kg) treatment **(E).** Divya Swasari Vati treatment (6 µg/kg) **(F).** Divya Swasari Vati treatment (28 µg/kg) **(G).** Divya Swasari Vati treatment (142 µg/kg). *[Courtesy:* (Balkrishna, Solleti, Verma, *et al.*, 2020b)*; Under CCBY License].*

Dexamethasone treatment resulted in a gradual restoration to normal morphology, with an arborized kidney network displaying a packed head region with glomerular tufts and tubular segments indicating typical renal architecture. This was not as noticeable as with DSV administration when all three drug concentrations demonstrated a packed network of mesonephros with strongly pigmented melanocytes that could be seen scattered throughout the kidney, indicating typical renal morphology.

The disease control at the 7-day time point showed structural anomalies with the loss of tubular segments and vascular degeneration indicating renal necrosis, and this was more widely distributed throughout the kidney compared to the 4-day. Dexamethasone treatment did not completely reverse the illness phenotype, as seen by disorderly melanocyte pigmentation, which suggested the presence of irregular glomerular tufts. DSV treatment completely reversed the anatomical abnormalities and restored normal renal shape. The anatomical study revealed a dense network of the mesonephros and strongly pigmented melanocytes throughout the tissue. This rescue event was observed with all three Divya Swasari Vati dosages.

4.6.5. Cytological Examination of the Kidney for Necrosis Induced by SARS-CoV-2 Spike Protein

The tubular configuration of renal epithelial cells in the kidney whole mount stained with hematoxylin and eosin distinguishes them. The normal control and HZF groups both had a well-organized and wide tubular network of the mesonephros with equally distributed erythrocytes and glomerulocytes, indicating typical renal pathology (Fig. **4.20**). Cytological analysis of kidney smears from the disease control group revealed disordered glomerular tufts as well as degenerative and necrotic cells that were considerably greater ($p < 0.0001$) than in the normal control group (Table **4.4**). The degenerative cells were identified by the presence of basophilic cytoplasm with very lightly stained nucleus. There was a higher aggregation of erythrocytes also indicating necrosis.

Table 4.4. Cytological profile of the renal tissue to determine necrotic and degenerative cells.

Study Groups	4th Day		7th Day	
	% Necrosis	% Degenerate cells	% Necrosis	% Degenerate cells
Normal control	0	0	0	0
HZF	0	0	0	0
Disease control	8.04 ± 4.7	40 ± 5.9	20.33 ± 6.5	49.54 ± 5.3
Dexamethasone	2.17** ± 1.7	19.92** ± 6.0	10.25** ± 6.5	34.71** ± 5.8
DSV-6 μg/kg	1.75** ± 1.2	19.63** ± 5.2	20.04* ± 5.4	44.75** ± 6.6
DSV-28 μg/kg	1.96** ± 1.2	12.33** ± 5.5	13.04** ± 6.9	19.29** ± 5.8

(Table 4.4) cont.....

Study Groups	4th Day		7th Day	
	% Necrosis	% Degenerate cells	% Necrosis	% Degenerate cells
DSV-142 µg/kg	1.46** ± 1.0	6.96** ± 4.7	3.08** ± 2.3	6.96** ± 3.5

Renal epithelial cells in a Hematoxylin and Eosin-stained slide from each fish were identified by their tubular form, and the percentage of degenerative and necrotic cells was computed. The data are represented as mean S.D., and ANOVA was used for statistical analysis. Significant differences, when compared with the HFZ-CoV-2-S group, were denoted by (**) when p <0.0001 and by (*) when p <0.05.

After four days of treatment with dexamethasone (0.08 g/kg), the distribution of erythrocytes (recognized by their defined nucleus), epithelial podocytes, and endocrine cells was normal. The percentage of degenerative cells and total necrosis were reduced significantly (p <0.0001). The DSV treated group showed dose-dependent rescue of cytological features. Treatment with 6 µg/kg and 28 µg/kg body weight showed mildly stained basophilic renal epithelial cells with a significantly (p <0.0001) lower percentage of necrotic and degenerative cells. The group treated with 142 µg DSV at 4-day showed the best cytological profile with well-defined erythrocytes and tubular epithelial cells distributed throughout, with very low cellular necrosis and degeneration.

The presence of the SARS-CoV-2 spike protein for a longer period of time enhanced kidney damage, as seen by disrupted internal architecture at the 7-day disease control time point (Fig. **4.20**). In the cytology smears, there was erythrocyte aggregation and a larger percentage of mainly basophilic degenerative and necrotic renal epithelial cells with faintly stained nuclei. Dexamethasone treatment resulted in weakly basophilic epithelial cells and erythrocytes with faintly stained nuclei, indicating a loss of typical cytological characteristics. When compared to the disease control group, there was a significant (p<0.0001) drop in the percentage of degenerative and necrotic cells (Table **4.4**). The DSV-treated group demonstrated dose-dependent cytological damage rescue. The 6 g/kg treatment group had a loss of renal epithelial cell architecture, with necrotic and degenerative cells that were widely dispersed. When compared to the disease control, the low dose resulted in a non-significant decrease in the percentage of nephrotic cells and a marginally significant (p<0.05) decrease in degenerative cells. The 28 g/kg treatment resulted in moderately distributed degenerative cells with an aggregated erythrocyte network. The fraction of necrotic and degenerative cells was reduced significantly (p <0.0001). The group was given 142 g/kg body weight DSV had the most robust phenotype, with normal kidney epithelial cytology similar to that of the normal control fish and considerably lesser degeneration.

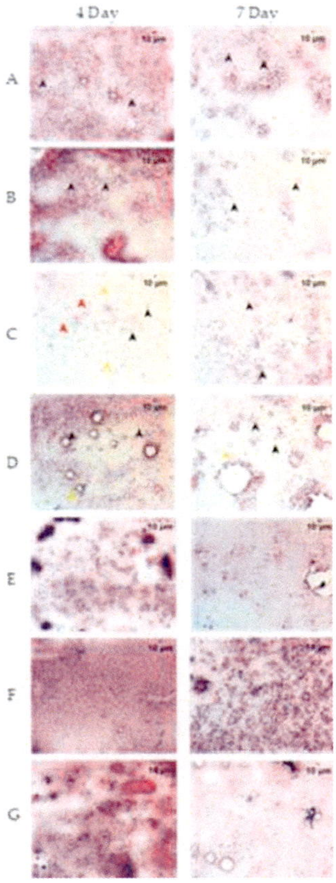

Fig. (4.20). At 200X magnification, a cytological examination of the kidney following staining with Hematoxylin and Eosin is performed. **(A).** Normal Control **(B).** Humanized zebrafish with xeno-transplanted A549 cells (HZFCTL) **(C).** Diseased fish with SARS-CoV-2 spike protein (DCTL) **(D).** Dexamethasone (0.08 μg/kg) treatment **(E).** Divya-Swasari- Vati treatment (6 μg/kg) **(F).** Divya Swasari Vati treatment (28 μg/kg) **(G).** Divya Swasari Vati treatment (142 μg/kg). Black arrowheads depict the nuclei of normal cells, yellow represent degenerative cells, while the red arrowheads depict necrotic cells. *[Courtesy:* (Balkrishna, Solleti, Verma, *et al.*, 2020b)*; Under CCBY License].*

4.6.6. Divya Swasari Vati Reversed the Skin Hemorrhage caused by the Induction with the Recombinant Spike Protein of SARS-CoV-2

Another symptom of SARS-CoV-2 infection is a loss of vascular integrity caused by infection of the endothelial cells that line the blood vessels (Varga, *et al.*, 2020). In zebrafish, this was observed as hemorrhagic patches on the skin in all fish injected with the recombinant spike protein. The presence or absence of hemorrhagic patches under the skin of zebrafish was assessed, as well as the total area of the hemorrhagic region was quantified. Only the disease control fishes in our study had skin haemorrhages, and all of the fish in that group had haemorrhage regions. There were hemorrhagic areas in the pelvic, anal, dorsal, and caudal fin areas. Neither the Dexamethasone nor the DSV therapy groups (at all three dosages) showed any skin bleeding, indicating that the clinical symptom had been completely resolved. indicating complete recovery from clinical indications of skin haemorrhage (Fig. **4.21**).

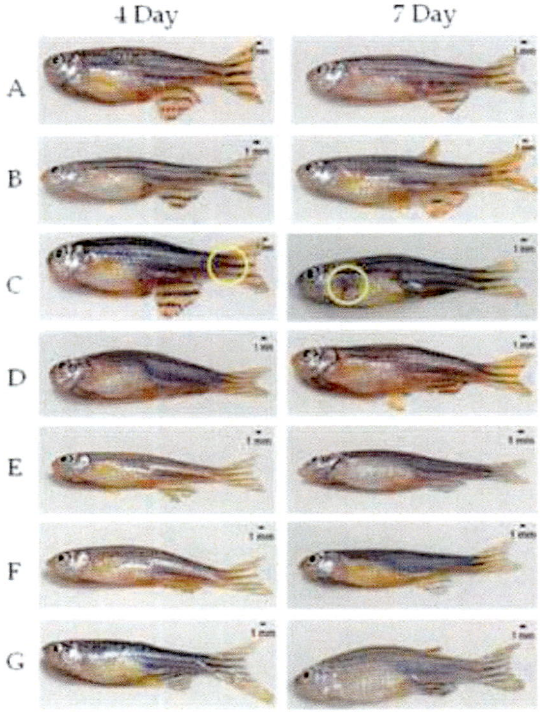

Fig. (4.21). The presence of hemorrhagic regions on the skin is detected using whole-animal imaging. **(A).** Normal Control **(B).** Humanized Zebrafish with xeno-transplanted A549 cells (HZF) **(C).** Diseased fish with SARS-CoV-2 spike protein **(D).** Dexamethasone (0.08 μg/kg) treatment **(E).** Divya Swasari Vati treatment (6 μg/kg) **(F).** Divya-Swasari- Vati treatment (28 μg/kg) **(G).** Divya Swasari Vati treatment (142 μg/kg). *[Courtesy:* (Balkrishna, Solleti, Verma, *et al.*, 2020b)*; Under CCBY License].*

The areas of bleeding in seven individual fish were measured, and the mean area was calculated. The average area of the 4-day disease control group was 21.23 0.6 mm^2, which was considerably ($p<0.0001$) greater than the HZF control and normal control groups, which did not show any symptoms of bleeding. The average area of cutaneous bleeding following a 7-day induction was 9 mm^2. The average area of skin haemorrhage after 7-day induction was slightly lower at 9.43 ± 0.6 mm^2 and was still significantly higher than the control groups.

4.6.7. Divya Swasari Vati Rescued Changes to the Behavioral Fever Phenotype Post Induction with Spike Protein of SARS-CoV-2

Behavioural fever is a synergic response to infection in zebrafish in which the fish travel to locations with the same temperature as their body. The normal control and HZF groups spent the majority of the observed time at 29 degrees Celsius, indicating healthy persons without behavioural fever. The disease control fish with the recombinant spike protein were observed to spend more time at 37 °C indicating changed behaviour due to the induction of disease phenotype. This was depicted as a heat map, with the higher the intensity of the colour indicating more time spent at a certain temperature (Fig. **4.22**). When compared to the infected group, 3 days of dexamethasone treatment dramatically reduced the duration spent by the fish 37 °C. (Table **4.5**). However, the behavioural fever was distinctly dissimilar to the normal control group suggesting that the symptom of induction was still persistent even on 4th day of treatment.

Table 4.5. Behavioral fever as a reflection of the body temperature.

Study Groups	4th Day			7th Day		
	23 °C	29 °C	37 °C	23 °C	29 °C	37 °C
NCTL	35.6 ± 3.0	129.6 ± 1.4	14.9 ± 2.7	24.1 ± 0.7	130.0 ±0.8	25.8 ± 0.7
HZFCTL	37.8 ± 1.5	134.0 ± 1.5	8.2 ± 2.0	25.8 ± 1.3	135.7 ± 1.5	18.3 ± 1.3
DCTL	15.9$^{\#}$ ± 1.6	7.0$^{\#}$ ± 1.3	157.1$^{\#}$ ± 1.6	2.4$^{\#}$ ± 1.1	4.7$^{\#}$ ± 1.3	172.8$^{\#}$ ± 1.3
Dexamethasone	21.1* ± 2.3	30.4* ± 2.3	128.3* ± 1.9	45.5* ± 1.6	57.5* ± 2.0	76.9* ± 2.1
DSV-6 µg/kg	0*	129.7* ± 2.0	50.3* ± 2.0	3.5* ± 1.5	151.5* ± 1.9	25.0* ± 2.0
DSV-28 µg/kg	0*	133.9* ± 1.8	45.8* ± 1.8	9.0* ± 2.1	132.2* ± 2.2	38.8* ± 1.8
DSV-142 µg/kg	0*	170.0* ± 1.7	9.9* ± 1.8	22.3* ± 1.7	125.8* ± 2.1	31.8* ± 2.1

The amount of time fish spend in each of the temperature chambers reflects their body temperature. A single fish was introduced to the 29°C chamber, and the time spent in each of the temperature chambers was measured. Results are shown as mean ± S.D for each group of fish. (#) denotes p <0.0001 when compared to the normal control while (*) denotes p <0.0001 when compared to the disease control.

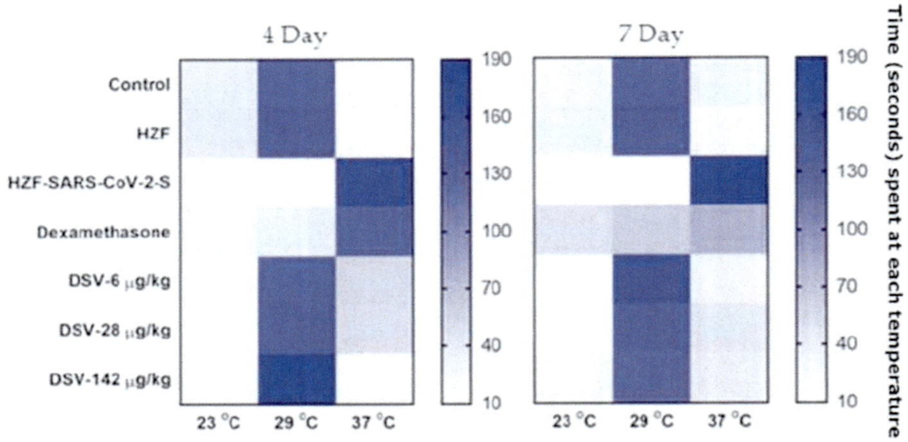

Fig. (4.22). In a SARS-CoV-2 induction model, Divya Swasari Vati alleviates behavioural fever. Behavioural fever heat maps. The intensity of the colour reflects how much time each fish spent in each temperature chamber; the darker the colour, the more time spent. Divya Swasari Vati ameliorates behavioural fever in the SARS-CoV-2 induction model. Data are presented as a mean of the observations, n = 24. *[Courtesy:* (Balkrishna, Solleti, Verma, *et al.*, 2020b)*; Under CCBY License].*

When treated with DSV, the fish showed a dose-dependent reduction in the time spent at 37°C and a corresponding increase in the time spent at 29°C. This is a very strong indication of the rescue of behavioural fever with DSV within 7 days.

After 7 days of dexamethasone therapy, the fish with the spike protein was seen to spend almost similar time in each of the three temperature chambers, indicating a reduction in behavioural fever. The fish treated with Divya Swasari Vati spent a majority of time in the 29°C chamber when compared to the 23°C or 37°C chamber showing a reversal of the behavioural fever seen in the infected fish. At 7 days, the duration spent in each of the three temperature chambers by the 142 g/kg treatment group was comparable to that of the normal control fish, indicating a complete reversal of the symptoms of induction with the recombinant spike protein. At 7 days, the duration spent in each of the three temperature chambers by the 142 g/kg treatment group was comparable to that of the normal control fish, indicating a complete reversal of the symptoms of induction with the recombinant spike protein.

4.6.8. Vati Enhanced Survival of Zebrafish after Induction of Disease Symptoms with the Recombinant Spike Protein of SARS-CoV-2

The survival of fish in each of the seven groups was plotted against the number of days after starting treatment with either dexamethasone or DSV. The survival analysis was completed, and the results were shown as a Kaplan-Meier Survival

Curve. The normal control and A549 xeno-transplanted fish both survived until day 10 after the disease phenotype was induced. During the same time period, just 80% of the disease control group survived. Fish treated with a single dose of dexamethasone and three separate doses of DSV exhibited 100% survival with no observed mortality, comparable to the normal control group (Fig. **4.23**).

The normal control and A549 xeno-transplanted fish both survived until day 10 after the disease phenotype was induced. During the same time period, just 80% of the disease control group survived. At low and medium doses (6 g/kg and 28 g/kg), the formulation demonstrated moderate baseline rescue, as well as complete recovery of preclinical endpoints, such as kidney degeneration and necrosis, improvement of behavioural fever, absence of skin bleeding, and survival rate at 142 g/kg dose. At the end of the study period, the phytochemical-rich formulation exhibited increasing recovery of immune cell infiltration with very few pro-inflammatory infiltrates, indicating that it is an efficient immunomodulator. The published preclinical study suggested that Divya Swasari Vati be tested in human subjects infected with SARS-CoV-2.

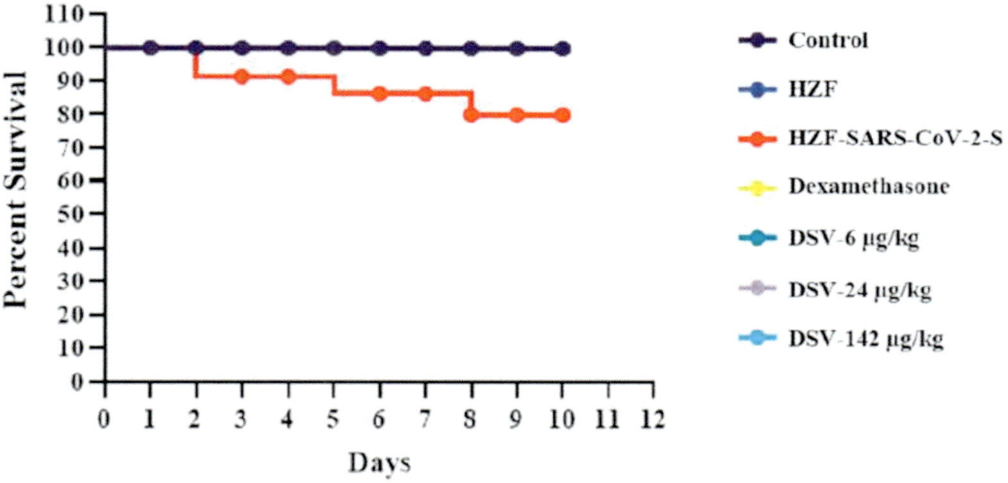

Fig. (4.23). Survival analysis of the different groups of zebrafish presented as a Kaplan-Meier survival curve. *[Courtesy:* (Balkrishna, Solleti, Verma, *et al.*, 2020b)*; Under CCBY License].*

CONCLUDING REMARKS

In conclusion, pre-clinical investigations support the efficacy of Coronil and Divya Swasari Vati in treating SARS-CoV-2 spike protein-induced diseases in zebrafish. The suitability of the model organism utilised was also validated. These studies serve as models for confirming the *in vivo* efficacy of various herbal medications.

CHAPTER 5

Importance of Studying Adverse Effects of High Doses of Drugs Using Toxicology Studies

Abstract: This chapter highlights the requirements for conducting an adverse effect study involving laboratory animals. Though this study is not required for Ayurvedic formulations, we are conducting these studies to follow the requirements in order to make the medicinal formulation acceptable by modern medical practitioners. The maximum tolerance limit for the formulation needs to be tested in toxicology studies using a rat and a rabbit model under the 'New Drugs and Clinical Trials Rules,' Ministry of Health and Family Welfare, Government of India, and the 'Organization for Economic Co-operation and Development (OECD)' guidelines. These two animals are the species accepted by regulatory agencies for conducting safety and toxicity studies. The acute toxic class method is a stepwise procedure using 3 animals of a single-sex per step. Depending on the mortality and/or the moribund status of the animals, on average, 2-4 steps may be necessary to allow judgement on the acute toxicity of the test substance. This procedure is reproducible, uses very few animals, and can rank substances based on their toxicity. The acute toxic class method is based on biometric evaluations with fixed doses, adequately separated to enable a substance to be ranked for classification purposes and hazard assessment. The objective is to determine the possible health hazards of the formulation after repeated daily oral administration for 28 consecutive days. In a second set, the animals were allowed to recover for a further 14 days after a 28-day drug administration to test for reversibility, persistence, or delayed occurrence of toxic effects. The study will provide information on major toxic effects, target organs, if any, and determine the No-Observed- Adverse-Effect-Level (NOAEL) of the Ayurvedic formulation. We tested Coronil and Divya Swasari Vati in both rats and rabbits. Preliminary studies showed that either formulation did not show any toxic effects for 28-day administration followed by a 14-day recovery period. We will present data obtained in the toxicity studies in an appropriate forum once the study is completed. This chapter mentions the protocols and standard procedures to be followed while conducting such studies. This is critical since the clearance for clinical studies is based on these toxicological observations, as is described in the next chapter.

Keywords: Acute toxicological study, Sub-acute toxicological study, NOAEL, New Drugs and Clinical Trials Rules, Organization for Economic Co-operation and Development' (OECD) guidelines.

5.1. BACKGROUND

After conducting lots of research to establish the efficacy of our investigational Ayurvedic formulation through pre-clinical studies as per different guidelines, methods, and protocols, we proceeded for safety/toxicity evaluation as per Central Council for Research in Ayurvedic Sciences guidelines. However, our case is exempted from such requirements (as per page no: 6, The Gazette of India: Extraordinary (Part II-Section 3-Sub-section (i)). Since this book is intended to serve as a comprehensive guideline for developing Ayurvedic formulations into medicines acceptable by modern practitioners, so, continuing along the sequence of requirements, we conduct toxicological studies as per Organization for Economic Co-operation and Development (OECD) and Drugs and Cosmetics Act, Government of India, following the principles of Good Laboratory Practices (GLPs) in compliance with Committee for the Purpose of Control and Supervision of Experiments on Animals (CPCSEA) guidelines. This chapter mainly aims to lay out the prerequisites for conducting an adverse effect study. The guidelines for a 28-day repeated dose toxicity study in rats are as per the OECD guideline for testing chemicals, No. 407, titled 'Repeated Dose 28-Day Oral Toxicity Study in Rodents'. The guidelines for repeated dose toxicity in rabbits are as per the guidelines of 'Schedule Y' of the Drugs and Cosmetics Act, 1945, Govt. of India. The toxicology studies are also in line with the International Council of Harmonization (ICH) guidelines 'M3R2'.

5.2. RATIONALE BEHIND THE USE OF TOXICOLOGY STUDIES

Once the efficacy of the Ayurvedic formulation was tested by *in vitro* and *in vivo* studies, the maximum tolerance limit for the formulation needs to be tested in toxicology studies using a rat and a rabbit model. These two animals are the species accepted by regulatory agencies for conducting safety and toxicity studies.

The repeated dose toxic class method is a stepwise procedure using 3 animals of a single-sex per step (Schlede *et al.*, 2005). Depending on the mortality and/or the moribund status of the animals, on average, 2-4 steps may be necessary to allow judgement on the acute toxicity of the test substance. This procedure is reproducible, uses very few animals, and is able to rank substances based on their toxicity. However, for an Ayurvedic formulation, such a ranking system has not been established and, in most cases, may not be needed or relevant. The repeated dose toxicity method is based on biometric evaluations with fixed doses, adequately separated to enable a substance to be ranked for classification purposes and hazard assessment. The method, as adopted in 1996, was extensively validated *in vivo* against LD_{50} data obtained from the literature, both nationally and internationally. When the method was adopted, it replaced the oral LD_{50}

method. As such, in the case of using Ayurvedic formulations, specific guidelines for LD_{50} data might not be relevant. However, the oral LD_{50} test is no longer accepted by the OECD, the European Union, and the USA, making the use of alternatives to the oral LD_{50} test mandatory.

The objective is to determine the possible health hazards of the formulation after repeated daily oral administration for 28 consecutive days. The study will provide information on major toxic effects, target organs, if any, and determine the No-Observed-Adverse-Effect-Level (NOAEL) of the Ayurvedic formulation.

In a second testing set, the animals will be observed for further 14 days after 28-day drug administration to evaluate reversibility, persistence, or delayed occurrence of toxic effects.

5.3. INSTITUTIONAL REQUIREMENTS

The testing for toxicity of a test drug, or in this case, a formulation, must be performed by experts of the field under some very strict guidelines. These guidelines ensure that all parameters of toxicity can be adhered to and carried out in a way such that no ambiguity exists, either in the testing conditions or in the results obtained. All the certifications for the facility have to be current before the start of such toxicity studies.

(i) All the study procedures must be carried out based on standards set forth by the government of India, under the 'New Drugs and Clinical Trials Rules, Ministry of Health and Family Welfare, Government of India (Department of Health and Family Welfare), Gazette of India, (extraordinary) Part-II, Section 3(i) vide G.S.R. 227(E), dated 19th March 2019.

(ii) In addition, the toxicity study will have to comply with 'Good Laboratory Practice' (GLP) norms set out by 'Organization for Economic Co-operation and Development' (OECD) [(revised 1997, issued January 1998) ENV/MC/CHEM (98) 17 Environment Directorate, Organization for Economic Co-operation and Development, Paris, 1998].

(iii) The facility where such testing is carried out has to be a certified GLP laboratory under the principles set by the 'National GLP Compliance Monitoring Authority' (NGCMA), Department of Science & Technology, Govt. of India, for compliance to OECD-GLP.

(iv) Clearance from 'Committee for the Purpose of Control and Supervision of Experiments on Animals' (CPCSEA) must be obtained for conducting experiments on small laboratory animals (CPCSEA, 2003).

(v) A team of experts in the particular field is needed for quality assurance and should inspect/audit various phases of the study. The team is charged with maintaining high standards in the study and preventing any changes to the study protocol without prior approval and proper justification.

5.3.1. Principles of Good Laboratory Practice (GLP) and Compliance Monitoring As

Mandated by OECD

This short description was adopted from the publication of OECD Principles on Good Laboratory Practice (Series 1, revised in 1997).

The criteria for a set of standardized principles to be followed by various governments and industries to maintain standards in the quality of non-clinical health and environmental monitoring were set by the OECD member countries. This regulatory guideline was issued to prevent differences in quality standards among different countries in an effort to promote equality in this era of globalization. The OECD members implemented the harmonization of test methods and good laboratory practices towards achieving this goal. The principles of GLP were adopted by the OECD Council in 1981, following the recommendations of an international group of experts established under the 'Special Programme on the Control of Chemicals' using the common scientific practices, as an 'Annex to the Council Decision on the Mutual Acceptance of Data in the Assessment of Chemicals [C(81)30(Final)]'.

The original set of principles adopted in 1981 was replaced by the revised and updated set of principles in 1997, following the recommendations of a new group of experts. These principles of GLP were to promote the development of quality test data and promote acceptance of data among the member countries. This ensures time-saving and resources to prevent multiple testings by each country, avoid the creation of technical trade barriers, and further improve the health and safety of the population as well as safeguard the environment.

The use of these principles is limited to non-clinical safety testing of test items, such as pharmaceuticals, pesticides, cosmetics, veterinary drugs, including food additives and industrial chemicals. These items may often be synthetic but may also be of biological origin, and in special instances, maybe live organisms. These principles cover the work done in laboratories, greenhouses, and the field. It is necessary to obtain data on the safety, properties, and/or safety concerning human health and/or their impact on the environment during their use and disposal. Unless specifically exempted, these principles on GLP apply to all non-clinical health and environmental safety studies required for licensing pharmaceuticals, food and feed additives, cosmetic products, veterinary drug products, and industrial chemicals.

Each registered test facility should ensure compliance with the principles of GLP within their facility. The test facility should be of adequate size, and segregation of the test systems to special rooms and conditions as specified by the manufacturer should be followed. Cross-contamination of the test material and reference standard should be avoided at all costs, and separate areas should be designated for their storage and preparation before testing. Personnel involved in testing should ensure that such carryover of materials is avoided. The disposal of all the reagents and materials used for quality testing also ensures that cross-contamination does not occur and errors are avoided.

In the case of biological material, ambient or below ambient storage of the materials should be ensured as needed. Newly received plants or animals should be isolated until the required duration to not only ensure their health but also to overcome any undue stress encountered during the transportation process. Disposal of such living organisms should be according to the health and environmental norms of the area the test facility is located in. In the case of live animal testing, all ethical norms should be followed as set by the institutional ethics committee and appropriate governmental agencies.

The onus is on the facility to ensure that each of the personnel is sufficiently qualified and trained to conduct the study in a timely manner and follow the Standard Operating Procedures (SOPs). The SOPs are related to both the instruments used and the actual process of testing. Any deviations from the set principles should be adequately justified and recorded.

The head of the team involved in such studies (or the study director) should ensure that the qualified personnel are assigned to the study and ensure that the proper procedures are followed. The OCED Test Guideline or other approved test guidelines or methods should be followed during the testing process. The instruments used in the study are of standard make and should be certified for the nature of work being done in the particular laboratory. The records for any maintenance and calibration should be up to date and maintained at the testing facility for easy access and availability to audit. All data generated by such instruments should also be maintained in their raw form, and any derivations of the data should be performed on duplicated data rather than the original.

The team should have dedicated quality assurance to assure compliance at all stages of the study. All copies of data generated should be properly recorded and maintained even after the completion of the study. The quality assurance members should conduct regular inspections to ensure that all studies are being conducted according to the SOP, and records of such inspections should be maintained. A final report should be generated for each study in a standardized format, and it should be properly signed and dated by the study participants. Once the final report is generated and signed, no changes should be made, and any necessary changes to the report should be made as amendments to the original report. The report should also contain the historical records of the SOPs used, the date of any instrument calibration and their report if necessary, the data in an easily readable format while referencing the raw data wherever needed, and a concise conclusion to the study.

All records pertaining to the study should be properly archived, and any test or reference material should be stored under appropriate conditions until their expiry period. Once the expiry date is over, they should be properly disposed of, and a record of their disposal should be maintained. Only authorized personnel should have access to the archives, and any movement of material out of the archive should be minimized. If the material needs to be accessed, the movement of the material in and out of the archives should be recorded. All such records should be maintained according to the local rules and regulations.

5.3.2. Terms and Conditions of 'National GLP Compliance Monitoring Authority' (NGCMA), for Obtaining and Maintaining GLP Certification by a Test Facility

These guidelines are issued by the NGCMA under the Department of Science and Technology, Government of India, for compliance with the OECD-GLP norms. The latest issue of guidelines is under Document number GLP-101, Issue number 08, dated 25th October 2019. The document can be obtained from the NGCMA website (http://www.dst.gov.in/ngcma).

A test facility is eligible to apply for a GLP certification if it is involved in non-clinical health or environmental safety studies. Organizations, such as a contract research organization, research, and development laboratories, universities or deemed universities, institutes of national importance, an industry, company, government organization, PSU, or a registered organization can apply for the GLP certification. The certification is awarded only to a particular division, section, department, or laboratory of a larger organization and is valid only for that specific division performing the specific function as per the GLP norms. The certification is valid for three years unless revoked in consonance with Document number GLP-113, 'Policies and procedures of NGCMA for taking adverse and other decisions against test facilities.' This three-year period is subject to continued compliance to OECD Principles of GLP and is termed a GLP certification cycle.

Each testing facility needs to apply for acquiring the GLP certification or re-certification using the online portal of the NGCMA (ngcma.qci.org.in) and paying the appropriate fees. The applicant is required to enclose all organizational documents, such as floor plans, master schedule, and others, during the application process. All such documents should be accompanied by dated signatures by all the members of the test facility management.

If a test facility is involved in multisite studies, the details of all such test sites, including the location and address, management structure, and the type of studies carried out at that site, should be mentioned. It is the onus of the facility to ensure that all the OECD Principles of GLP are adhered to by the off-site facility also.

Once the initial application is found to be complete and all the eligibility criteria for GLP certification are met, a team from the NGCMA will conduct an on-site examination of the test facilities' buildings, procedures, and practices to ascertain compliance. The inspection planning will be carried out as specified in Document number GLP-109, 'Scheduling of GLP inspections by NGCMA' at a mutually convenient date. The inspections to be carried out are defined in the Document Number GLP-111 'Definitions of General Terms Used in NGCMA' and GLP-104 'Procedures of NGCMA Secretariat'. Once the GLP certification is issued, the facility is subjected to a 'Surveillance Inspection at 18 months (± 3 months) from the date of issuance. The re-certification process beyond the existing cycle should be started at least 6 months before the expiry of the existing GLP certification. The status of each test facility with regard to its compliance with OECD Principles of GLP is published on the website of NGCMA (http://www.dst.gov.in/ngcma).

The NGCMA may also conduct an inspection(s) or audit(s) at the request of a Regulatory Authority, the GLP Compliance Monitoring Authority (CMA) of OECD Mutual Acceptance Data (MAD) adherent country or countries. Joint inspections with any of the above-mentioned bodies may also be conducted following NGCMA procedures for such inspections.

In case of any serious discrepancies, the NGCMA may take appropriate actions such as issuing a statement highlighting the details of the inadequacies or faults, issuing a recommendation for termination of a particular study, suspension of the GLP compliance certificate, or in an extreme case, legal action where warranted by circumstances.

The test facility can file a complaint/ grievance/ appeal against any adverse decision of NGCMA, and this will be processed as per Document Number GLP-108 'Procedure for the Handling of Complaints, Grievances, and Appeals. All disputes arising out of NGCMA decisions that remain unresolved, even though the mechanisms provided by the NGCMA, are subjected to the exclusive jurisdiction of the Courts and New Delhi.

5.3.3. CPCSEA Guidelines for Laboratory Animal Facility

These guidelines are issued by the 'Committee for the Purpose of Control and Supervision on Experiments on Animals' Thiruvanmiyur, Chennai-600041. (www.cpcsea.com).

The guidelines follow Good Laboratory Practices (GLP) for animal facilities to assure quality maintenance and safety of animals that are used for biomedical and behavioural research and product testing.

GLP for animal facilities is intended to assure quality maintenance and safety of animals used in laboratory studies while conducting biomedical and behavioural research and testing of products. The guidelines provide specifications needed to enhance the wellbeing of all animals used in studies, assure quality in the pursuit of advancement of biological knowledge relevant to humans and animals. The guidelines deal with all the aspects of animal care, including procurement, design of the animal house and housing requirements of different species, feed and water containers, surveillance, prevention and treatment of diseases, procedures for the administration of test substance, surgeries, anaesthesia and euthanization of animals, and the protocols and personnel involved in ethical handling of animals.

Institutional ethics committee should be constituted to ensure compliance with all ethical norms involved in handling and experimentation of the animals. The ethics committee should review all the protocols and procedures involved not only for handling and upkeep of the animals but also the feasibility and necessity of animal use for a particular study. Once the IEC approves the study protocol, the procurement of the animals can be initiated. All animals should be procured lawfully according to the CPCSEA guidelines, and each consignment must be inspected for compliance.

The transport of animals should be according to the guidelines specified in the document, and all incoming animals should be inspected for overt health problems. The newly acquired animals have to be quarantined and stabilized according to species-specific procedures.

Adequate veterinary care must be provided at all times by either a practising veterinarian or a technician trained in laboratory animal science and medicine. The animals need to be observed daily, even during the non-study period, for changes in health, behaviour, or changes in dietary habits. Appropriate methods for disease surveillance and diagnosis must be in place, including equipment and surgical suites if needed. Unexpected deaths and signs of illness, distress, or other deviations from the normal health condition of the animals should be reported promptly, and causes for the deviations should be investigated. Protocols should be in place to mitigate such unforeseen problems in the future. Special policies should be in place governing experimentation with hazardous agents, and such obvious agents should be avoided in animal experimentation.

Animal living areas should be kept separate from experimentation areas, and the animal house areas should have designated areas for handling different aspects of animal handling and experimentation. Constant temperature and humidity should be maintained to reduce animal discomfort and avoid deviations in experimental protocols. The animal house should be constructed keeping in mind that only 50 to 60% of the available space is occupied by animal housing spaces, and the rest is left for assorted functions, including cage washing, feed storage, and waste disposal.

Animals should be fed palatable feed free of contaminants and should be nutritionally adequate. Animals should be fed daily unless the experimental protocol requires otherwise. The feed and water should be made available in easily accessible containers so that the animals can access them whenever needed. The diet and water should be free of heavy metals, and perishable items should be free of biological and chemical contamination. Waste should be removed regularly and frequently, and disposed of in a safe and sanitary manner, preferably by incineration. The incinerators should comply with all environmental regulations.

All records of animal procurement, health records of animals, any diseases or procedures done to maintain animal health, and finally, the disposal should be maintained not just throughout the study period but also as mandated by the Institutional Ethics Committees and local regulatory bodies. All procedures for animal care and handling should be followed according to established SOPs, and any deviations from the SOP should be recorded. The reasons for the deviations should also be recorded as per the accepted procedures.

5.4. STUDY REQUIREMENTS

A short description for the different aspects of the toxicity testing was adapted from the OECD guideline for testing of chemicals, No. 407, titled 'Repeated Dose 28-day Oral Toxicity Study in Rodents' and the guidelines outlined in 'Schedule Y' of the Drugs and Cosmetics Act, 1945; Govt. of India.

Before a study can commence, a study plan/protocol has to be prepared and approved by the Institutional Animal Ethics Committee (IAEC) (Appendix 5.1). The study protocol has to be prepared by the sponsor of the study with details regarding the composition of the test drug or formulation and a vehicle in which the test drug has to be mixed. Data of stability and homogeneity of the drug should be mentioned along with the storage stipulations. The required dosage and route of administration should be based on the intended clinical route of administration and should be provided in detail.

The study protocol should contain details of the type of animals, their gender, age, body weight, and any other relevant information.

Once the protocol has been approved, the animal characteristics and all study parameters have to be strictly adhered to and any deviations in the protocol must be communicated to the study director and recorded.

5.5. DESCRIPTION OF HUSBANDRY CONDITIONS AND ANIMAL REQUIREMENTS

5.5.1. Animals

The acute toxicity method recommends the use of 3 rabbits or 5 rats of the same gender per group, divided into different groups based on the study requirement. In most cases, a single-gender is used and could either be male or female, but a specific requirement for a specific gender or both genders can be justified. One such example is the SARS-CoV-2 virus, wherein emerging global data suggests that men appear to have a higher risk of infection and mortality than women. This sex-based disparity is seen in incidence and hospitalization, as well as in mortality from COVID-19. Such observations or evidence-backed data may be useful in the use of a specific gender for the toxicity assays to focus on. If females are to be used in the study, they should be nulliparous and non-pregnant.

In general, all animals should be tested free of pathogens and housed in airy and spacious cages in a stress-free condition.

The parameters for testing, such as housing conditions, observations, and their frequency, along with the final termination and collection of different organs for analysis, remain constant irrespective of the animal used. The only change is the dosage of the drug being given and the animal housing density.

5.5.1.1. Rabbits

The New Zealand white rabbit is the most popular choice for toxicological studies. Healthy young adults between 2 and 4 months (the exact age of each animal has to be recorded) and body weight between 1500 and 3000 g are generally recommended. At the commencement of treatment, the weight variation of animals should not exceed ± 20% of the mean weight of each sex, and the exact body weight of each animal should be recorded. The repeated dose toxicity testing for adverse effects of Coronil and Divya Swasari Vati on rabbits were according to the guidelines in 'Schedule-Y' of the Drugs and Cosmetics Act, 1940. For this, the mentioned doses were 50, 150, and 500 mg/kg/day for the main study and at 500 mg/ kg/day for the treatment, followed by a 14-day recovery study. The control animals are administered vehicle alone. The route of administration in this study was oral, using an oral gavage tube fitted with a graduated syringe. The dose volume was maintained at 10 ml/kg body weight and the actual volume to be administered was calculated based on the recent body weights of each animal.

5.5.1.2. Rats

Any species of laboratory rats can be used, but mainly lines derived from albino Wistar rats, such as Sprague-Dawley, Wistar, or Long Evans, are the most popular. Animals between 6 and 8 weeks of age and weighing between 150 and 250 gm are chosen for the studies (The precise age and weight of the rats have to be recorded).

The repeated dose toxicity studies for Coronil and Divya Swasari Vati were in accordance with the OECD guideline for testing of chemicals, No. 407. The doses that were chosen for rats in this study were 100, 300, and 1000 mg/kg/day for the main study and 1000 mg/ kg/day for the 14-day recovery group. The control animals are administered vehicle alone. The drug and vehicle were administered to the animals orally, as described previously. The acute toxicology study is currently underway, and the results of the study will be published when done.

5.5.2. Housing Conditions

Animals are housed, and all testing procedures are carried out in specialized housing termed 'animal houses.' These animal houses are generally away from the main laboratory work area and have specialized air handling systems to minimize pathogen entry. Only specially designated personnel can enter the animal housing area, and anyone needing to handle laboratory animals requires training in the safe and ethical handling of animals.

In the case of rabbits, each animal is housed at a maximum of 3 animals of the same sex per cage (approximately 58.0 cm x 58.0 cm x 58.0 cm). The cage is made of sterilized mesh bottom, standard stainless steel having provision for holding pelleted food and drinking water in a bottle with stainless steel sipper tube throughout the study period. The environment of the housing area is automatically controlled to be comfortable to the animals, with a temperature of 22 ± 3 °C and humidity of 30% to 70%. The photoperiod will be 12 h light and 12 h dark, and 10 to 15 air changes per hour will be maintained throughout the in-life phase of this study. The feed is in the form of standardized pellets, UV sterilized and provided to the animals in feed boxes that can be eaten whenever needed. Water is mainly reverse osmosis water provided in autoclaved sipper bottles.

Each animal is temporarily marked with a non-toxic marker pen on the left inner pinna and is allowed to acclimatize to the housing conditions and the food. The animals are observed at least once a day for any changes in their general health and behaviour for up to 5 days. Once the acclimatization period is done, a detailed clinical evaluation is performed on the animals. These include serum biochemistry and ophthalmic examinations. Once the animals pass the criteria set for acceptance, they are randomized into different treatment groups, ensuring that each group contains animals from the same gender. During randomization, the animals are assigned a permanent animal number and will be marked on the right inner pinna using a non-toxic marker pen throughout the study period. Body weights will be taken before randomization. At the commencement of the study, the weight variation of the animals used will be minimal and will not exceed ± 20% of the mean body weight for each sex. The animals not selected for study following randomization will be returned to the facility without any further investigations.

5.5.3. Preparation of the Dose Formulation

The required quantity of the test item will be weighed on butter paper and crushed to a fine powder using a mortar and pestle. Subsequently, a small volume of 0.5% Methyl Cellulose (MC) solution will be added by using a syringe with continuous stirring. After the test item has been properly wetted, the remaining volume of MC will be added dropwise by using a syringe, with continuous stirring to obtain a stable suspension. The exact amount of the test item and the vehicle should be recorded. The test drug is generally given in three different doses; low dose, medium dose and high dose.

5.5.4. Observations

Following observations will be recorded from all the animals. Additional observations, if any, will be performed and recorded depending upon the requirement and at the discretion of the study director.

(i). Mortality and Clinical Signs Observations

All the animals will be observed carefully at least once daily throughout the study period for clinical signs and at least twice daily for morbidity and mortality. Onset, severity, duration, and the reversibility of clinical signs, if any, will be recorded. Moribund animals will be isolated and/or euthanized and subjected to the post-mortem examination, and organs will be collected for histopathology at the discretion of the study pathologist and study director.

(ii). Detailed Clinical Observations

All animals will be observed for detailed clinical observations at least once a week till terminal sacrifice. Examinations include changes in the skin, fur, eyes, and mucous membranes, the occurrence of secretions and excretions, and basic observations of autonomic activity (e.g., lacrimation, piloerection, pupil size, and unusual respiratory pattern) if any.

(iii). Functional Observation Battery

If the treatment-related clinical observations are observed, the functional observation battery will be performed in all animals during the last week of treatment and observation period for the main and recovery groups, respectively. Examinations include changes in gait, posture, and response to handling as well as the presence of clonic or tonic movements, stereotypes (e.g. excessive grooming, repetitive circling) or bizarre behaviour (e.g., self-mutilation, walking backwards), sensory reactivity to stimuli of different types (e.g., auditory, visual and proprioceptive stimuli), assessment of grip strength and motor activity assessment.

(iv). Body Weight

Body weight will be recorded a minimum once a week till the terminal sacrifice of the main group and continued for recovery group animals. Additionally, fasting body weights will be recorded before terminal sacrifice. Bodyweight gain will be calculated for the individual animals.

(v). Feed Consumption

Feed consumption of all the groups will be recorded at weekly intervals till the terminal sacrifice of the main group and continued for recovery group animals. The quantity of average feed consumed by each animal per cage in a week will be recorded.

(vi). Ophthalmoscopic Examination

The ophthalmological examination will be performed during the last week of treatment for vehicle control and high-dose group animals. If treatment-related changes are noticed, the examination will be extended to lower-dose groups. A suitable mydriatic agent (used to dilate the pupil) will be used if required, and details will be included in a raw data file. Examination of ocular lesions will be performed along with ophthalmoscopic examination.

(vii). Clinical Pathology Observations

Clinical pathology examinations will be performed in all surviving fasted main group and recovery animals on Day 29 and Day 43, respectively. The blood samples will be withdrawn from marginal ear veins. If any of the organs show gross pathological changes, the representative organs mentioned above from the control and high dose group will be processed routinely and embedded in paraffin. Sections of 3-5 μm thickness will be cut, stained with hematoxylin-eosin stain, and will be examined microscopically. Organs showing gross pathological lesions from any group will also be subjected to histopathological evaluation. If the treatment-related changes are observed in the high dose group, then the identified target organs will be processed into low (G2) and mid (G3) groups.

CONCLUDING REMARKS

To sum it up, this chapter has provided detailed requirements for toxicological studies, which are mandatory for drug development. Although herbal medicines are exempted from this requirement, toxicological studies will add acceptability to these medicines.

CHAPTER 6

Designing Clinical Research: Application on Evidence-based Practice

Abstract: This chapter is a guide on designing and executing clinical trials for traditional medicines. It includes the guidelines to be followed during protocol designing and study execution. Patanjali Research Institute combines deep therapeutic and scientific knowledge of Ayurvedic medicines with unmatched clinical trial design execution. Every patient who participates in a clinical trial plays a critical role in conquering disease and discovering cures for COVID-19 on behalf of all of us. Thus, with an in-depth understanding of the issues related to the clinical trial, Patanjali Research Institute has conducted human clinical trials and studies as per the ethical codes of biomedical research.

Keywords: Clinical study, Trial design, Clinical trial document, CTRI, Randomized clinical trial, Observational study.

6.1. BACKGROUND TO CLINICAL RESEARCH

Owing to millions of cases and thousands of deaths that have occurred due to this present devastating pandemic, COVID-19, the healthcare system is at the hilt and being tested for effective management of COVID-19. Understanding the importance of clinical trials as a premier method for validating new drugs and therapies, Patanjali Research Institute has been working proactively in advance due to the evident public concern since late February 2021. We take pride in addressing the fact that we had developed a formulation when no specific vaccine or treatment was approved for COVID-19. After conducting preclinical studies as per the standard procedures while addressing all the challenges, we moved forward with the quest of conducting clinical studies in order to find an effective treatment regime against a virus.

The meaning of clinical research may appear to be self-evident. However, some researchers have narrowly defined clinical research to refer to clinical trials (*i.e.*, intervention studies in human patients), while others have broadly defined it to include any research design that studies humans (patients or subjects) or any materials derived from humans. Altogether with the above considerations, clinical

Acharya Balkrishna

studies are also conducted with the aim to obtain knowledge on the safety, efficacy, and mechanism of action of investigational new drugs on human subjects and to obtain regulatory approval. Numerous statements describe clinical research, some of which are valid and while some are not. We have opted for a 'middle of the road' approach that comprehends the term **'patient-oriented research**,' which is defined as research conducted with human subjects or on human-derived material, in which the investigator directly interacts with the human subjects at some point throughout the initiation to termination of the study (Hoffmann *et al.*, 2020).

Clinical research, in essence, serves as a connection to bridge the gap between research and clinical practice, which is handled with our evidence-based approach (EBP). The EBP framework entails the amalgamation of research findings with clinical knowledge and traits, values, and preferences, and so serves as an important basis for undertaking clinically relevant research as well as empiric research based on sensitive clinical practice (Hershenberg, Drabick, and Vivian, 2012), which is reproduced in evidence-based practise (EBP) (Fig. **6.1**).

6.1.1. Patanjali Research Institute Quest to the Map-Design

With the above background, our major purpose at the clinical research division is to reduce assumptions and seek universal truth. In fact, little, if anything, is clear in science, and the interpretation of data does not imply truth but rather an opinion on what the data signify. Nonetheless, in our quest, this is the standard body of knowledge, and this may raise additional questions that will invariably generate further research. Recently, in our ongoing research with COVID-19, we have addressed all the aforementioned components for the development of therapeutic management that can address the gap between research and practice (Fig. **6.2**).

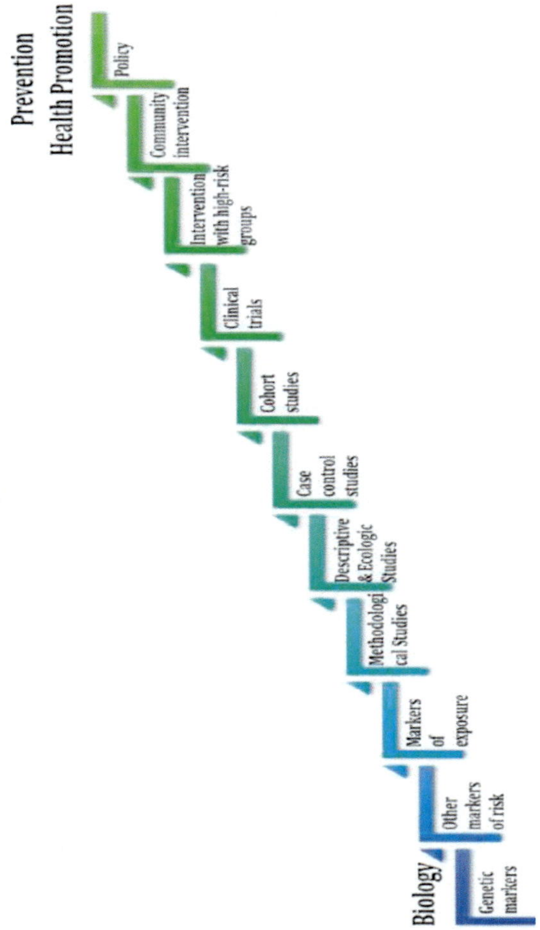

Fig. (6.1). Bridge which Patanjali Research Institute encompasses under term "clinical research".

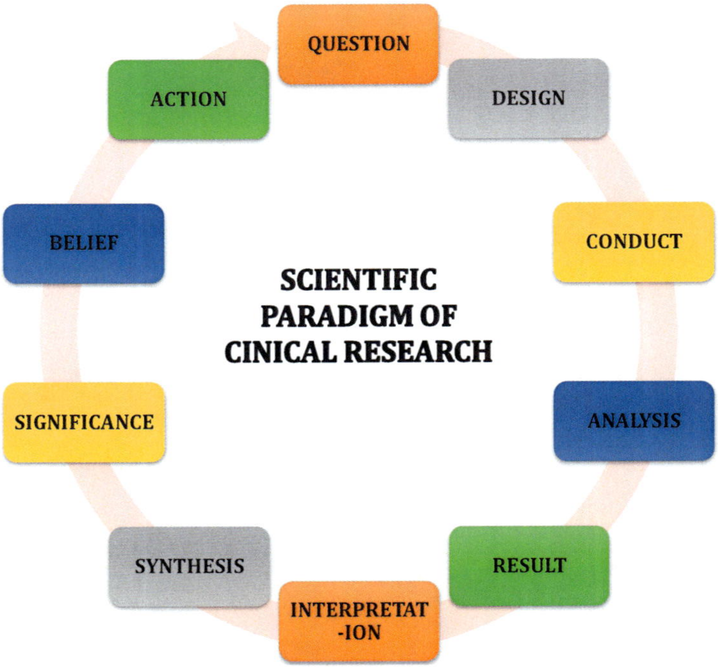

Fig. (6.2). Scientific method of Clinical Research Paradigm.

6.2. CLINICAL STUDY DESIGN: THE ESSENTIALS

A study design is a precise strategy or process for conducting the study that permits the conceptual possibility to be translated into an operational one. In other words, "the rule or method that governs the process of collecting and arrangement of knowledge for analysis is called **"research designing."** It is very critical to understand that a "poor study design cannot be salvaged by good statistics." The epidemiologic study designs are broadly classified into "Observational" and "Experimental" study designs (Chidambaram and Josephson, 2019). Our goal is to construct a study that will allow us to reach a legitimate and relevant scientific conclusion by employing proper statistical methodologies. The outcomes of a research study might either enhance health care or result in inadvertent harm to patients. As a result, this necessitates a well-designed clinical research study built on a solid foundation of comprehensive methodology and governed by ethical clinical principles. The conclusions derived from a research study can either improve health care or result in inadvertent harm to patients. Hence, this requires a well-designed clinical research study that rests on a strong foundation of a detailed methodology and is governed by ethical clinical principles.

6.2.1. OBSERVATIONAL STUDY DESIGN

The observational study design is qualitative research to explore the causal-effect relationship in which the investigators/scientists only monitor the participants involved through their clinical records, questionnaires, and measurable parameters. The differentiating characteristics between an observational study and experimental study design are that, in the latter, the presence and absence of ongoing intervention categorize the groups. The followings are examples of observational studies:

Case reports: A study design in which the likelihood of a relationship between an observed impact and a specific environmental exposure is investigated using extensive clinical evaluations and individual histories. There is a lack of control groups which decreases the statistical validity or conclusion about the causal association.

Case series studies: One of the most fundamental types of study design is the case series (also known as clinical series), in which researchers report the experiences of a small number of people. The case series provides a detailed narrative of individual research subjects' clinical experiences, as well as evaluates and explains the potential success and effectiveness of any novel intervention.

Case-control studies: In a case-control study (CCS), the researcher first identifies a certain outcome in the population, then pairs the "diseased group" with a "healthy group," and then identifies and compares the two groups exposures. As no intervention is tried and no attempt is made to influence the course of the disease, a case-control study can be called an observational study. The purpose is to identify the exposure to the risk factor of interest in each of the two groups of people: cases and controls, retrospectively. The practice of the terminology 'trohoc design' cohort spelled and written backward is used for CCS studies due to its retrospective study design.

Cohort studies: In this study design, one or more study samples (called cohorts) are tracked prospectively, followed by subsequent status evaluations of a disease or its outcome. Therefore, a cohort study helps to identify risk factors. Results from each cohort's participants are measured as the study progresses, and correlations with specific characteristics are examined. As the study progresses, the outcomes of each cohort's participants are measured, and correlations with specific characteristics are examined.

Cross-sectional studies: In a cross-sectional study, the investigator simultaneously evaluates the outcome and the research participants' exposures. Unlike in case-control studies (participants are chosen based on their outcome status) or cohort studies (participants are chosen based on their exposure status), participants in a cross-sectional study are chosen solely based on their inclusion and exclusion criteria (Thaker, Gogtay and Thatte, 2015) (Fig. **6.3**).

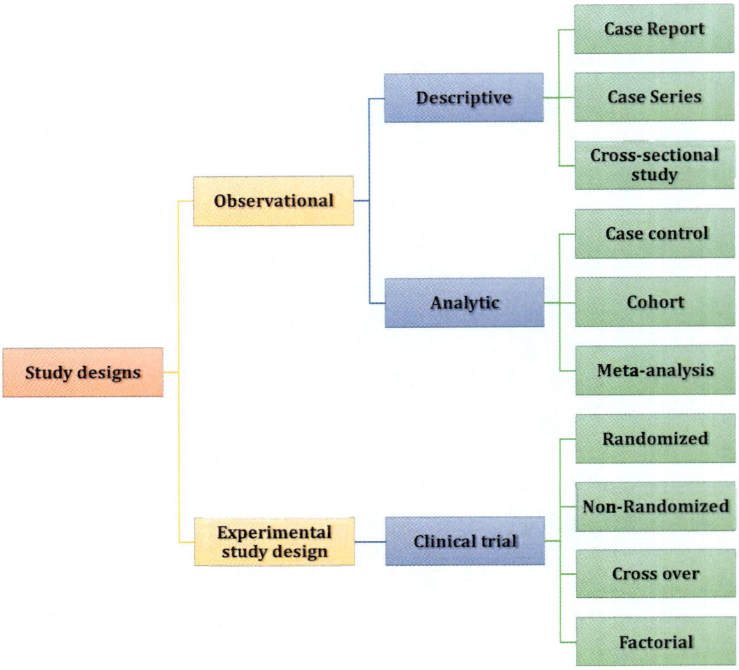

Fig. (6.3). Types of clinical research design.

In conclusion, observational studies (*e.g.*, cross-sectional, case-control, and cohort studies) play an important role in research. Despite their critical significance, there is a lack of vital information that is either missing or unclear in some of the previously published observational studies; and this is why lack of information leads to the development of a guideline document for reporting observational studies, *i.e.*, STROBE (Strengthening and Reporting of Observational Studies in Epidemiology) and CHERRIES (Checklist for Reporting Results of Internet E-Surveys).

Following the standard guidelines and principles, recently, we have conducted our two observational studies (case-control and cross-sectional) in COVID-19 to establish the importance of treatment regimen, Divya Swasari Coronil Kit manufactured as per the government license (Government of Uttarakhand, India) by Divya Pharmacy, Haridwar, India.

6.2.2. EXPERIMENTAL STUDY DESIGN

These studies are ones where researchers introduce an intervention and study the effects. In these studies, the risk factors/exposure of interest are pre-defined. Experimental studies are usually randomized, which means that the subjects are grouped by chance; if not, they are non-randomized, factorial, or cross-over. The Randomized Controlled Trial (RCT) remains the "gold standard" study design, and its results are rightfully regarded as providing the highest level of scientific evidence (greatest likelihood of causation)(Schulz and Grimes, 2002). The STROBE statement is designed after the CONSORT (Consolidated Standards of Reporting Trials) statement that outlines the guidelines for reporting RCTs (Lepage *et al.*, 2001). These criteria should be closely followed for any experimental study (Fig. **6.4**).

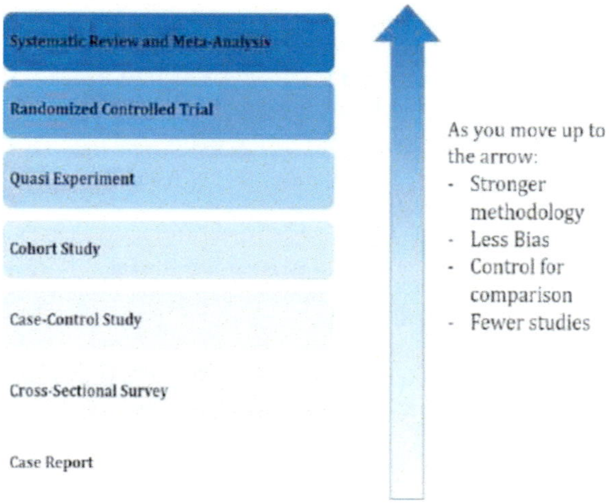

Fig. (6.4). Hierarchy representing the strength of clinical study design.

This study broadly comprises clinical trials, which are conducted to test the new drug or treatment. In the case of COVID-19, due to its nature of transmissibility and aetiology of virus and with the unavailability of treatment, it has evolved as a global threat. Many clinical trials are underway to find effective management against COVID-19. Patanjali Research Institute has conducted "Randomized Placebo-Controlled Double-Blind Clinical Trial on the Efficacy of Ayurvedic Treatment Regime" in the specialized COVID-19 ward of National Institute of Medical Sciences and Research, Jaipur, India (CTRI No. CTRI/2020/05/025273) and Chhatrapati Shivaji Subharti Hospital, Meerut, Uttar Pradesh (CTRI/2020/09/027882), with few more underway to establish Divya Swasari Coronil Kit as a first and foremost traditional medicine to fight SARS- CoV-2.

6.3. PRINCIPLES FOR CONDUCTING THE RESEARCH

Principles for the conduct of biomedical research are outlined in internationally recognized documents mentioned below. Strict processes as per the code of conduct should be followed to conduct biomedical research on human participants.

6.3.1. Ethics and Good Clinical Practice

- **The Declaration of Helsinki**, The World Medical Association's Declaration of Helsinki, promulgated in 1964 and revised as needed, is the fundamental document in the field of ethics in biomedical research and has had a significant influence on the formulation of international, regional, and national legislation and codes of conduct.

In short, most interventions in medical practice and research involve risks and burdens. Medical advancement and development are based on research, which must eventually include human subjects' studies. The major goal of medical research with human beings is to better understand the causes, progression, and effects of diseases, as well as to enhance preventive, diagnostic, and therapeutic interventions (methods, procedures).

6.3.2. Important principles for conducting medical research in brief:

- Protection of life, health, dignity, integrity, right to self-determination, privacy, and confidentiality.
- Acceptable scientific principles described in a detailed protocol.
- Protocol must be reviewed by an Ethical Committee.
- Taking into account local rules and regulations.
- Evaluation of predictable risks, burdens, and their consequences.
- The investigator's training and qualifications are adequate.
- Participation must be entirely voluntary.
- Participants must be given appropriate information and must consent to participation.

The **International Conference on Harmonization** E6 guidelines for **Good Clinical Practice** (ICH GCP E6) were issued in 1996. The European Union, Japan, and the United States met at the International Conference on Harmonisation of Technical Requirements for Registration of Pharmaceuticals for Human Use (ICH). The ICH aims to eliminate unnecessary delays in the global development and availability of new medicines while retaining quality, safety, and efficacy precautions, as well as regulatory commitments to protect public health. The ICH GCP was first introduced in 1997, and the original version is still in use today (See Table **6.1**).

Table 6.1. The principles of ICH-GCP.

• Clinical trials should be conducted in accordance with the ethical principles that have their origin in the Declaration of Helsinki and that are consistent with GCP and the applicable regulatory requirement(s).
• Predictable dangers and inconveniences should be evaluated against the expected benefit to the individual trial subject and society before a trial begins. A trial should be initiated and continued only if the anticipated benefits justify the risks.
• The rights, safety, and well-being of the trial subjects are the most important considerations and should prevail over the interests of science and society.
• The available nonclinical and clinical information on an investigational product should be adequate to support the proposed clinical trial.
• Clinical trials should be scientifically sound and described in a clear, detailed protocol.
• A trial should be carried out in accordance with the protocol that has acquired previous approval/favourable opinion from an institutional review board (IRB)/independent ethics council (IEC).
• Medical care provided to subjects, as well as medical decisions made on their behalf, should always be the duty of a trained physician or, where appropriate, a qualified dentist.
• Each individual involved in conducting a trial should be qualified by education, training, and experience to perform his or her respective task(s).
• Freely given informed consent should be obtained from every subject before clinical trial participation.
• All clinical trial data should be recorded, processed, and maintained in such a way that it can be accurately reported, interpreted, and verified.
• The confidentiality of records that could be used to identify persons shall be preserved according to the applicable regulatory requirement(s). Investigational items must be created, handled, and stored properly.
• Investigational products must be created, handled, and kept in conformity with good manufacturing practices (GMP). They must be used in accordance with the protocol that has been approved.
• It is necessary to develop systems and procedures that ensure the quality of all aspects of the trial.

The **International Conference on Harmonization (ICH)** "Good Clinical Practice" (GCP) is an international ethical and scientific quality standard for the design, conduct, performance, monitoring, auditing, recording, analyses, and reporting of clinical trials that ensure that the data and reported results are credible and accurate, as well as the rights, integrity, and confidentiality of trial subjects. Ethical and scientific quality criteria for planning, conducting, documenting, and reporting trials involving human beings to ensure that the trial subjects' rights, safety, and well-being are protected, ascertaining the validity of clinical study data.

The International Conference on Harmonization of Good Clinical Practice (ICH GCP) has emerged as the most widely used international standard for clinical trial conduct. It is more of an operational guideline than a policy document, laying out the operational details and obligations associated with clinical trials.

- The principles of these and other standards are translated into legal requirements through laws and regulations with other national-level guidelines, such as the **Central Council of Research in Ayurvedic Sciences (CCRAS) and National Ethical Guidelines for Biomedical and Health Research involving Human Participants (ICMR); New Drugs and Clinical Trials Rules, 2018.** The socio-cultural ethos of India, as well as the country's different healthcare standards, present distinct problems in applying universal ethical norms to biomedical and health research. These recommendations have covered some newer fields, like public health research, social and behavioural sciences, research for health and responsible conduct of research, and research during humanitarian catastrophes and disasters involving human participants. Patanjali Research Institute follows guidelines to validate the safety and efficacy of ayurvedic formulation through fundamental, and all of the above-mentioned principles and diverse approaches of drug development (Standardization and quality assurance), safety and toxicity, and clinical evaluation as a ready reference (Mathur and Swaminathan, 2018; MoHFW, 2019; Series-iii, n.d.)

6.4. STUDY CENTERS: THE BACKBONE OF DRUG DEVELOPMENT

According to Good Clinical Practice (GCP Sections 4.2.3, 5.6.1, and 5.18.4), the sponsor should choose a trial site with adequate resources, qualified staff, and facilities as per the requirement (Wright, 2017). It also defines the characteristics that a site should have, as well as the need for appropriate, qualified employees for the duration of the trial. Normally, sponsors would appoint a Clinical Research Organization (CRO) to organize the clinical trial. In the case of COVID-19-based clinical investigations, only those sites should be chosen that meet the fundamental criteria, such as the availability of COVID-19 wards. The conduct of clinical trials in accordance with SOPs (Standard Operating Procedures), requirements of sample size, and demography require a lot of monetary investment and time of the sponsor (Rajadhyaksha, 2010; Abu-Arafeh and Andrews, 2016).

In the case of investigator trial site visits by industry sponsors, the sponsor investigates the feasibility and potential of the trial site after a non-disclosure agreement, which is signed where necessary.

There are certain key factors taken care of by Patanjali Research Institute as a checklist before optimal trial site selection while finalizing the trial site for COVID-19 related clinical studies (Fig. **6.5**):

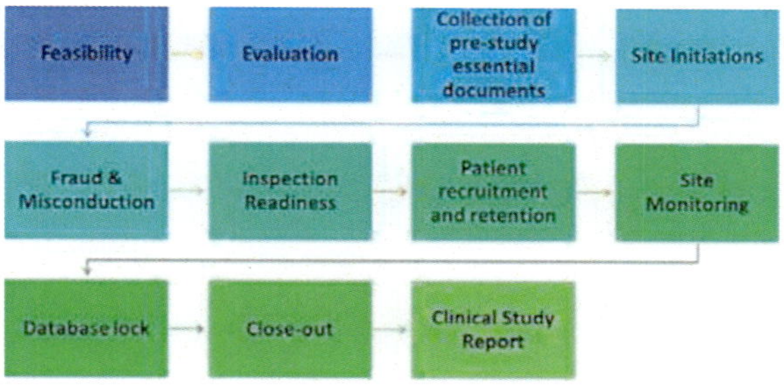

Fig. (6.5). Typical sequence to check the site and project feasibility.

- Trained and experienced staff who understand the complexity of research protocols and regulatory requirements, especially the professional career of the PI is also important.
- Recruitment capabilities and strength of database.
- Well-efficient to coordinate with Institutional Review Board and regulatory requirements.
- The site has the feasibility to conduct specialized lab procedures, collection, and shipping methods for samples (Example: RT-PCR testing).

In addition, unless it is professionally or ethically objectionable, there is no justification to decline a study during the feasibility stage.

6.5. REGULATORY REQUIREMENTS AND AGREEMENTS

The regulatory requirement submission varies depending upon the type of intervention. The Ministry of AYUSH, Government of India, acts as the national medical authority for ayurvedic drugs. Although ICH-GCP is the fundamental guideline to review for the conduct of any clinical trial, an Institutional Ethical Committee acts as a representative on the national or state levels, which reviews the Clinical Trial Application (CTA) in accordance with the Declaration of Helsinki 2013 and ICH-GCP. The major pre-requisites required prior to the enrollment of even the first participant in the clinical trial are approval from the AYUSH ministry for ayurvedic drug, approval from a registered IEC/IRB, and CTRI registration (national clinical registry) which can be accessed by the general public (Table **7.2**).

Clinical trials have immense potential for benefiting participants, improving therapy regimens, and ensuring evidence-based progression in medical practice. Trial registration will assure clinical studies' transparency, accountability, and accessibility. The Clinical Trials Registry-India (CTRI), which is housed at the ICMR's National Institute of Medical Statistics (NIMS, New Delhi), is a registry for clinical trials in India. Today, any investigator planning to conduct a trial involving human participants of any intervention, such as drugs, surgical procedures, preventive measures, lifestyle modifications, devices, educational or behavioural treatment, or rehabilitation strategies, as well as trials conducted under the auspices of the Ministry of AYUSH (http://indianmedicine.nic.in/), is required to register the trial in the registry. Trial registration entails making a public declaration and identifying trial Investigators, Sponsors, Interventions, Participant population, Trial site, and so on. For trial registration in the CTRI, Ethics approval and Ministry of AYUSH permission (if necessary) are required. Multi-country trials in which India participates that have been registered in an international registry are also expected to be registered in the CTRI. Details on Indian investigators, trial venues, Indian target sample size, and enrollment date are recorded. After registering a trial, investigators are expected to regularly update the trial status or other aspects as the case progresses. After registering a study, investigators are expected to keep the trial status or other aspects up to date regularly. All upgrades and modifications will be documented and made available to the public.

Patanjali Research Institute has registered two trials on intervention studies on COVID- 19 patients on Ayurvedic regimen on Clinical Trials Registry- India (CTRI), which has been approved and ensured that the research is complete, authenticated, and thus readily available data on research is made public. This improves transparency, accountability, and accessibility (Appendix 6.1).

6.5.1. IRB/IEC Ethics Committees

The IEC/IRB is an independent committee of medical, scientific, and non-scientific members who review, evaluate and approve proposed trial protocol to ensure the rights, safety, and well-being of all trial subjects. In addition, IEC also reviews and discusses essential documents relating to the trial and determines the impact the trial will have on the study population. Regardless of the status of regulatory bodies, the Institutional ethical committee is registered under the national body **Central Drugs Standard Control Organization** (**CDSCO**) to ensure that review procedures are standardized according to the global processes and national regulations. Patanjali Research Institute strictly follows these regulatory requirements for all the approvals of a new drug trial (Fig. **6.6**). Our recent IEC approval and CTRI registration documents procured for investigational drug Divya Swasari Coronil Kit are in Appendix 6.1.

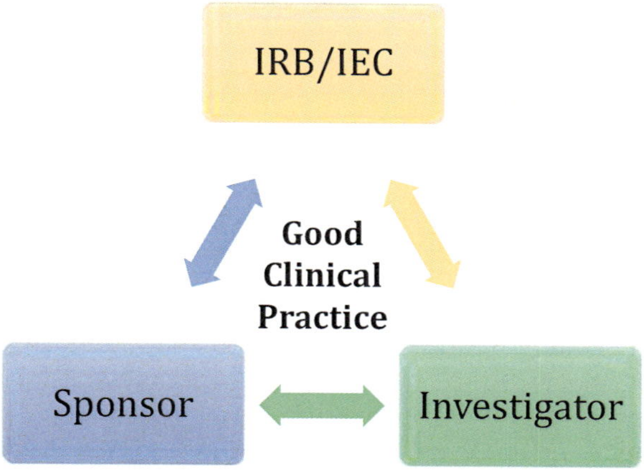

Fig. (6.6). Ethical Network.

Table 6.2. The legislation, regulations, and guidelines of India for Research involving drugs and devices.

Country	National Regulatory Body	Legislation	Regulation	Guidelines
India	Central Council for Research in Ayurvedic Sciences	Clinical Establishment (Registration and Regulation), Act 2010	-	General guidelines for safety/ toxicity Evaluation of Ayurvedic formulations. General guidelines for clinical evaluation of Ayurvedic interventions
	Indian Council of Medical Research (ICMR)	Drugs and Cosmetics Act, 1940 (2005)	Permission for a clinical trial: General Statutory Rules 63(E)	Ethical Guidelines for Biomedical Research on Human Participants Chapter IV: Drug trials
	Central Drugs Standard Control Organization (CDSCO)		Ethics Committee Registration: General Statutory Rules 72 (E)	

6.5.2. Clinical Trial Agreements and Contracts

All the clinical trial contracts and agreements should be signed by all the involved parties. The agreements or contracts should contain procedures with a line of communication and individuals' roles and responsibilities following standards of clinical trial regulations (Canada, 2018).

ICH-GCP E6 Section 1: A contract is a written, dated, and signed agreement between two parties that outlines any arrangements for delegation and distribution of tasks and obligations, as well as, if applicable, financial considerations. The protocol could form the basis of a contract.

A clinical trial agreement is signed between the sponsor and the legal body of the trial site that is in charge of the clinical trial's execution (Principal Investigator signs as third party or acknowledgement of agreement).

There are standard contract terms that should always be described in the CTA: parties to the agreement: roles and responsibilities of principal investigator involved in the clinical trial, study details as per mentioned or followed in accordance with the trial protocol, compliance of protocol and procedures as per ICH-GCP and identified standard operating procedures, timelines considers regarding the initiation and termination of trial with the submission of final status reports and interim analysis reports, data, confidentiality briefs on the right of access, removal, and delivery of data with details on data intellectual property, insurance/indemnity, termination, general consideration, payment details (Mihajlovic-Madzarevic, 2010).

6.6. PRE-REQUISITES FOR RESEARCH PROTOCOL

To draft a sound scientific design of a clinical research study, the clinical research team at the Patanjali Research Institute recommends that the following information should be included in a research protocol. It will help facilitate the application submission process and study approval from IRB/IEC and the regulatory check.

6.6.1. Protocol: General Information and Protocol Synopsis

- Protocol title, protocol number, protocol date, and protocol version.

- Name and address of the sponsor

- Name and title of principal investigator and co-investigator, address, and contact details of the site.

- Name and address (es) of laboratories/technical departments or other institutions involved (Table **6.3**).

Table 6.3. Protocol summary.

Protocol title	(The title of relevant IEC proposals (*e.g.*, applications for new studies, process amendments, research progress reports) must match the title of the protocol).
Objectives	Include study objectives: Primary and Secondary objectives
Outcome measures	Include primary/secondary outcome measures and the method by which outcome will be determined. Primary outcome: Secondary outcome:
Phase	Discuss the phase of the study (I, II, III, IV)
Number of sites	Single/Multi-centric
Study design	Open-label, Randomized, Masking, etc.
Study duration:	Allow time between the start of the study and the end of the study with a closeout.
No of participants /Participant's duration	Provide the total number of statistically verified sample sizes, and the time it will take to complete the study for each participant.
Description of study intervention:	Include the intervention's name, reference, dose, dosage form, mode of administration, and references, as well as the intervention's name.
Estimated time to complete the enrollment	Duration of project completion.
Principal Investigator (PI) and Co-Principal Investigator	Name, title, address, and telephone number of the PI, Co-PI, sponsors and study coordinators, investigator's affiliation

6.6.2. Background/Rationale

WHO (World Health Organization) recommends below-mentioned descriptors to be included as a significant rationale in the clinical trial study protocol;

• The rationale explains why the research is being conducted in light of current knowledge. It should include a well-documented statement of the need/issue that is the project's foundation, the cause of this problem, and potential solutions. It is analogous to the opening of a research paper in that it contextualizes the proposal.

• Summary of results from prior clinical studies and clinical data to date.

• Name and description of the investigational product, and in case of retrospective reviews, the justification for the chart and medical record reviews.

• Description of the population to be studied.

• The dosing regimen and treatment period are described and justified.

• A statement that the clinical investigation would be carried out in accordance with the protocol, SOPs, and international, state, and local regulations.

• Citations from references and data pertinent to the study also serve as a context for the trial.

In our protocol submission for initiating clinical trials for Divya Swasari Coronil Kit, we rigorously followed those objectives.

6.6.3. Clinical Trial Outcome/Endpoint

The clinical trial endpoint is an indicator that can be monitored in a participant or in a sample collected from the participant in order to assess the clinical trial's purpose. A trial's endpoint measure might be of several forms.

• Include a full description of the study's primary and secondary objectives, as well as its purpose, and clearly describe your research hypothesis or question.

• Give details of resources, skills, and experience to complete the study. The three-time points for assessment of trial participants are:

Screening: Prior to the start of a trial, participants are typically assessed to check their health state in respect to specified trial inclusion/exclusion criteria. Such screening values can be calculated using the results of laboratory test samples, for example.

Baseline: Once a person has met the inclusion/exclusion criteria, the trial endpoint measures' baseline value is recorded. The baseline is the point at which a clinical trial begins, just before any treatment is administered.

End of Trial: At the conclusion of the experiment, the trial endpoint measure is repeated. The research team frequently compares the baseline endpoint results to those at the end of the experiment to determine how well the treatment worked (Please view our graphic from our recent clinical trial for more information). (Fig. **6.7**).

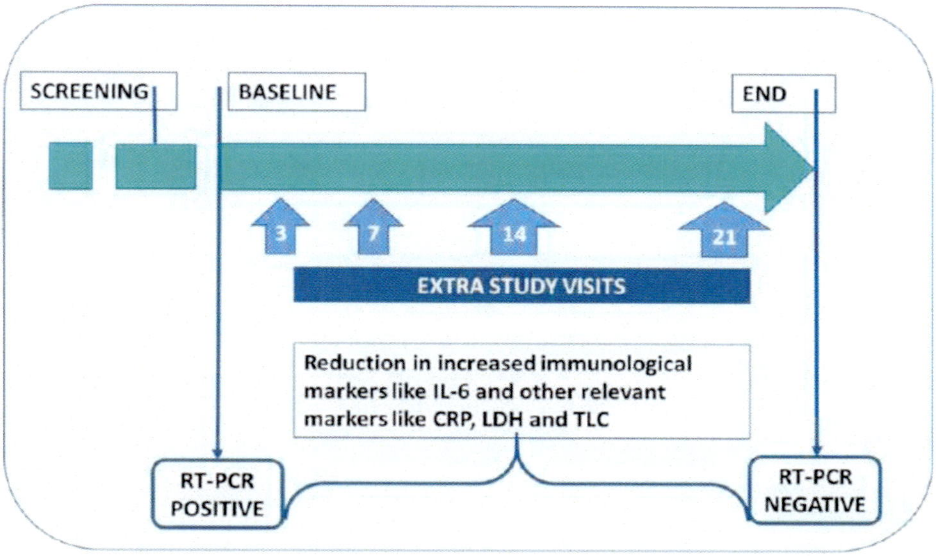

Fig. (6.7). Typical sequence of visits during a clinical trial: screening of participants and informing them about the trial details.

Participants, who agree to participate, attend a screening visit; eligible participants recorded under baseline criteria, an extra study site visit to assess changes in parameters, endpoint assessment, and adverse event recording, for instance.

At the conclusion of the experiment, the trial endpoint measure is repeated. The research team frequently compares the baseline endpoint results to those at the end of the experiment to determine how well the treatment worked (Please view our graphic from our recent clinical trial for more information).

Example: COVID-19, confirmatory phase, sample size: 150 patients (see the illustration on the following page (Fig. **6.8**)).

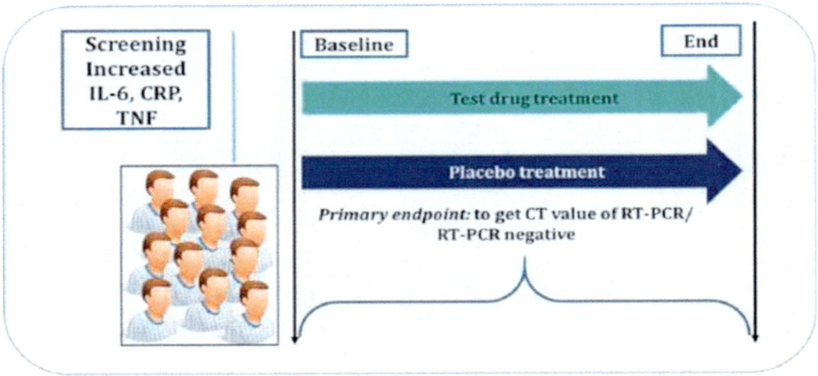

Fig. (6.8). Baseline and the primary endpoint.

• Objective: "Evaluate the effect of an Ayurvedic Regimen (Divya Swasari Coronil Kit) administered to nCoV-2 (COVID – 19) Patients."

• Trial design: Treatment, randomized, double-blind, placebo-control, parallel assignment, safety/efficacy trial.

• Primary Objectives

- To render the proportion of patients showing clinical improvement in mild, moderate, and severe COVID-19 cases.

- Mean duration (days) for clinical recovery.

• Secondary Objectives

- To restore health and reduction in serum viral load.

- Rate of patients with negative SARS-CoV2 on nasal or throat swab RT-PCR test.

- Reduction in increased immunological markers, like IL6, and other relevant markers, like quantitative C-reactive protein, serum lactate dehydrogenase, total leucocyte count.

- Drug-related side effects and toxicity, and tolerability.

- Health status improvement in quality of life through WHO QOL brief questionnaire (Fig. **6.9**).

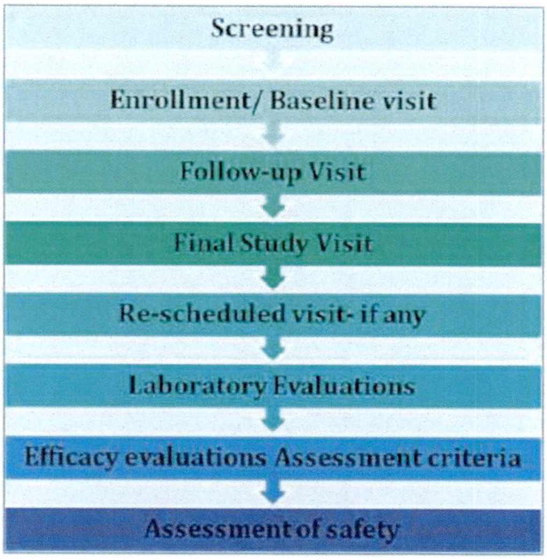

Fig. (6.9). Study procedures.

6.6.4. Clinical Trial Study Design

The following are the descriptions that should be included as study design in the protocol:

• Include the study design, *e.g.*, single, double-blind, observational, randomized, retrospective, etc. A schematic diagram of the study design would be helpful (See the example of CONSORT guidelines in Fig. (**6.10**)).

• An explanation of the study population (*e.g.*, healthy/sick, in-patient/out-patient).

• A discussion of the rationale for design features.

• Phase of the trial.

• Trial site description: single or multi-center

• The number of study groups/arms.

• Include the amount of dosage, dosing regimen of the drug, packaging, and labelling of the experimental drug.

• Describe how the research drug will be stored and distributed.

• Include the projected duration of the study and the subject's participation, and a description of the chronology and duration of all study periods.

• Discuss any follow-up visits.

• Describe when a subject's participation in the trial may be discontinued.

• Maintenance of randomization codes and confidentiality.

• Describe the potential risks and steps taken to minimize the risks.

• Identify possible benefits of the study.

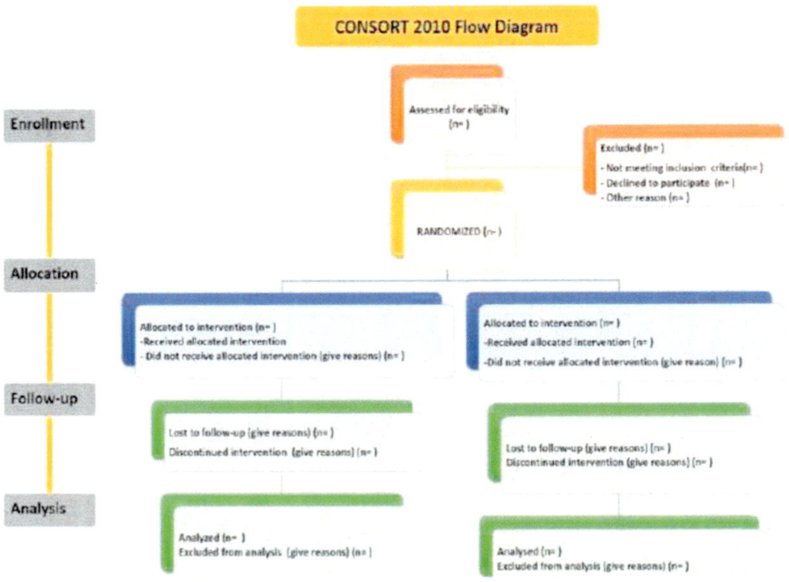

Fig. (6.10). Transparent reporting of trials.

6.6.5. Randomization

Randomization is a treatment allocation approach that involves the distribution of study subjects at random (*i.e.*, by chance). As a result, randomization gives all randomized units (*e.g.*, subjects) an equal and independent chance of being assigned to any of the treatment groups, and it is difficult to comprehend or predict which group a subject will be assigned to in advance (Lachin, Matts and Wei, 1988; Zheng and Zelen, 2010). Randomization and blinding are two key strategies that are typically used in conjunction during a clinical experiment. Randomization of trial participants lowers selection bias, which occurs when specific people are preferentially enrolled in one treatment group over another. (ref ICH E9).

6.6.5.1. Methods of Randomization

Simple Randomization: This is a procedure in which each individual in a population has an equal chance, similar to tossing a coin: Heads = Active, Tails = Placebo. External validity is provided by a simple random sample that is representative of a population. The acquired results may be deemed as near to reality as possible. Random number generators are widely available online, and they can also be generated using Microsoft Excel.

Block Randomization: This randomization approach aids in the achievement of the same sample size in two or more groups. Block randomization is accomplished by creating random permuted blocks (blocking). Possible treatment allocations within each block for two treatments options- A, B and Block size of 2 x 2= 4; AABB, BBAA, ABAB, BABA, ABBA, BAAB Block size depends on the number of treatments; it should be short enough to prevent imbalance, and long enough to prevent guessing allocation in trials.

Stratified Randomization: Imbalanced randomization reduces statistical power, but imbalanced prognostic factors are also more likely to be inefficient for predicting treatment effects. Pre-randomization stratification is done based on requirements such as age, gender, prognostic variables, and so on to avoid confounders among baseline characteristics (Suresh, 2011).

6.6.6. Blinding

The word blinding refers to the act of ensuring that those involved in a research project (participants, investigators, or assessors) are unaware of the treatment they are getting. In the conduct and interpretation of a clinical trial, blinding or masking is used to limit the occurrence of bias due to treatment or the evaluator/investigator who is carrying out the study. (Schulz and Grimes, 2002).

There are three different levels of blinding:

i. The term "single-blind" usually refers to the fact that one of the three groups of people is unaware of the intervention being used during the experiment.
ii. During a double-blind experiment, participants, investigators, and assessors are usually all uninformed of the intervention allocation.

iii. Triple blind usually indicates that the subjects, investigator, and data analyzer are all unaware of the treatment.

Most trials use double-blind randomization for the investigator and participants — for example, drugs are pre-packaged by a pharmacist in accordance with the randomization schedule. The investigational medicinal product supplied to the study/trial site is labelled only with a participant number and treatment period and looks identical (placebo) for all treatment groups. As a result, trial site investigators or personnel are uninformed of the specific therapy assigned to any given participant. During the trial planning stage, the randomization list is created and delivered to the person in charge of creating the test article. As a result, trial site investigators or personnel are uninformed of the specific therapy assigned to any given participant. During the trial planning stage, the randomization list is created and delivered to the person in charge of creating the test article.

Randomization should be undertaken by a third party/CRO (Clinical Research Organization) that is not involved in the study's conduct, monitoring of trial data, or patient recruitment. Except for the person responsible for manufacturing the trial medicines and the Data and Safety Monitoring Committee, the randomization list is kept confidential by all parties during and after the experiment (in case of adverse events). Generally, a computerized randomization code is generated by the designated person who will provide a password-protected study randomization code *via* a secure file transfer before the start of the study. A copy of the treatment code should be kept on hand at all times in case the code needs to be broken for a participant, for as by unblinding a sealed envelope or *via* an electronic telephone-based unblinding technique. We mandated the aforementioned randomization and blinding methods during the conduction of clinical trials, and the same can be found in our recent COVID-19 multicentric study (Fig. **6.11**).

6.6.7. Participants Inclusion and Exclusion Criteria:

- Subject's inclusion criteria.

6.6.7.1. Example:

- Willing to engage in and follow all study procedures for the duration of the trial term.
- According to the study protocol, age and gender are required.
- Clinical signs and symptoms correspond to the conventional diagnostic criteria of the specific illness condition being studied in a clinical trial.
- Laboratory parameters within a specific range.
    - Subject's exclusion criteria.

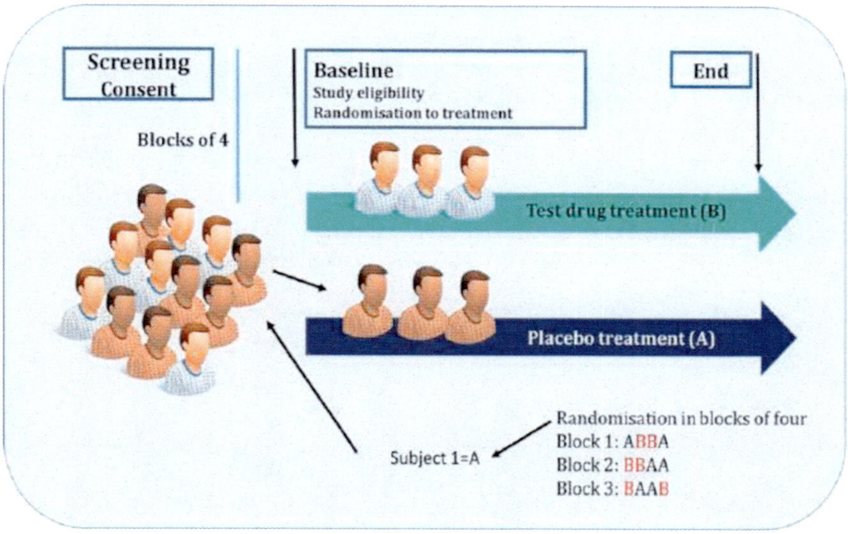

Fig. (6.11). Randomization of study participants is performed after informed consent and assessing baseline criteria. Example: Subject 1- following placebo treatment.

6.6.7.2. Example:

- Women of childbearing potential should not be regularly excluded from the study; nevertheless, pregnant women should be excluded if there is a compelling reason.
- A medical issue, laboratory finding, or physical exam finding that prevents participation (*e.g.*, vital signs outside of a certain range).
- Patients on any concurrent medications or any other AYUSH drugs.
- Anything that, in the opinion of the investigator, is a risk or precludes the participant's full compliance with or completion of the study.
- Enroll people from a variety of racial and ethnic backgrounds to guarantee that the advantages of the research study are dispersed fairly.
- Withdrawal Criteria: If a participant voluntarily withdraws, the Investigator must persuade him or her to complete an end-of-study evaluation.
- Participants may also choose to discontinue receiving the research intervention for any reason.

For instance, if any clinical adverse events (AE), laboratory abnormalities, concurrent illness, or other medical condition or circumstance develops, continuing participation in the study would not be in the participant's best interests.

- The participant meets any exclusion criteria (either newly developed or not previously recognized).

6.6.8. Collection of Adverse Events/SAE

With an in-depth understanding of the importance of drug safety in patient care and disease management, we follow a standard chronological method of adverse drug reaction reporting. From the time informed consent is obtained until the last appointment for the follow-up, the Investigator must monitor the patient's condition throughout the experiment.

The sources of adverse events cover:

- The patient's reaction to health-related queries (a basic non-leading query such as "How have you been feeling since your last day?")
- Symptoms reported by the patient on their own initiative.
- Investigations and examinations in which the findings are deemed clinically significant changes or anomalies by the investigator.
- Other information about the patient's health becomes available to the Investigator (*e.g.*, hospitalisation).

6.6.9. Recording of Adverse Events/SAE

- The investigator must record all adverse events in the Adverse Event Log provided in each patient's CRF with information about:
- Adverse event
- Date of onset (time can be recorded, if applicable)
- Intensity
- Causal relationship to Investigational drug
- Action taken regarding Investigational drug
- Other action taken
- Date and time of outcome
- Seriousness

According to the Indian Good Clinical Practice Guidelines, the investigator must notify the sponsor of any SAEs/AEs as soon as possible (within 24 hours). The investigator has a legal and ethical obligation to notify the IEC that approved the study protocol within seven days. The investigator will follow the regulatory procedures for reporting safety to the regulatory body, the Institutional Ethics Committee, and the co-investigators. All adverse events, whether connected to the experiment or not, must be listed, examined, and addressed in length in the final report at the conclusion of the trial. The investigator is responsible for the medical management of the adverse event, and the procedure for adverse event management, including an allocation of responsibilities, must be pre-defined in the protocol and submitted to the Institutional Ethics Committee. The sponsor shall supply the Investigator(s)/Institution with ADR/AE reporting forms (s). All serious and/or unexpected adverse medication responses should be reported to all parties involved (including the Ethics Committee and regulatory authorities) as soon as possible (Fig. **6.12**). Any unexpected SAE, as defined in the Indian GCP (Good Clinical Practice) Guidelines, that occurs during a clinical trial shall be disclosed to the licensing authority and the investigator(s) of other trial sites participating in the study within 14 calendar days by the sponsor.

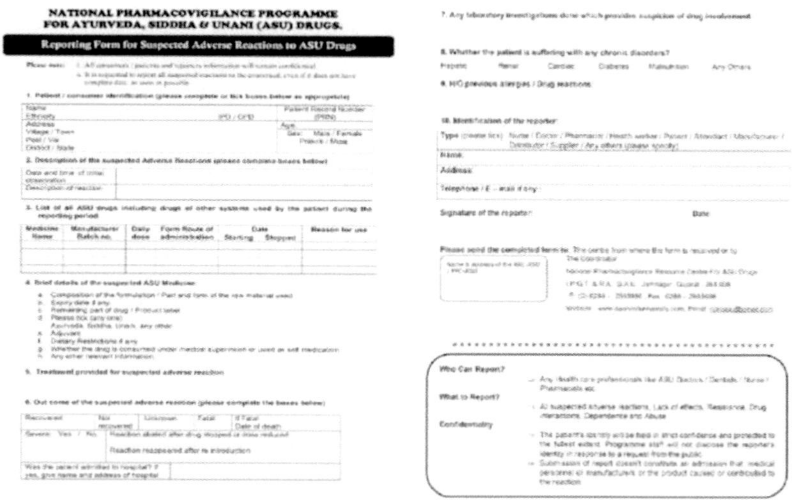
NATIONAL PHARMACOVIGILANCE PROGRAMME
FOR AYURVEDA, SIDDHA & UNANI (ASU) DRUGS.

Reporting Form for Suspected Adverse Reactions to ASU Drugs

Medicine Name	Manufacturer Batch no.	Daily dose	Form Route of administration	Date Starting	Date Stopped	Reason for use

Reaction reappeared after re introduction

Who Can Report?

What to Report?

Confidentiality

Fig. (6.12). Adverse Drug Reaction form for Ayurveda, Siddha, and Unani Drugs.

6.6.10. Investigational Product Management

- Provide a description of the experimental product as well as its packaging (stating all ingredients and the formulation of the investigational drug and any placebos used in the study).
- The precise dose needed for the study.
- Packaging and labelling of research substances.
- Treatment assignment method and subject identification code numbering system.
- Storage conditions for study substances.
- Accountability for experimental products: Describe procedures for receiving,

storing, dispensing, and returning investigational products to guarantee a comprehensive accounting of all investigational items received, dispensed, returned, or destroyed.
- Outline the policy and procedure for dealing with unused investigational goods.

The chemical characterization of the Ayurvedic regimen for the clinical trial has been briefed in the chemistry section of this booklet, which ensures that Patanjali Research Institute follows strict guidelines as per mandate under good clinical practices.

6.6.11. Data Analysis

Provide information about the statistical methodology that will be used, such as sample size, how the sample size was established, including assumptions used in making this determination, efficacy objectives (primary and secondary), and safety endpoints.

Statistical analysis: Give full details on how the data will be analyzed and presented, as well as a description of the statistical tests that will be used to examine the primary and secondary endpoints stated above. Describe the degree of significance, statistical tests to be performed, and techniques for missing data; method of data evaluation for treatment failures, noncompliance, and subject withdrawals; rationale and conditions for any planned interim analysis.

For example, Clinical symptoms, Subjective parameters, and Laboratory parameters will be subjected to Univariate and multivariate analysis using Statistical Package for Social Sciences (SPSS) 15.0 version with appropriate statistical methods. Unless specified otherwise, all statistical testing will be two-sided and will be performed using a significance level (α) of 0.05.

6.6.12. Risk and Benefit Balance

In the notion of risk and benefit analysis in clinical trials, the risk-benefit ratio and risk-benefit balance are equivalent terminologies. When a new chemical entity emerges from the drug discovery process, it is thoroughly evaluated in animals (pre-clinical research) and humans (clinical trials) to determine its risk-benefit profile. Efficacy data for a new chemical entity are gathered in pre-clinical research from specific animal models of the target disease among numerous species and strains of animals, whilst safety data are gathered from diverse toxicological studies. In the form of an investigational new drug application, the sponsor submits all information from pre-clinical trials to regulatory authorities.

The risk-benefit balance issue is handled judiciously by the ethical committee at the start of the clinical research. In general, while doing research that poses a greater than minimal risk of harm to participants, the investigator must show that the potential benefit clearly surpasses the risk of harm: "In medical research involving human subjects, the well-being of the individual research subject must take precedence over all other interests." "Medical research involving human subjects may be done only if the value of the goal outweighs the inherent risks and disadvantages on the research subjects." (Declaration of Helsinki).

It is the Ethical Committee's obligation to determine if a clinical study has an ethically acceptable risk-benefit balance, while potential participants must decide if it suits their interests and welfare or not. The Ethical Committee must ensure that the research is correctly conceived and conducted while also ensuring that participants are not being exposed to hazards that are unjustifiably or unnecessarily. The advantage is not strictly associated with the persons participating, but rather with the benefit to society, *i.e.*, discovering new knowledge and contributing to society's progression in terms of drug development. Both the risks of harm and the potential benefits of a clinical trial are largely dependent on the phase of the trial, the type of medicinal agent examined, the disease under testing, the current best treatment, and the standard of care offered. (Table **6.4**).

Table 6.4. Scientific evaluation of a Clinical Trial Protocol.

("Reviewing Clinical Trials: A Guide for the Ethics Committee," 2010) Any study protocol that has a few minor or substantial concerns might be suggested for adjustment and alteration as needed and then re-assessed. This is the list of content in the study protocol that demands special attention and evaluation.	
Major Attention	**Potential Questions**
Third-party review	Has the current version of the procedure been evaluated and formally accepted by any regulatory or scientific bodies? Has the procedure been evaluated by any other ECs?
Protocol development:	Are the identities of those involved in protocol development, as well as their qualifications and duties, provided?
Pre-clinical information:	What is the test article's safety and effectiveness profile?
Test article manufacturing:	Is the product made in accordance with GMP?
Study objective:	What is the scientific basis for the study?
Clinical rationale:	What are the predicted benefits of the test article in routine clinical care?
Study design – treatment:	What is the argument for using a placebo comparison rather than the best standard treatment?

(Table 6.4) cont.....

(“Reviewing Clinical Trials: A Guide for the Ethics Committee,” 2010) Any study protocol that has a few minor or substantial concerns might be suggested for adjustment and alteration as needed and then re-assessed. This is the list of content in the study protocol that demands special attention and evaluation.	
Major Attention	**Potential Questions**
Study design – outcome:	Is the research exploratory or confirmatory? Is the trial's primary outcome a clinical result or a surrogate result? Is the result of the most recent and valid internationally acknowledged outcome? Is the study utilizing the best available comparison groups for its intended purpose?
Study design – randomization:	Is the experiment using treatment group randomization? How will this be done if it is randomized?
Study design – blinding:	Is blinding used for the investigator, participants, and trial outcome evaluator? How is this ensured if blinding is used?
Study design – sample size:	Has a proper sample size calculation been made? Who calculated the sample size? What were the assumptions behind the sample size calculation?
Participant availability:	Are there enough participants available? What is the anticipated duration of patient recruitment? Are there other clinics or hospitals available to secure the anticipated sample sizes?
Resources:	Are enough financial and manpower resources available for the completion of the trial?

One of the benchmark trials carried out following the gazette notification, Ministry of AYUSH (F. No. L.11011/8/2020/AS) to address the test formulation as an intervention for the management of COVID-19 infection was carried out by Patanjali Research Institute, governed by Patanjali Foundation Trust after institutional ethical committee clearance and CTRI registration, validates the statement of “benefit strictly does not associate with the participants involved but more relates with the beneficence to the society.” The findings of the double-blind, randomized, placebo-controlled trial, in which we discovered a reduction in major inflammatory markers and in the meantime of recovery from COVID-19, formed cornerstone evidence during this critical time when medical science is battling to break the cycle of this tough and mutating virus.

6.6.13. Policy of Publication

If not handled in a separate agreement, a publication policy should be described in the protocol.

The International Committee of Medical Journal Editors (ICMJE) defines authorship as the following criteria:

- Significant contributions to the work's conception or design, or the acquisition, analysis, or interpretation of data for the work;
- Drafting the work or revising it for important intellectual content;
- Final approval of the version to be published;
- Agreement to be accountable for all aspects of the work and ensure that questions related to the accuracy or integrity of any part of the work are appropriately investigated and resolved.

6.7. ESSENTIAL TRIAL DOCUMENTS

The informed consent document is a summary of the trial prepared in layman's terms for the general public's understanding. According to section 4.810 of the ICH-GCP standards, the paper should include a brief purpose of the study as well as complete treatment protocols and events. The ICD is divided into two sections: (i) the patient/participant information sheet (PIS) and (ii) the informed consent form (ICF). The PIS contains information on known facts about the research relevant to involvement. This is followed by the ICF, in which the participant acknowledges that she or he has understood the material in the PIS and agrees to engage in the research. Before using trial site patients, the attached informed consent was approved by the IEC/IRB.

6.7.1. Documentation of Informed Consent Process

As stated in Principle 1 of the Nuremberg Code, "the voluntary consent of the human subject is essential." Each prospective participant should sign the informed consent form after going through an informed consent process of receiving information, understanding it, and voluntarily agreeing to participate in the research.

In case the patient/participant is incompetent (medically or legally) to give consent, the Legally Authorized Representative's (LAR) consent must be documented.

- The process of consent for an illiterate participant/LAR should be witnessed by an impartial literate witness who is not a relative of the participant and is unrelated to the conduct of research, such as other patients on the ward who are not in the study, social service department staff, and counsellors.

- The witness should be literate and able to read the participant information sheet and permission form as well as understand the participant's language.
- If the participant cannot sign due to any certain conditions, then a thumb impression must be obtained.
- The investigator who administers the consent must also sign and date the consent form.
- In the event of institutionalized individuals, authorization to perform the research should be sought from the director of that institution/department in addition to the individual/LAR agreement.
- In some situations, the partner/spouse may be required to grant further consent. The lead investigator must explain the risks and benefits to the possible participant and the legal representation, as well as allow ample time for the participant and family members to ask questions and discuss.
- The consent process should be documented in the participant source, including a summary of how consent was gained, the participant's level of comprehension, the start and end time of the consent procedure, and questions and answers provided to the participant (Box **1**).

Box 1: ICH GCP quote on Informed Consent of Trial Participants

ICH GCP and Informed Consent The essentials of informed consent are addressed in Section 4.8 Informed Consent of Trial Participants. In a nutshell, it states: "The Investigator should have the EC's written approval of the written informed consent document as well as any other written information to be presented to participants; any revised written informed consent document and written information should have the EC's approval prior to use; It should not include language that allows the participant to relinquish any legal rights or free the investigator, institution, or sponsor from liability for carelessness; and language used during the informed consent procedure should be as non-technical as possible; The written informed consent statement should be signed and personally dated by the participant, or their legally authorized agent, as well as whoever conducted the informed consent talk, before to participating in a trial."

6.7.2. Investigator Brochure

The investigator brochure contains a synopsis of information about the investigational novel product. The pamphlet contains information on preclinical studies and other clinical trials, with the goal of providing investigators with the information they need to manage the clinical study. The primary issues discussed in the investigator brochure are drug dose, delivery procedures, and medication safety monitoring.

6.8. OVERVIEW OF RCT CONDUCTED AT NIMS HOSPITAL, JAIPUR, RAJASTHAN

6.8.1. Objective

To evaluate the impact of traditional Indian ayurvedic treatment regimen on asymptomatic patients with COVID-19 infection.

6.8.2. Study Design

Treatment regimen developed on the principles of Ayurveda (traditional Indian medicinal system) was evaluated for efficacy through a randomized, placebo-controlled double-blind clinical trial on 100 patients in the COVID-19 ward at the Department of Medicine in National Institute of Medical Sciences and Research, Jaipur, India. The clinical trial was registered with the Clinical Trial Registry-India (CTRI) (CTRI No. CTRI/2020/05/025273). The protocol for the study was approved by the Institutional Ethical Committee (IEC) (Ref. No. NIMSUR/IEC/2020/036). Fig. (**6.13**) depicts a complete study strategy. The study was registered with Clinical Trial Registry-India (CTRI) (CTRI No. CTRI/2020/05/025273).

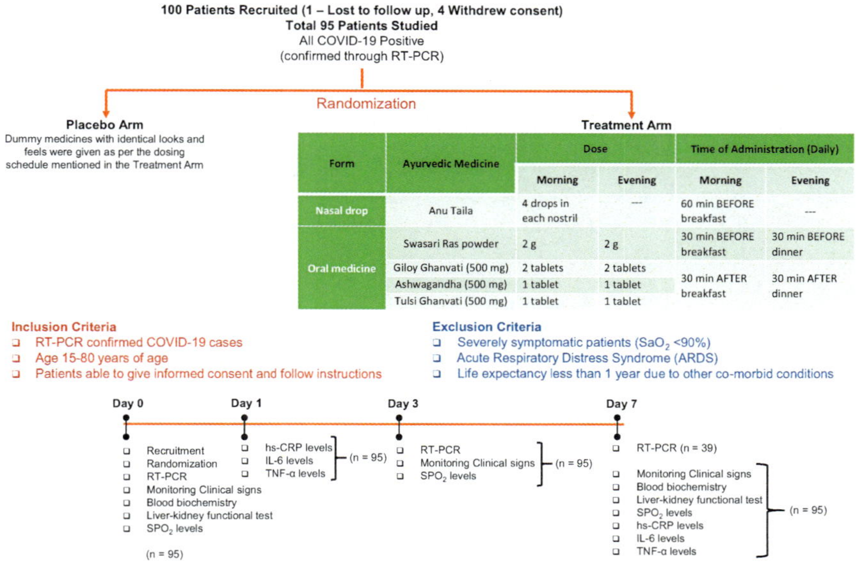

Fig. (6.13). A detailed study plan of Randomized Clinical Trial*[Courtesy:* (Devpura *et al.*, 2021)*; Under CCBY License].*

6.8.3. Interventions

The treatment comprises of 2 g/day each of Swasari Vati (twice before meals) and Giloy Ghanvati (twice after meals) and 1 g/day each of Ashwagandha and Tulsi Ghanvati (both twice after meals) were given to the patients in the treatment group for 7 days. They also received 4 drops of Anu taila in each nostril every day

1 h before breakfast.

6.8.4. Results

By day three, 71.1 and 50% of patients in the therapy and placebo groups, respectively, recovered. By day 7, the treatment group recovered completely, whereas the placebo group had only recovered 60%. The treatment group's average fold changes in serum levels of C-reactive protein (CRP), interleukin-6 (IL-6), and tumour necrosis factor (TNF-) were correspondingly 12.4, 2.5, and 20 times lower than the placebo group. There was a 40% absolute risk reduction in the treatment group, with the number needed to treat was noted to be three by day 7.

6.8.5. Conclusion

This randomized, placebo-controlled trial is the first of its kind and showed that Ashwagandha, Tulsi, Giloy, Swasari, and Anu Taila can promote faster clearance of the virus. Ayurvedic treatment can expedite virological clearance and concomitantly reduce the risk of viral dissemination. Reduced inflammation markers suggested less severity of COVID-19 infection in the treatment group. Overall, the ayurvedic treatment was associated with faster recovery from COVID-19 infection in asymptomatic and mildly symptomatic cases (Fig. **6.14**) (Devpura *et al.*, 2021).

6.9. EVIDENCE-BASED STUDY OF PATANJALI AGAINST COVID-19

COVID-19, an illness with influenza-like symptoms in mild to moderate cases and ARDS-like symptoms in severe cases, was first reported in December 2019 and quickly spread as a pandemic worldwide (Lu, 2020; Zhu, *et al.*, 2020). The human cost of COVID-19 alone is appalling, not to mention the socioeconomic and psychological constraints that have exacerbated the problem. In the absence of specific medicine or vaccination, the only way to cure COVID-19 is through supportive care and non-specific therapy. The World Health Organization (WHO) has recognized the lengthy history of Traditional Medicine (TM) and defines it as an inherited heritage of a repertoire of knowledge, skills, and practices local to a community. TMs might or might not be explicable; nevertheless, they are used in the maintenance and improvement of health. China has reported several studies claiming the efficacy of Traditional Chinese Medicine (TCM) against COVID-19. In fact, three formulations, Lianhua Qingwen Capsule, Jinhua Qinggan Granule, and Xuebijing Injection, have been made commercially available (Koe, 2020). These TCMs, however, are not without skepticism, as scientists outside of China believe that these treatments may not be acceptable, especially in the lack of solid clinical data (Cyranoski, 2020). As a result, efforts are being undertaken to make TCM evidence-based by examining and meta-analyzing entries from various databases (Li *et al.*, 2020), as well as case reports (Ling Ren, Zhang, and Wang, 20). However, such zealous efforts to investigate the potentials of Ayurveda, the 5000-year-old system of Traditional Indian Medicine (TIM), against COVID-19 are woefully lacking, even though the National Centre for Complementary and Integrative Health has reported the effectiveness of this system against diseases such as osteoarthritis and rheumatoid arthritis based on pilot studies and short-term clinical trials (*Ayurvedic medicine: In depth*, 2019). Interestingly, one of the classic texts of Ayurveda, Charak Samhita, acknowledges epidemic as *janapadodhwamsa vikara*, which literally translates into a disease that can demolish human habitations due to a high death rate. Ayurveda employs natural-source medicines (Rastogi, Pandey and Singh, 2020). During the 2006 Chikungunya Epidemic in India, Ayurvedic medications were employed to treat patients (Girija and Sivan, 2020). COVID-19 is also considered an epidemic in Ayurvedic medicine. However, except for a single case study report on Ayurvedic treatment alleviating COVID-19 illness, no current scientific data is showing a potential role for Ayurveda in preventing, treating, or curing COVID-19 illness (Girija and Sivan, 2020).

Although there are government guidelines on employing Ayurvedic treatments as immune boosters and pragmatic planning for Ayurvedic intervention against COVID-19, there is a dearth of evidence developed *via* planned clinical research on the curative impact of TIM on COVID-19 positive patients (Ministry AYUSH, 2020; Rastogi, Pandey and Singh, 2020).

Following the canonical teachings of Charak Samhita, Patanjali prepared a prescription combining natural medications to cure COVID-19 using Ayurvedic principles during the start of the COVID-19 epidemic. Among these are Divya Swasari Ras (DSR), Giloy Ghanvati (GG), Ashwagandha capsule (AC), Tulsi Ghanvati (TG), and Anu Taila (AT). Constituents of these medicines are listed in Table **6.5**.

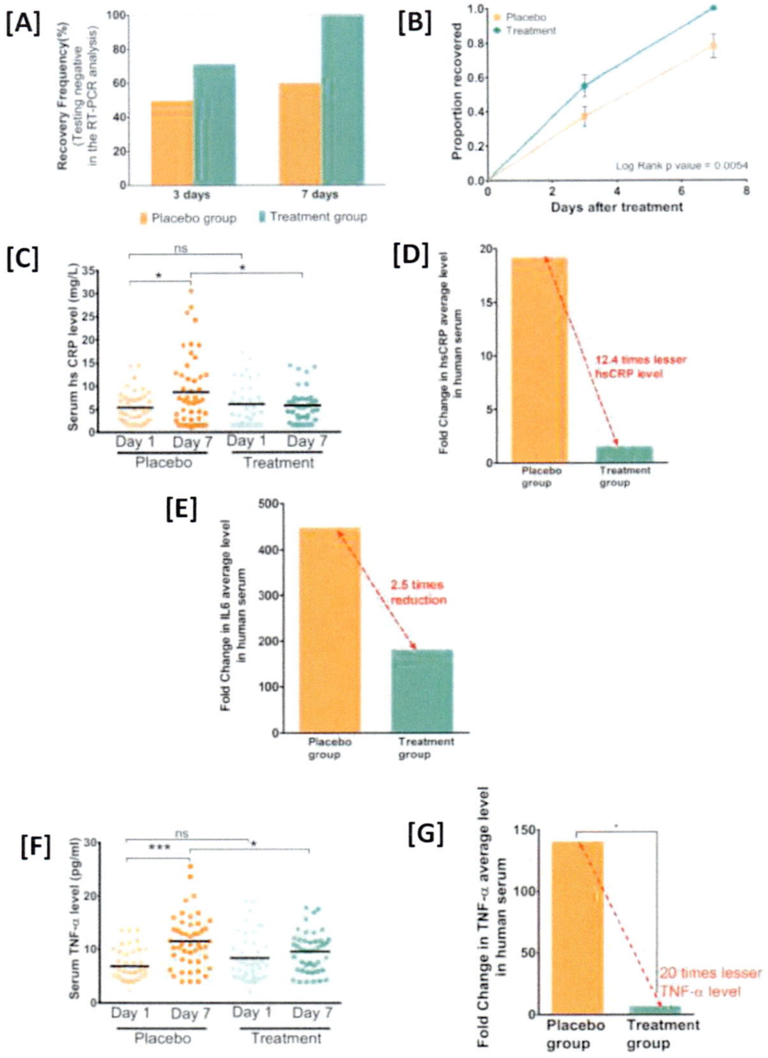

Fig. (6.14). Outcomes of the Randomized Clinical Trial. **[A]** Recovery efficiencies in the placebo and treatment arms after 3 and 7 days of treatments. **[B]** Kaplan Meier Curve showing the proportion of the recovery. **[C]** Serum levels of hs-CRP on day 1 and day 7 after commencement of treatment in placebo and treatment groups. Statistical significance of the differences between the two groups was determined by an unpaired two-tailed *t-test.* **[D]** Fold change in serum hs-CRP in placebo and treatment groups. **[E]** Fold changes in serum IL-6 levels in placebo and treatment groups. **[F]** Serum levels of TNF-α on day 1 and day 7 after commencement of the treatment in placebo and treatment groups. **[G]** Comparison between the fold changes in serum TNF-α in placebo and treatment groups. Statistical significance of the differences between the two groups was determined by an unpaired two-tailed *t-test. [Courtesy:* (Devpura *et al.*, 2021)*; Under CCBY License].*

Table 6.5. Constituents of the Ayurvedic medicines surveyed in this study.

Ayurvedic/ Natural Medicine	Scientific Name of the Constituent	Traditional Name (in Hindi)
	Glycyrrhiza glabra L.	Mulethi
	Syzygium aromaticum (L.) Merr. & L.M.Perry	Lavang
	Cinnamomum zeylanicum Blume	Dalchini
	Pistacia integerrima J.L. Stewart ex Brandis	Kakdasinghi
	Cressa cretica (L.)	Rudanti
	Zingiber officinale Rosco	Sounth
Divya Swasari Ras (DSR)*	*Piper nigrum* (L.)	Marich
	Piper longum (L.)	Chhoti pipal
	Anacycluspyrethrum (L.) Lag.	Akarkara
	Herbally processed calcined mica ash	Abhraka bhasma
	Herbally processed calcined shell of Pearl oyster ash	Mukta-shukti bhasma
	Herbally processed calcium-rich gypsum ash	Godanti bhasma
	Herbally processed calcined cowry shell ash of *Cypraea moneta* Linn.	Kapardak bhasma
Giloy Ghanvati (GG)#	*Tinospora cordifolia*	Gudduchi
Ashwagandha Capsule (AC) #	*Withania somnifera*	Ashwagandha
Tulsi Ghanvati (TG)	*Ocimum sanctum*	Tulsi

(Table 6.5) cont.....

Ayurvedic/ Natural Medicine	Scientific Name of the Constituent	Traditional Name (in Hindi)
Anu Taila (AT)[@]	*Leptadenia reticulate* (Retz.) Wight & Arn.	Jivanti
	Phyla nodiflora	Jala
	Cedrus deodara	Devdaru
	Cyperus scariosus	Nagarmotha
	Cinnamomum zeylanicum Blume	Dalchini
	Vetiveria zizanioides	Sevya (Useera)
	Hemidesmus indicus	Anantmool (Sareeva)
	Santalum album	Swet Chandan
	Berberis aristate	Daruhaldi
	Glycyrrhiza glabra L.	Mulethi
	Cyperus scariosus	Plawa
	Aquilaria agallocha	Agaru
	Asparagus racemosus	Satavari
	Boerhavia diffusa	Punarnava
	Aegle marmelos	Bel
	Nymphaea stellata Willd	Utpala
	Solanum indicum	Brahati
	Solanum virginianum	Kantkari
	Pluchea lanceolata	Surbhi (Rasna)
	Desmodium gangeticum	Salparni
	Uraria picta	Prashanprani
	Embelia ribes	Vidang
	Cinnamomum tamala	Tejpatra
	Amomum aromaticum Roxb.	Truti (Suksmaila)
	Vitex negundo	Renuka
	Mallotus philippensis	Kamala Kinjala
	Goat milk	Ajadugdha
	Sesame oil	Till taila

DSR is a poly herbo-mineral formulation; its ingredients have been confirmed through pre-clinical trials for the treatment of respiratory tract problems such as cough, bronchitis, asthma, rhinitis, and excessive mucus formation (Balkrishna, Solleti, Singh, *et al.*, 2020a). DSR has been employed in clinical settings in numerous Ayurvedic hospitals across India on thousands of patients as recorded in Patanjali Electronic Medical Records (PEMR).

GG is made up of natural chemicals isolated from *Tinospora cordifolia* (also known as 'Giloy' or 'Guduchi' in India). Computational studies have revealed that Tinocordiside, one of *T. cordifolia's* key phytocompounds, docks into the ACE2-RBD complex and hence has the potential to disrupt this crucial interaction (Balkrishna, Pokhrel, and Varshney, 2020). *T. cordifolia* is also a great immunostimulant and effective against a variety of microbiological diseases (Sinha *et al.*, 2004). Tinosporine, diterpenoid furano lactone, tinosporaside, cordifolide, cordifol, syringin, clerodane furano diterpene, tinosporidine, columbin, heptacosanol, -sitosterol, and tinosporide are other important phyto-components found in T. cordifolia. Tinosporin, a diterpenoid, has been specifically claimed for the treatment of viruses such as all subgroups of retroviruses (HIV-1, HIV-2), HTLV, and Herpes Simplex Virus (HSV) (Ghosh and Saha, 2012). Ashwagandha Capsules (AC) are made up of natural components derived from the Withania somnifera plant (traditionally, known as Ashwagandha in India). Docking and molecular dynamic modelling studies reveal that Withanone, one of the key phytochemicals present in W. somnifera, could also dock into the binding interface of the SARS-CoV-2 spike (S) protein receptor-binding domain (RBD) and host ACE2 receptor complex, similar to Tinocordiside. This damaged the ACE2-RBD connection, which is required for virus entry into the host cell (Balkrishna, Pokhrel, *et al.*, 2021). Withania somnifera had unique effects on the viral RBD and the host ACE2 receptor complex. Thousands of phytochemicals were screened *via* molecular docking against the ACE2-RBD complex, as well as molecular dynamics-based screens. According to some recent computational studies, Withanone can also target the SARS-CoV-2 major protease (M^{pro}) and the host transmembrane TMPRSS2 (Kumar, Dhanjal, Bhargava, *et al.*, 2020; Kumar, Dhanjal, Kaul, *et al.*, 2020). The epidemic spread from China to the rest of the world, causing high fatalities and disrupting regular life to the point where the world came to a halt. Severe Acute Respiratory Syndrome Coronavirus 2 (SARS-CoV-2/2019-nCoV) is the causative agent.

Ocimum sanctum (Tulsi) is an important part of India's spiritual and traditional living practices. These rituals and behaviours have begun to receive scientific support based on data (Cohen, 2014). *O. sanctum* has a wide range of health advantages, one of which is antiviral activity (Priyashree, Jha and Pattanayak, 2010; Mahajan, *et al.*, 2013). Phytochemicals abound in *O. sanctum*. We observed that Scutellarein, a naturally occurring flavone found in *O. sanctum,* docks into the active site of the SARS-CoV-2 coronavirus's RNA-dependent RNA Polymerase (RDRP) enzyme, which is required for viral replication.

COVID-19 infection causes nasal congestion, anosmia, runny nose, sneezing, fever, and overall weariness. Anu taila is used in Ayurvedic medicine for Nyasa procedures (nasal drops) to relieve inflammation in the nose canal and respiratory tract. The polyherbal components of Anu Taila, *Aegle marmelos* (Nicolis, *et al.*, 2009; Pynam and Dharmesh, 2018; Rajaram *et al.*, 2018), *Asparagus racemosus* (Gautam *et al.*, 2009; Kanwar and Bhutani, 2010; Tiwari, Dwivedi and Kakkar, 2014), *Aquilaria agallocha* (D. Yadav, *et al.*, 2013), *Cedrus deodara* (Gupta, Walia and Malan, 2011), *Cinnamomum verum* (Hagenlocher, *et al.*, 2013), *Coleus vettiveroides* (Ma, *et al.*, 2019), *Cyperus esculentus*, *Cyperus rotundus*, *Desmodium gangeticum* (A. K. Yadav, *et al.*, 2013), *Elettaria cardamomum*(Majdalawieh and Carr, 2010), *Embelia ribes* (Shirole, Shirole and Saraf, 2015), *Glycyrrhiza glabra* (Lee, *et al.*, 2019), *Nelumbo mucifera* (Zhao, *et al.*, 2010), *Ocimum sanctum* (Choudhury, *et al.*, 2014), and *Pogostemon cablin* (Yang, *et al.*, 2018) have anti-inflammatory potential and can ameliorate pro-inflammatory cytokines such as IL-1β, TNF-α, IFN-γ, IP-10, MCP-1, IL-4, and IL-8.

6.9.1. Study Population and Design of the Study

We collected, with an informed agreement, the medical data of 59 patients who opted to receive Allopathic treatment in combination with Ayurvedic medicines ('AlloAyur' group) (n = 41) or Ayurvedic medicines alone ('Ayur' group) (n = 18) between May and June 2020. These patients were admitted to various COVID-19 care centres in Ahmedabad, Gujarat, India, after being confirmed to be COVID-19 positive using RT-qPCR of nose swab samples. Data were obtained from health care centres' medical record departments (MRDs). Clinically, these individuals ranged from asymptomatic to mildly symptomatic. None of these patients had a history of international travel. The primary goal of this trial was to see if COVID-19 infection symptoms might be resolved.

6.9.2. Inclusion and Exclusion criteria

Patients between the ages of 10 and 80, of either gender, who were asymptomatic (had contact with a COVID-19 positive individual within the previous 72 hours but had not developed any symptoms) or had any of the clinical symptoms, namely fever, cough, headache, fatigue, sore throat, nasal congestion, dyspnea (mild to moderate), and who tested positive on RT-qPCR for nasopharyngeal swab tests, were included. Other vital inclusion criteria included the ability to provide informed consent and a willingness to follow-up on the fourteenth and thirtieth days after being found COVID-19 positive. Patients with severe symptoms, ARDS symptoms, or a life expectancy of less than one year as a result of other co-morbidities were excluded from the trial.

6.9.2.1. Study Completion Criteria

The participating patient had to have a normal body temperature and should not suffer from ailments, such as cough, headache, weariness, sore throat, nasal congestion, and dyspnea in order to be discharged from the care centre and the study.

6.9.2.2. Treatment

The allopathic drugs prescribed were based on the symptoms displayed by the patients. Azithromycin, as well as Vitamin C and anti-histamine, were administered as part of the Allopathic treatment regimen. The attending physician also provided acetaminophen on an emergency basis. Total daily doses of DSR and GG of 2 g each, and AC and TG of 1 g each, were delivered orally with lukewarm water. DSR was administered 30 minutes before meals, whereas the rest were administered 30 minutes after meals. 1 hour before breakfast, 4 drops of Anu taila were applied to each nostril. Table **6.6** shows a daily dosing schedule for Ayurvedic medicines. These drugs were made by Divya Pharmacy in accordance with a government license (Government of Uttarakhand, India) and were subjected to routine quality control (QC) analysis. Azithromycin, as well as Vitamin C and antihistamines, were supplied as part of the contemporary medical treatment regimen. Patients in either group were monitored for COVID-19 clinical signs.

Table 6.6. Recommended daily Ayurvedic treatment regime for COVID-19 infection.

Ayurvedic Medicine*	Daily Dose #		Time of Administration (Daily)	
	Morning	Evening	Morning	Evening
Divya Swasari Ras [1] (500 mg)	2 tablets	2 tablets	30 minutes before breakfast	30 minutes before dinner
Giloy Ghanvati [2] (500 mg)	2 tablets	2 tablets		
Ashwagandha Capsule [3] (500 mg)	1 capsule	1 capsule	30 minutes after breakfast	30 minutes after dinner
Tulsi Ghanvati [4] (500 mg)	1 tablet	1 tablet		
Anu Taila 5	4 drops in each nostril	---	60 minutes before breakfast	---

* Composition of these Ayurvedic medicines are provided in detail in Table **6.6**.

[#] Half dose for patients below 15 years

6.9.3. Patient Evaluation

The patients' clinical symptoms, such as body temperature, cough, weariness, headache, sore throat, nasal congestion, and dyspnea, were monitored at the start. Following that, these indicators were constantly checked, along with any other observable indicator of treatment side effects. At the start of the study, nasopharyngeal swabs were obtained for RT-qPCR.

6.9.4. Data Representation

The distribution of age and gender was recorded and graphed as bar graphs. Gender distribution throughout each age group is displayed as a proportional bar graph as a percentage of male/female of the total patients within that age group. Proportional bar graphs depict percent healing within and after 13 days in the Allopathic + Ayurvedic intervention and Ayurvedic intervention groups. The Kaplan-Meier curve was used to compare the recovery trends in both groups. Log-rank p-value was calculated using the in-built statistical software of GraphPad Prism 7.0.

6.9.5. Results

6.9.5.1. Freedom to Choose Treatment Options Affected the Sample Sizes of Study Groups

Although we aimed to include individuals who were asymptomatic to mildly symptomatic, the patient pool we reviewed only comprised mildly symptomatic individuals. We wanted to cover a broad age range, so we selected patients ranging in age from 10 to 80. As a result, the dosages were changed. Half of the dose listed in Table **6.6** was given to kids under the age of 15. Most significantly, we included patients who consented to return in 14 and 30 days. These follow-ups allowed for continuous surveillance of the patients for any indication of side effects. We eventually had 41 patients in the Allopathic + Ayurvedic intervention group and 18 in the Ayurvedic intervention group since the patient agreement was the primary modulator in the grouping. Fig. (**6.15**) depicts the inclusion and exclusion criteria, as well as the study plan.

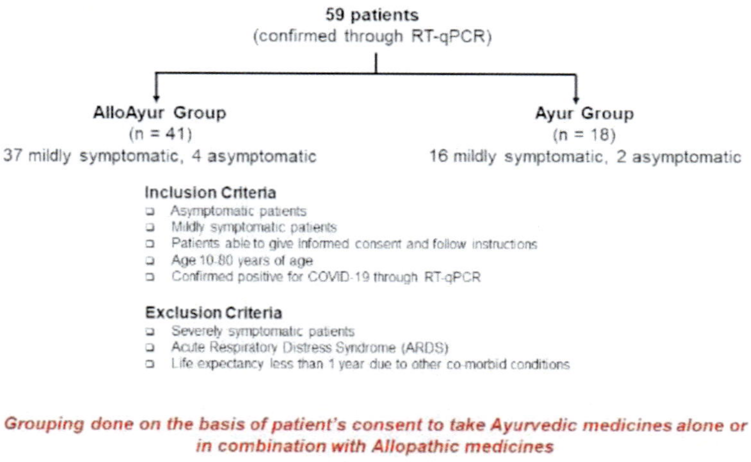

Fig. (6.15). The inclusion and exclusion criteria.

This was an observational study, and categorization was essentially a result of the patients' choice. We did not include any patients who had severe symptoms and needed breathing assistance. Such patients would be unable to give informed permission or make any decisions. We also excluded patients with acute respiratory distress syndrome (ARDS) for the same reasons as we did those with severe symptoms. We also omitted individuals with co-morbidities that resulted in life expectancies of less than a year in order to keep the readouts of our observations as clean and noise-free as feasible.

6.9.5.2. Age and Gender Distribution Among the Observed Patients

We examined the age distribution of the COVID-19 cases in this study and discovered that the vast majority (62.71 percent) were between the ages of 30 and 55, with 20.34 percent and 11.86 percent being between the ages of 18 and 30 and > 55, respectively. Only 5% of the incidences were found in patients under the age of 18. (Fig. **6.16 A**). There was no death reported. We discovered that male patients were more likely to become infected with COVID-19 in all age groups except those over 55, where the trend shifted, with 57.14 percent of patients being female and 42.86 percent being male. Males accounted for 66.67 percent of all patients under the age of 18 and between the ages of 18 and 30, while females accounted for 33.33 percent. Similarly, males made up 62.16 percent of overall patients aged 31 to 55, while females made up 37.84 percent (Fig. **6.16 B**). We examined the male-female ratios in the Allopathic + Ayurvedic intervention and Ayurvedic intervention groups to rule out the possibility of skewed gender distribution influencing our primary observation on the therapeutic benefits of natural medicines on COVID-19 infection. Within these groups, the gender distribution was similar; the Allopathic + Ayurvedic intervention group had 68 percent male and 32 percent female, while the Ayurvedic intervention group had 72 percent male and 28 percent female (Fig. **6.16 C**).

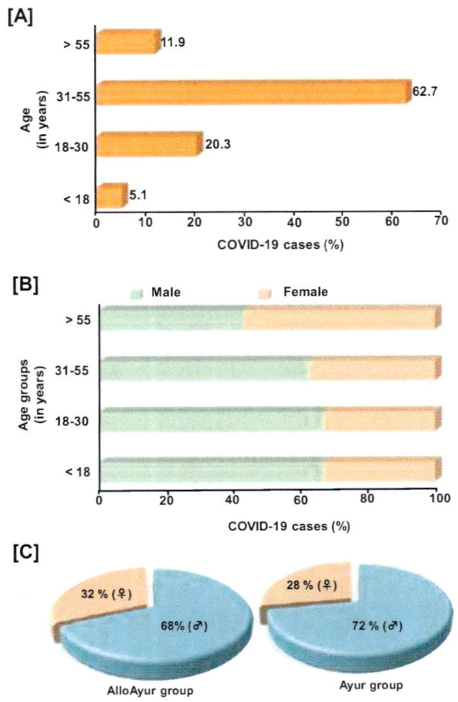

Fig. (6.16). Age and gender distribution of the study population [A, B, C].

6.9.5.3. Patients on Natural Medicines Alone Exhibited Faster Recovery

The most positive finding is the tendency of a faster recovery in the Ayurvedic intervention group, where patients were exclusively given natural medicines. 15 of the 18 patients in this group were cured within the first 13 days of treatment, resulting in an 83.33 percent recovery rate. In comparison, out of 41 patients in the Allopathic + Ayurvedic intervention group, 20 got cured, making a 48.78% recovery within the first 13 days (Fig. **6.17 A, B**).

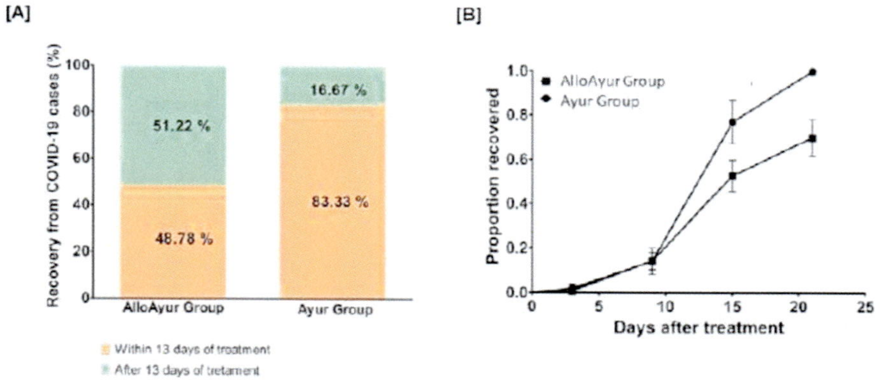

Fig. (6.17). Recovery comparison between Allopathic + Ayurvedic Intervention and Ayurvedic intervention group (A, B).

To statistically visualize the pattern of recovery efficiencies within the Allopathic + Ayurvedic Intervention and Ayurvedic Intervention groups, we generated a Kaplan Meier curve. We observed a similar percent of improvement in both groups after 9 days of treatment. By day 15 of the treatment, the recovery proportion was clearly higher in the Ayurvedic intervention group than in the Allo + Ayur intervention group. This fraction became 1 on day 21, suggesting 100 percent recovery by this time in the Ayurvedic intervention group. In contrast to the Ayurvedic intervention group, the Allopathic + Ayurvedic intervention group had a recovery proportion of 0.7 by day 21, indicating considerable lag. The computed Mantel-Cox log-rank p-value, on the other hand, was 0.0854, indicating that the difference between the two curves is not statistically significant. This is most likely due to the non-uniformity of the group sizes as well as the overall short sample size. Presumably, because the sample sizes of the groups were influenced by the bias of patients' treatment combination selection, a statistically significant remedial effect on COVID-19 infection in the Ayurvedic intervention group in comparison to the Allo+ Ayur intervention group could not be demonstrated. As a result, a larger sample size with uniform patient distribution is required to establish statistical significance and verify these findings. Nonetheless, the efficacy of natural medications against COVID-19 is clear from these findings.

We did not stop here; scientists at Patanjali Research Institute, with their relentless effort under the guidance of Swami Ramdev Ji and Acharya Balkrishna Ji, recently carried out Randomized, Placebo-Controlled Double-Blind, Clinical Trial on the Efficacy of an Ayurvedic Treatment Regime on Patients with COVID-19 Infection and the results from the treatment group with the herbal formulation were astounding, with 69 percent and 52 percent of patients recovered in the treatment and placebo groups, respectively, by day three. By day 7, the treatment group had recovered completely, whereas the placebo group had recovered only partially.

This study found that, when compared to Allopathic and Ayurvedic combined intervention, Ayurvedic treatment alone can reduce the time to symptomatic recovery in COVID-19 individuals who are asymptomatic or slightly symptomatic. This study also suggests that Ayurvedic medicine may be effective against COVID-19 infection. These discoveries have provided a ray of light to the society that has been devastated by COVID-19, as well as stating that phytochemicals found in Ashwagandha, Giloy, and Tulsi have the ability to combat COVID-19. Patanjali Research Institute has been unwavering in its efforts to make significant contributions to bolstering our capacities to deal with this epidemic.

CONCLUDING REMARKS

This chapter projects the technical requirements, protocols, and other regulatory fulfilments towards providing scientific authentication for traditional medicines. The two clinical studies shared here exemplify the appropriate satiation of these requirements.

CHAPTER 7

Public Health Research and Development

Abstract: This chapter essentially discusses the contribution of Patanjali Research Institute, Haridwar, in conducting research for human ailments in general and COVID-19 in particular. We strive to enhance the quality and understanding of healthcare and traditional medicine globally. We are committed to harnessing the power of Ayurvedic knowledge resources in order to discover, comprehend, and resolve unmet public health requirements. It can be assumed that by harnessing the power of Human Data Science, we can create new approaches to solving the world's most challenging health problems.

Keywords: Correlation matrix, Demographic variables, HR-QoL, Human Data Science, Public health, Psychosomatic study, TSQM.

7.1. BACKGROUND OF PUBLIC HEALTH

As a cutting-edge research institute, Patanjali works to enhance the quality and understanding of healthcare and traditional medicine globally. Patanjali Research Institute is dedicated to playing its part by pooling resources and expertise to find, comprehend, and resolve unmet public health issues. We think that by combining the power of scientific research with tried-and-true disease-prevention strategies, we can envision new ways to solve the world's most difficult health problems and improve people's lives.

From a precautionary perspective, public health highlights a complicated relationship between the state/country, its policies, and society, involving individuals and organizations (Fig. **7.1**).

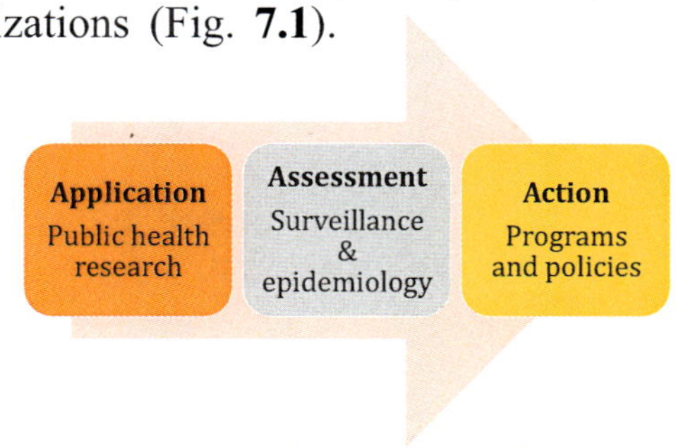

Fig. (7.1). Integrative approach in Public Health.

Ethics in public health apply to both practice and research, which rely on epidemiology and other methodologies to improve societal conditions and lead to healthier lives.

As a result, public health protects both individuals and the general public because the benefits and risks affect not only individuals but also communities, populations, and the environment. It is crucial to understand that public health interventions have the ability to reveal and exploit the vulnerabilities of communities and populations.

We firmly believe that public health research investigations and interventions should therefore be conducted through a process of ethical reflection, together with the establishment of appropriate protections, oversight procedures, and governance mechanisms. We have recently started interdisciplinary work to understand the impact of Ayurvedic formulations as health-related quality of life predictors and other critical health matters. We develop a research plan to understand health situations and assess health trends, as well as setting norms and standards.

7.2. PRINCIPLES OF PUBLIC HEALTH RESEARCH ETHICS

We strongly believe in the following concepts, which are outlined in the Indian Council of Medical Research (ICMR) guidelines for public health research:

- ***Principle of respect for autonomy, right, and dignity***: Autonomy is a Latin word that means 'self-rule,' which gives the right of decision, confidentiality, and respect to human dignity. Because the interests of an individual as part of Public Health Research and the society as a whole are related, the principle of respect for autonomy is relational. As a result, individual autonomy may not always be appropriate as a stand-alone concept for use at the community level. Understanding this superlative connection, all individuals should be respected in terms of individuality to outreach and inter-relate the whole community. The method to address this principle is the informed consent process which should be addressed from one to all in addition to ethical committee approval (Mathur and Swaminathan, 2018).
- ***Principle of beneficence:*** Public health research attempts to fulfil a moral commitment by maximizing social benefit over individual benefit while maintaining an adequate risk/benefit balance.
- ***Principle of non-maleficence:*** This principle entails a responsibility to minimize the harm caused to persons, such as the community, particularly in the collecting of data and the conduct of any interventional pharmacological trial.

As noted in the guidelines, "harm" can take the form of stigma, poverty, and discrimination that affect people living with diseases, such as HIV, mental illness, and the current COVID-19 pandemic, among other things. There should be safeguards in place to ensure secrecy, as there could be indirect harm to the individual, community, or relationships, as well as a loss of benefits. The ideas listed below may overlap with those in public health and research.

- Harm principle: If an individual's or a group's liberty is rightfully restrained against their choice to protect others, the choice should be supported by solid ethical reasons. In short, one person's actions should be limited to not damage other people.
- **Principle of least infringement**: When liberty is restricted, the least restrictive measures should be used as much as practicable.
- **Principle of proportionality**: This principle demands public health officials to reduce risks and improve public health. Individual autonomy and privacy should be weighed against the likelihood of public benefits and the necessity of such intervention. It must justify the costs borne by participants and communities.

- ***Principle of social justice***: As a result of this principle, public health authorities are required to reduce hazards and promote public health. Individual liberty and privacy should be weighed against the potential public good and the need for such intervention. It should justify the hardships that participants/communities have to bear.
- ***Principle of reciprocity:*** This principle urges public health officials to reduce dangers while also promoting public health. Individual autonomy and privacy should be weighed against potential public advantages and the necessity of such intervention. It must justify the costs borne by participants/communities.
- ***Principle of solidarity:*** Intra- and inter-dependence as a key principle based on sharing both the benefits, such as wealth and the burdens equally among members of communities, leading to solidarity for collective welfare or the common good, should be respected in public health research.
- ***Principle of accountability and transparency*:** The conduct of research must be open, honest, and transparent in every aspect. The outcomes should be made available to the general public.

According to the ICMR guidelines, PRI being a public health representative, strictly follow these guidelines. For conducting any research, these principles should be stringently followed during the conduction of any public health research (Mathur and Swaminathan, 2018) (Fig. **7.2**).

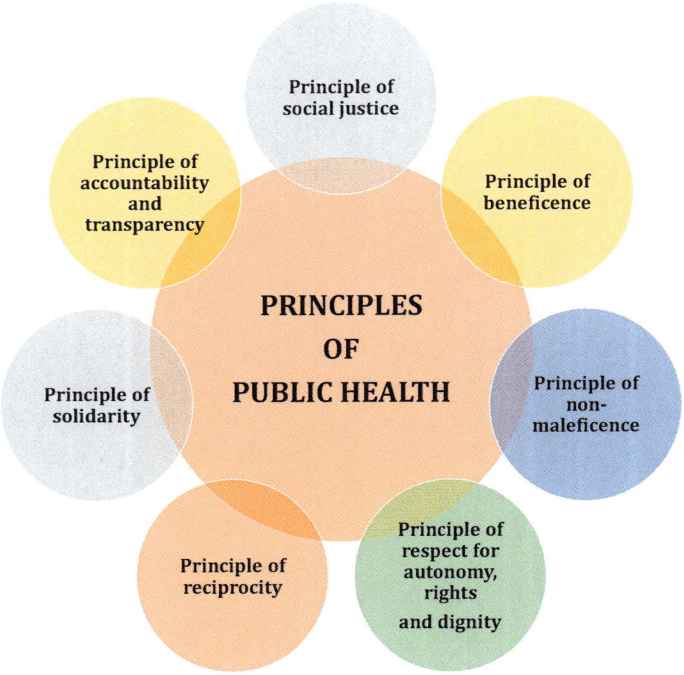

Fig. (7.2). Principles of Public Health.

7.3. OUR CLINICAL STUDIES BASED ON PATIENT-REPORTED OUTCOMES

7.3.1. Role of Traditional Ayurvedic Regime in Relation to Treatment Satisfaction on Psychological Health and Quality of Life

COVID-19 pandemic, first reported in Wuhan city of China, is posing as an unforeseen public health crisis that has plunged the world into a "crisis like no other," resulting in more than one million deaths and economic disruption among 213 countries and territories. The pandemic is well-known for being more than a medical emergency; it impacts individuals and society, causing disruption, worry, stress, stigma, and xenophobia (Jakovljevic, *et al.*, 2020). Individual conduct as a unit of society or a community has a significant impact on the dynamics of a pandemic, including the intensity, flow, and aftereffects. Because of the rapid human-to-human transmission of SARS-CoV-2, regional lockdowns were imposed to prevent the disease from spreading further (Lee, 2020). Isolation, social alienation, and the shutdown of educational institutions, employment, and entertainment venues forced people to stay at home in order to assist break the transmission cycle. The restrictive measures, on the other hand, have clearly had a negative impact on people's social and mental health (Jakovljevic, *et al.*, 2020). Several cross-sectional studies and longitudinal studies have demonstrated the psychological impact of COVID-19 (Serafini, *et al.*, 2020) to address this extremely contagious virus-induced psychopathology, such as depression and anxiety disorders in persons, in addition to jeopardizing our physical health and life.

The availability of the 'Divya Swasari Coronil Kit,' which combines Swasari Vati, Coronil Tablet, and Anu Taila, has been repurposed as a combined therapy regimen against the most severe and devastating COVID-19 pandemic. These drugs have been proven to inhibit inflammatory storm, modify immunological function, and reduce lung damage induced by SARS-CoV-2 in preclinical investigations. Preclinical research has proved to provide promising bi-directional control of symptoms associated with SARS-CoV-2 infection is possible.

In order to gain a better understanding of real-world experiences on treatment satisfaction and its impact on psychological health (PH) and quality of life (QoL), the Patanjali Research Institute undertook an exploratory, web-based survey under its scientific purview (Fig. **7.3**).

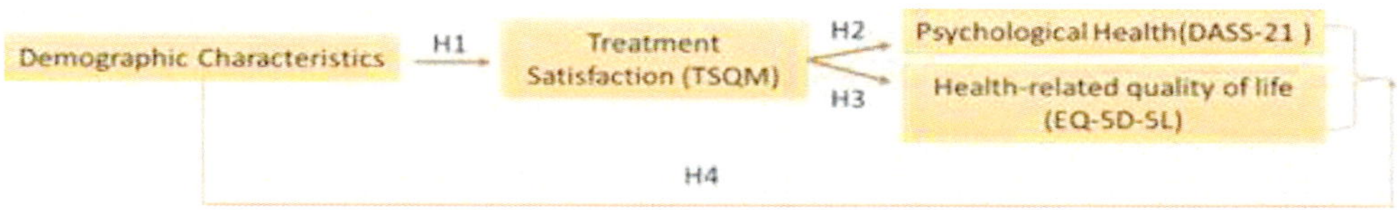

Fig. (7.3). Conceptual model: Each path is identified by the hypothesis with which it is associated.

Patients with age ≥18 years, access to the internet, willingness to participate in the online survey administered with Divya Swasari Coronil Kit were included in the study. The call of the invitation was sent to the participant *via* SMS and emails in both English (2nd widely spoken language) and Hindi language, according to the standard CHERRIES (checklist for reporting of Internet E-surveys) (most widely spoken language).

As the user clicks the shared link, they would be directed to a page with brief details of the survey and the required procedures. If they wish to continue, they were asked to click on the link to take them to the next page, which specifically mentions informed consent. After giving consent, one can proceed with the survey. They were then taken to the next section, which included questions based on sociodemographic details, clinical data from COVID-19, a psychological health questionnaire (DASS-21), a treatment satisfaction and confidence questionnaire (TSQM version 9), and a health-related quality of life questionnaire (EQ-5D-5L). The data were analyzed using IBM SPSS (Statistical Package for Social Sciences) statistics version 22.0. For demographic variables and clinical characteristics, descriptive statistics were used. The association between DASS-21, TSQM, HR-QoL, and demographic information was determined using Pearson correlation. Multicollinearity tests were conducted using factor analysis, and demographic variables and TSQM were investigated using multiple linear regression analysis. The p0.05 significance level was chosen.

7.4. RESULTS

7.4.1. Demographic Characteristics

Of the 680 invitations sent for participation in the survey, 259 patients were excluded (invitations returned undelivered and subjects who did not meet the assigned eligibility criteria. The remaining 421 individuals were included in the survey if they responded, were verified eligible based on the inclusion criteria, gave informed consent, completed the entire survey, and were using the Divya Swasari Coronil Kit. The total response rate was 53.9%. The detailed patient socio-demographics and clinical characteristics are shown in Table **7.1** and Fig. **(7.4)**.

Table 7.1. Demographic Characteristics and Frequencies at the Study's Commencement.

Socio-Demographic Details		
Variables		**N (%)**
Gender	Male	260 (70.8)
	Female	107 (29.2)
	Others	None
Age	18-28	118 (32.2)
	29-38	150 (40.9)
	39-48	67 (18.3)
	49-58	25 (6.8)
	59-68	7 (1.9)
Marital Status	Single	91 (24.8)
	Married	276 (75.2)
	Widowed/Separated/Divorced	None
Modified Kuppuswamy Scale		

(Table 7.1) cont.....

Socio-Demographic Details		
Education	Post-Graduation	194 (52.9)
	Graduate	144 (39.2)
	Intermediate	12 (3.3)
	High School	7 (1.9)
	Middle School	2 (0.5)
	Primary School	5 (1.4)
	Illiterate	3 (0.8)
Occupation	Professional	222 (60.5)
	Semi-professional	70 (19.1)
	Clerical/shop/farm	15 (4.1)
	Skilled	3 (0.8)
	Semi-skilled	10 (2.7)
	Unskilled	5 (1.4)
	Unemployed	42 (11.4)
Monthly Income	≥ ₹31,507	105 (28.6)
	₹15,754-₹31,506	124 (33.8)
	₹11,817-₹15,754	22 (6.0)
	₹7,878-₹11,816	2 (0.5)
	₹4,727-₹7,877	65 (17.7)
	₹1,590-₹4,726	5 (1.4)
	≤₹1,589	44 (12.0)
Socio-economic Cass	Upper class	117 (31.9)
	Upper middle	39 (10.6)
	Lower middle	172 (46.9)
	Upper lower	36 (9.8)
	Lower	3 (0.8)

(Table 7.1) cont.....

Socio-Demographic Details		
Physical Symptoms	Sore throat	Yes- 44 (12.3) No- 323 (88.0)
	Cold/Cough	Yes- 109 (29.7) No- 258 (70.3)
	Headache	Yes- 78 (21.3) No- 289 (78.7)
	Myalgia	Yes- 31 (8.4) No- 336 (91.6)
	Fever	Yes- 29 (7.9) No- 338 (92.1)
	Breathing Difficulty	Yes- 23 (6.3) No-344 (93.7)
	Fatigue	Yes-50 (13.6) No- 317 (86.4)

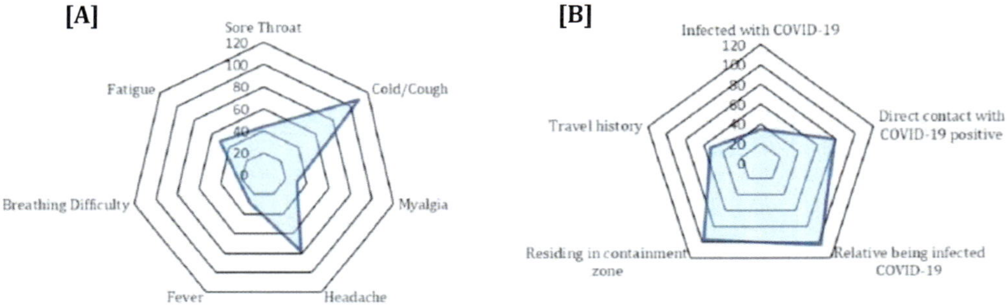

Fig. (7.4). [A] Self-reported clinical symptoms are presented; [B] The overall purpose of using the Divya Swasari Coronil Kit (N=367).

7.4.2. Correlation Matrix between Treatment Satisfaction, Quality of Life, Psychological Health, and Demographic Characteristic

Table **7.1** displays descriptive statistics (mean SD) for psychological health (depression, anxiety, and stress), health-related quality of life, treatment satisfaction from medication, demographic variables, and clinical characteristics, as well as correlation variables. Table **7.2** is the shaded part that comprises a statistically significant association ($P < 0.05$). Quality of life is favourably connected with effectiveness, convenience, and overall satisfaction, with all $r > 6.0$ at $p < 0.05$. All of the significant connections are highlighted. As a result, the Pearson analysis results confirm hypothesis 3, indicating that treatment satisfaction for medication has a positive impact on quality of life.

Table 7.2. Correlation matrix for the TSQM, HR-QoL, PH and demographic variables.

Predictor		M±SD	1	2	3	4	5	6	7	8	9	10	11
1	**Age**	33.61±9.47	1										
2	**Gender**	0.29±0.45	-.157**	1									
3	**Physical Symptoms**	1.12±1.69	.228**	-.059	1								
4	**Modified Kuppuswamy Scale**	21.85±3.94	.292**	-.124*	.113*	1							
5	**Depression**	7.40±3.89	-.017	-.005	.457**	.071	1						
6	**Anxiety**	8.24±4.26	-.073	.032	.468**	.062	.811**	1					
7	**Stress**	7.57±4.04	-.027	.048	.422**	.104*	.800**	.757**	1				
8	**Effectiveness**	88.49±7.41	.064	.010	.029	.117*	.013	-.033	.021	1			
9	**Convenience**	91.47±10.58	.047	-.070	.038	.295**	-.075	-.085	.067	.410**	1		
10	**Global Satisfaction**	83.86±8.57	.014	-.034	.207**	.141**	-.118*	-.113*	-.106*	.412**	.702**	1	
11	**EQ-5D-5L**	0.95±0.48	-.109*	.023	-.638**	-.024	-.547**	-.533**	-.509**	.643**	.551**	.590**	1

*. *Correlation is significant at the* $p<0.05$ *level (2-tailed).*
**. *Correlation is significant at the* $p<0.01$ *level (2-tailed).*

Global satisfaction is correlated with psychological health (depression, anxiety, and stress). This finding positively supports hypothesis 2 by demonstrating a negative correlation between treatment satisfaction and psychological illness. The lowest tolerance value in our analysis is 0.436, while the largest inflation variance is 2.345. Anxiety and depression have a correlation of 0.81, which is higher than 0.8. On all of the data, we performed a multi-collinearity test.

Multi-collinearity is often directly related to the variance of inflation. More specifically, if the tolerance value is more than 0.10 and the variance of inflation (VIF) is less than 10, multicollinearity is not an issue (de Carvalho, Draper, and Smith, 1981; Dowell, Hamilton and McLeod, 2000). The lowest tolerance value in our research is 0.436, while the maximum inflation variance is 2.345. As a result, in our datasheet, multi-collinearity does not appear to be a big issue. Physical symptoms are positively correlated with psychological health (depression, anxiety, and stress) but adversely associated with health-related quality of life, confirming hypothesis 4 that demographic characteristics are positively correlated with psychological health (Fig. **7.5**). The findings of the multiple linear regression analysis in Table 7.2 support hypothesis 1 to some extent. Marital status and socioeconomic class of socio-demographic characteristics are significantly associated with all domains of treatment satisfaction of medication (TSQM).

Physical symptoms are significantly correlated with global happiness and effectiveness, but age is significantly correlated with effectiveness (Table **7.3**).

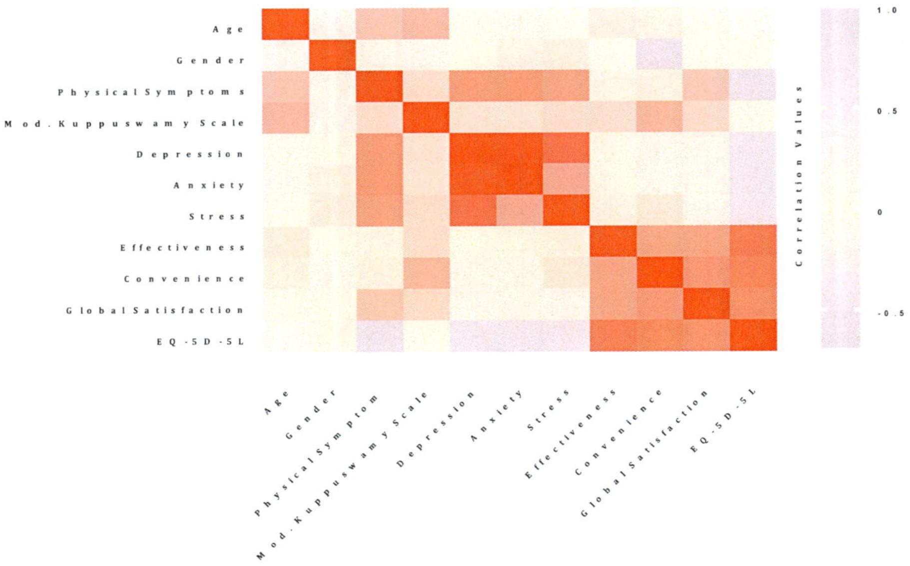

Fig. (7.5). Correlation matrix for the TSQM, HR-QoL, PH, and demographic factors is represented by a heat map.

Table 7.3. Multiple regression analysis between domains (demographic, physical symptoms, PH, and treatment satisfaction.

Predictor	Global Satisfaction		Effectiveness		Convenience	
	Coefficient β	SE	Coefficient β	SE	Coefficient β	SE
Age	0.05	0.071	0.18*	0.72	0.02	0.06
Gender	0.45	0.31	0.76	0.33	-0.99	0.17
Marital Status	0.76*	0.56	0.90**	0.59	-0.68*	0.40
Socio-Economic Class	0.32**	0.09	0.14	0.09	0.55**	0.08
Depression	0.13	0.01	-0.40	0.62	0.13	0.55
Anxiety	-0.21	0.481	-0.33	0.48	0.29	0.43

(Table 7.3) cont.....

Predictor	Global Satisfaction		Effectiveness		Convenience	
Stress	-0.14	0.53	-0.12	0.51	-0.21	0.45
Physical Symptoms	0.83*	0.47	0.80**	0.48	0.86*	0.42
HR-QoL	0.88	0.45	0.907	0.59	0.31	0.45
Adjusted R^2	0.284		0.224		0.228	
F	47.36***		31.8***		56.34***	

** Significant at the $p < 0.05$ level*
*** Significant at the $p < 0.01$ level*
****Significant at the $p < 0.001$ level*

In an Indian real-world scenario, our current study highlights patient-reported treatment experiences among patients on a preventative Ayurvedic regimen against COVID-19.

All dimensions of treatment satisfaction were positively correlated with quality of life, according to the results of our web-based survey. Furthermore, psychological health was negatively correlated with global satisfaction of the treatment satisfaction domain from the treatment regimen. From all the categories of socio-demographic details, marital status and socio-economic class correlated with treatment satisfaction from medication.

Treatment satisfaction from the Divya Swasari Coronil Kit has implications on psychological health, quality of life, and demographic characteristics, according to our pilot study. The afore-mentioned study is a unique study conducted in the field of public health addressing the importance of traditional medicines in this COVID-19 pandemic.

CONCLUDING REMARKS

With Ayurveda by our side, we stand in a hopeful position, as evident from the detailed narration provided in this book. We have been able to identify a remedy and validate it by understanding its mechanism of action as an antiviral and establishing its clinical efficacy through rigorous clinical studies conducted in compliance with strict regulatory guidelines. To the best of our knowledge, this journey has paved the path for developing an Ayurvedic formulation into medicines acceptable to modern practitioners. The journey has been an ardent one with enriching experience for us and others who are willing to learn and benefit from it. Believing truly that our experience can make a difference for those who sincerely wish to see Ayurveda as a paradigm of medical practice, we have summed up our journey pictorially in a schematic road map in Annexure I.

By sharing our experiences through this body of work, we wish to reach a wider readership and, in the process, hope to do our meagre part towards the well-being of mankind.

APPENDICES

Appendix - 2.1

सीएसआईआर - राष्ट्रीय विज्ञान संचार एवं सूचना स्रोत संस्थान
CSIR - National Institute of Science Communication and Information Resources
वैज्ञानिक एवं औद्योगिक अनुसंधान परिषद् Council of Scientific & Industrial Research
(विज्ञान एवं प्रौद्योगिकी मंत्रालय, भारत सरकार Ministry of Science & Technology, Govt. of India)

RAW MATERIALS HERBARIUM AND MUSEUM, DELHI (RHMD)

Authentication No.-NISCAIR/RHMD/Consult/2019/3453-54-179 27/06/2019

CERTIFICATE FOR CRUDE DRUG SAMPLE AUTHENTICATION

This is to certify that leaves sample of *Ocimum sanctum*, Tulsi Desi, received from Dr Suman Kumar Jha vide letter No. Nil, Dated 23rd April 2019 has been found **correct as dried aerial parts of *Ocimum tenuiflorum* L.** syn. *Ocimum sanctum* L. **which is commonly known as Tulsi Desi, Sacred Basil.** The identification has been done on the basis of macroscopic studies of the sample followed by detailed scrutiny of literature and matching the sample with authentic samples deposited in the Raw Material Herbarium and Museum, Delhi (RHMD).

Identification pertains to the quantity/quality of specimen/sample(s) received in RHMD. This certificate is not issued for any judicial purpose.

(Dr. Sunita Garg)
Emeritus Scientist, CSIR-NISCAIR
sunitag@niscair.res.in; sunita.niscair@gmail.com
Ph.: +91-11-25846001; 25846301, Ext. 263

(Mr. RS Jayasomu)
Chief Scientist
Head, RHMD

Dr Suman Kumar Jha
QMS (Advisor)
Divya Pharmacy
Unit A-1, Industrial Area
Haridwar-249401, Uttrakhand
Phone- 01334-265857

विज्ञान संचार भवन, डॉ. के.एस. कृष्णन मार्ग, पूसा, नई दिल्ली-110012, भारत Vigyan Sanchar Bhawan, Dr. K.S. Krishnan Marg, Pusa, New Delhi-110012, India
फोन Phone: +91-11-25846301, 25842303; 25846304-7, 25842990, 25840602, 25847544, 25847566 फैक्स Fax: +91-11-25847062, 25849949
Vigyan Suchna Bhawan, Satsang Vihar Marg, New Delhi-110067
फोन Phone: +91-11-26560141, 26560143, 26560165, फैक्स Fax: +91-11-25862228
ई-मेल E-mail: coa@niscair.res.in वेबसाइट Website: www.niscair.res.in

Appendix - 2.2

सीएसआईआर - राष्ट्रीय विज्ञान संचार एवं सूचना स्रोत संस्थान
CSIR - National Institute of Science Communication and Information Resources
वैज्ञानिक एवं औद्योगिक अनुसंधान परिषद् Council of Scientific & Industrial Research
(विज्ञान एवं प्रौद्योगिकी मंत्रालय, भारत सरकार Ministry of Science & Technology, Govt. of India)

RAW MATERIALS HERBARIUM AND MUSEUM, DELHI (RHMD)

Authentication No.-NISCAIR/RHMD/Consult/2019/3453-54-15 **11/06/2019**

CERTIFICATE FOR CRUDE DRUG SAMPLE AUTHENTICATION

This is to certify that roots sample of *Withania somnifera*, Ashwagandha, received from Dr Suman Kumar Jha vide letter No. Nil, Dated 23rd April 2019 **has been found correct roots of *Withania somnifera* (L.) Dunal which is commonly known as Ashwagandha, Punir, Asgandh.** The identification has been done on the basis of macroscopic studies of the sample followed by detailed scrutiny of literature and matching the sample with authentic samples deposited in the Raw Material Herbarium and Museum, Delhi (RHMD).

Identification pertains to the quantity/quality of specimen/sample(s) received in RHMD. This certificate is not issued for any judicial purpose.

(Dr. Sunita Garg)
Emeritus Scientist, CSIR-NISCAIR
sunitag@niscair.res.in; sunita.niscair@gmail.com
Ph.: +91-11-25846001; 25846301, Ext. 263

(Mr. RS Jayasomu)
Chief Scientist
Head, RHMD

Dr Suman Kumar Jha
QMS (Advisor)
Divya Pharmacy
Unit A-1, Industrial Area
Haridwar-249401, Uttrakhand
Phone- 01334-265857

Appendix - 2.3

सीएसआईआर - राष्ट्रीय विज्ञान संचार एवं सूचना स्रोत संस्थान
CSIR - National Institute of Science Communication and Information Resources
वैज्ञानिक एवं औद्योगिक अनुसंधान परिषद् Council of Scientific & Industrial Research
(विज्ञान एवं प्रौद्योगिकी मंत्रालय, भारत सरकार Ministry of Science & Technology, Govt. of India)

RAW MATERIALS HERBARIUM AND MUSEUM, DELHI (RHMD)

Authentication No.-NISCAIR/RHMD/Consult/2019/3453-54-63 18/06/2019

CERTIFICATE FOR CRUDE DRUG SAMPLE AUTHENTICATION

This is to certify that stem sample of *Tinospora cordifolia*, Giloy, received from Dr Suman Kumar Jha vide letter No. Nil, Dated 23rd April 2019 **has been found correct as stem pieces of *Tinospora cordifolia* (Willd.) Hook.f. & Thoms. which is commonly known as Giloy, Giloe, Guduchi, Amrita, Golancha.** The identification has been done on the basis of macroscopic studies of the sample followed by detailed scrutiny of literature and matching the sample with authentic samples deposited in the Raw Material Herbarium and Museum, Delhi (RHMD).

Identification pertains to the quantity/quality of specimen/sample(s) received in RHMD. This certificate is not issued for any judicial purpose.

(Dr. Sunita Garg)
Emeritus Scientist, CSIR-NISCAIR
sunitag@niscair.res.in; sunita.niscair@gmail.com
Ph.: +91-11-25846001; 25846301, Ext. 263

(Mr. RS Jayasomu)
Chief Scientist
Head, RHMD

Dr Suman Kumar Jha
QMS (Advisor)
Divya Pharmacy
Unit A-1, Industrial Area
Haridwar-249401, Uttrakhand
Phone- 01334-265857

विज्ञान संचार भवन, डॉ. के.एस. कृष्णन मार्ग, पूसा, नई दिल्ली-110012, भारत Vigyan Sanchar Bhawan, Dr. K.S. Krishnan Marg, Pusa, New Delhi-110012, India
फोन Phone: +91-11-25846301,25842303; 25846304-7, 25842990, 25840602, 25847544, 25847566 फैक्स Fax: +91-11-25847062, 25849949
विज्ञान सूचना भवन, 14, सत्संग विहार मार्ग, नई दिल्ली-110067 Vigyan Suchna Bhawan, Satsang Vihar Marg, New Delhi-110067
फोन Phone: +91-11-26560141, 26560143, 26560165; फैक्स Fax: +91-11-26862228
ई-मेल E-mail: coa@niscair.res.in वेबसाइट Website: www.niscair.res.in

Appendix - 2.4

प्रेषक,

लाइसेंसिंग अधिकारी,
आयुर्वेदिक एवं यूनानी सेवाएँ,
उत्तराखण्ड, देहरादून।

सेवा में

मैसर्स दिव्य फार्मेसी यूनिट– ।।,
खसरा नं0 210, 211 पतंजलि फूड एवं हर्बल पार्क,
लक्सर रोड, ग्राम पदार्था हरिद्वार।

संख्या–1371–72 / डी–431 / 2020–2021 दिनांक 12 जून,2020

विषय– अतिरिक्त योगों के निर्माणार्थ अनुमति दिये जाने के सम्बन्ध में।

महोदय,

उपर्युक्त विषयक आपके पत्रों दिनांक 06.06.2020 एवं दिनांक 09.06.2020 के साथ प्राप्त अतिरिक्त औषधियों की सूची इस पत्र के साथ संलग्न करते हुए निवेदन है कि औषधि नियंत्रक / लाइसेसिंग अधिकारी, आयुर्वेदिक एवं यूनानी सेवायें उत्तराखण्ड देहरादून द्वारा प्रेषित औषधि निर्माणार्थ लाईसेन्स संख्या **UK.AY-274/2013** में उल्लिखित शर्तों एवं प्रतिबन्धों के अधीन कमांक 01 से कमांक 03 पर अंकित स्वानुभूत योगों को आयुर्वेदिक औषधि के रूप में निर्माण करने की अनुमति प्रदान की जाती है।

1- DIVYA CORONIL TABLET
2- DIVYA SWASARI VATI 540MG
3- DIVYA SWASARI VATI 350MG

भवदीय

(डॉ0 यतेन्द्र सिंह रावत)
लाइसेंसिग अधिकारी

संख्या एवं दिनांक तदैव।

प्रतिलिपि–औषधि निरीक्षक / जिला आयुर्वेदिक एवं यूनानी अधिकारी हरिद्वार को उक्त की एक प्रति इस पत्र के साथ संलग्न करते हुए सूचनार्थ एवं आवश्यक कार्यवाही हेतु प्रेषित।

(डॉ0 यतेन्द्र सिंह रावत)
लाइसेंसिग अधिकारी

Appendix - 2.5

National Accreditation Board for
Testing and Calibration Laboratories

NABL

CERTIFICATE OF ACCREDITATION

CENTRAL LABORATORY, PATANJALI FOOD & HERBAL PARK PVT. LTD.

has been assessed and accredited in accordance with the standard

ISO/IEC 17025:2017

"General Requirements for the Competence of Testing & Calibration Laboratories"

for its facilities at

VILLAGE PADARTHA, LAKSAR-HARIDWAR ROAD, HARIDWAR, UTTRAKHAND, HARIDWAR, UTTARAKHAND, INDIA

in the field of

TESTING

Certificate Number: TC-7269

Issue Date: 18/05/2020 Valid Until: 17/05/2022

This certificate remains valid for the Scope of Accreditation as specified in the annexure subject to continued satisfactory compliance to the above standard & the relevant requirements of NABL.
(To see the scope of accreditation of this laboratory, you may also visit NABL website www.nabl-india.org)

ame of Legal Identity : Companies Act

Signed for and on behalf of NABL

N. Venkateswaran
Chief Executive Officer

Appendix - 2.6

AYUSH/Divya Pharmacy/Haridwar/03/2020-DC (Unit-II)
Government of India
Directorate General of Health Services
Central Drugs Standard Control Organization
(AYUSH Section)

FDA Bhawan, Kotla Road
New Delhi-110002
Dated:

0 5 NOV 2020

To,

M/s. Divya Pharmacy (Unit-II)
Khasra No.-210,211, Patanjali Food & Herbal Park,
Padartha, Laksar Road, Haridwar,
Uttarakhand -249404.

Subject: Issuance of additional Certificate of Pharmaceutical Product (CoPP) of Divya Coronil Tablet as per WHO Certification scheme – reg.

Sir,

With reference to your application on the subject matter, please find herewith the additional Certificate of Pharmaceutical Product (CoPP) dated of Divya Coronil Tablet as per WHO certification scheme.

Please acknowledge the receipt.

Yours faithfully,

(Dr. V.G. Somani)
Drugs Controller General (I)

Copy to: **1.** Dr. DC Katoch, Advisor (Ay.), AYUSH Bhawan, 'B' Block, GPO Complex, INA, New Delhi 110023.

2. Dr. Yatender Singh Rawat, Licensing Authority (Ay.), Directorate of Ayurvedic & Unani Services, Danda Lakhond, PO Gujradda, near IT Park, Sahastradhara Road, Dehradun, Uttarakhand.

Appendix - 2.7

Government of India
Directorate General of Health Services
Ministry of Health & Family Welfare
Central Drugs Standard Control Organization

Certificate of Pharmaceutical Product (Herbal)

(This certificate confirms to the format recommended by the World Health Organization.)			
No. of certificate		:	WHO-GMP/COPP/DP-II//70/2020
Exporting (certifying) country		:	INDIA
Importing (requesting) country		:	As per Appendix –I
1.	Name and dosage form of product	:	**DIVYA SWASARI VATI**
1.4	Active ingredient(s) and amount(s) per unit dose for complete composition including excipients sees attached.	:	As Per Appendix- II
1.2	Is this product licensed to be placed on the market for use in the exporting country?		YES
1.3	Is the product actually on the market in the exporting country? (If the answer to 1.2 is yes, continue with section 2A and omit section 2B.If the answer to 1.2 is no, Omit section 2A and continue section 2B)		YES
2. A.1	Number of product license And date of issue	:	Licence. Number: UK.AY-274/2013 Granted on 13.12.2013, Valid up to 12.12.2023
2. A.2	Product license holder (Name and address)	:	M/s Divya Pharmacy (Unit-II), Khasra No. 210-211, Patanjali Food & Herbal Park, Padartha, Laksar Road, Haridwar-249404, Uttarakhand, India.
2. A.3	Status of product-license holder*	:	A. The Applicant is the manufacturer.
2.A.3.1	For categories b and c the name and address of the Manufacturing producing the dosage form is:	:	Not Applicable
2. A.4	Is summary basis of Approval appended?	:	Not Applicable
2. A.5	Is the attached, officially approved product Information completed and consonant with the License?	:	YES
2.A.6	Application for certificate if different from license Holder: (Name and address)	:	Not Applicable
2.B.1	Applicant for certificate (name and address)	:	Not Applicable
2.B.2	Status of applicant* a / b / c	:	Not Applicable
2.B.2.1	For categories b and c the name and address of the Manufacturing producing the dosage form is*	:	Not Applicable
2.B.3	Why is marketing authorization lacking?	:	Not Applicable
2.B.4	Remark:	:	--------

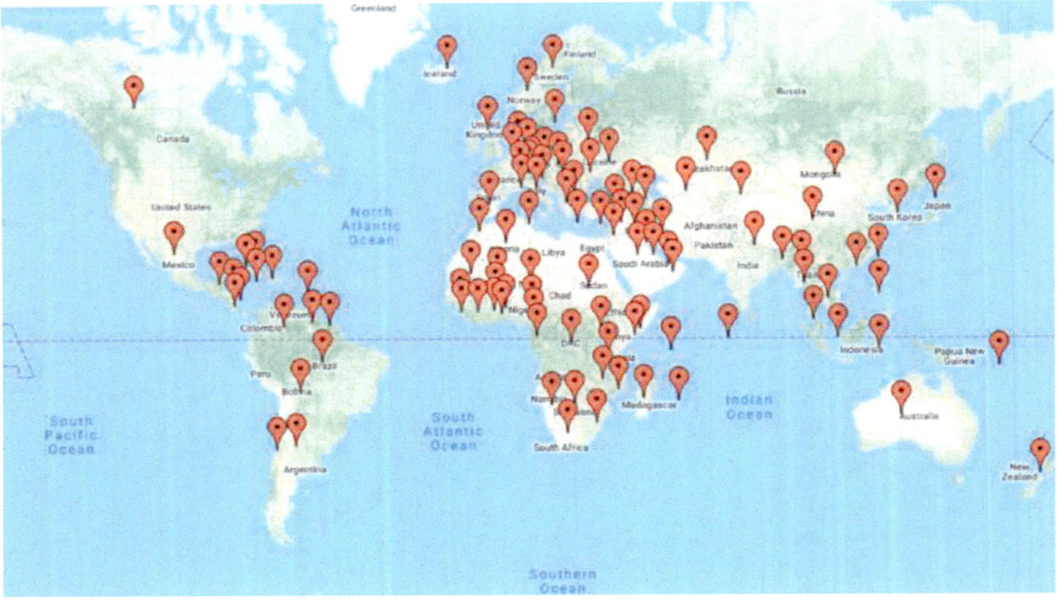
Greenland
Iceland
Finland
Sweden
Norway
Russia
Canada
United States
Mexico
North Atlantic Ocean
Libya
Egypt
Saudi Arabia
Afghanistan
Pakistan
India
China
Mongolia
South Korea
Japan
Chad
Sudan
Colombia
Peru
Bolivia
Argentina
South Pacific Ocean
South Atlantic Ocean
South Africa
Madagascar
Indian Ocean
Indonesia
Papua New Guinea
Australia
New Zealand
Southern Ocean

Appendix – 5.1

Pentagrit
Speed Unmatched

To whomsoever it may concern 11/6/2020

This is to confirm that Pentagrit will be offering facility for the study of, including, but not limited to Animal Modelling.

Study: "Humanized Zebrafish Covid-19 Spike Protein Model"

For:

Patanjali Research Foundation,

The study has been reviewed by us, in house Institutional Animal Ethics Committee and conducted with compliance to ICH harmonization principles for animal housing and handling.

IAEC Study No: 223/Go062020/IAEC.

Member of IAEC Pentagrit

1) Dr.Bibas Kar - Advisor at Center for Genetic Studies & Research, MMM
2) Dr. Kannan Maharajan – Professor, International Medical University, IMU
3) Dr. Charles Dhorni – National Institute of Nutrition, ICMR
4) Mr. Benin Joseph – Scientific Lead, Member of Institutional Animal Ethic Committee, Pentagrit
5) Ms. Kalaichitra – Registered Dietician & Scientific Director, Pentagrit
6) Mr.Preston Richard – Indian Patent Attorney
7) Mr.Manglesh – Group Leader for Animal and Environmental Welfare, CRY, NIZHAL

About Pentagrit: Pentagrit is a drug discovery and screening focused company with expertise in zebrafish and "Clinical Zebrafish Models". Academic research is a core principle in innovation towards being a scientific leader in drug discovery. Current services include ADMET, BABE and Animal Models for over 120 models offered to Academia/Research Institutions only as "Not for Profit" services. Currently for profit, clients include Biotech and Pharma outsourcing companies globally.

PENTAGRIT Chennai - 100

P.Kalaichitra
Scientific Director

Pentagrit Research

87, 3rd Floor Radhanagar First main road, Perumbakkum, Chennai-100
0091 8056156420, kal@pentagrit.com, www.pentagrit.com

Appendix – 6.1

NIMS UNIVERSITY RAJASTHAN, JAIPUR

Fully empowered & incorporated as a regular & full-fledged University under NIMS UNIVERSITY ACT, 2008 duly recognized by Government of India under the provisions of the Sections 2(f)and 22 of the UGC Act, 1956.

FACULTIES: • Medicine • Dentistry • Engineering • Advanced Engg. • Management • Law • Pharmacy • Nursing • Science & Technology • Physiotherapy • Allied Health Sciences • Fashion • Media • Mass Comm. • Hospitality • Aviation • Education • Library Sciences • Physical Education • Films & Television etc. • *multi-specialty 1130-bedded tertiary level Hospital on campus*

INSTITUTIONAL ETHICS COMMITTEE
NIMS UNIVERSITY RAJASTHAN, JAIPUR (INDIA)

Ref. No.: NIMSUR/IEC/2020/036 Date: 04th May, 2020

To

Name: **Prof. (Dr.) Ganpat Devpura**

Department of **Medicine**

Sub: **IEC (Institutional Ethics Committee) Approval for research project**

Institutional Ethics Committee had reviewed and discussed the research project titled **"Impact of Indian traditional Ayurvedic treatment regime for nCoV-2 (COVID-19)."** After review and discussion, members decided to accord ethical clearance and allowed the study to be undertaken at National Institute of Medical Sciences and Research, Jaipur (NIMS University Rajasthan, Jaipur)

This approval is valid till the completion of the study, please inform us in case of any serious event observed during the conduct of the study.

From

Member Secretary
Institutional Ethics Committee,
NIMS University Rajasthan, Jaipur

FULL DETAILS (Read-only) -> Click Here to Create PDF for Current Dataset of Trial

CTRI Number	**CTRI/2020/05/025273** [Registered on: 20/05/2020] **Trial Registered Prospectively**
Last Modified On:	20/05/2020
Post Graduate Thesis	No
Type of Trial	Interventional
Type of Study	Ayurveda
Study Design	Randomized, Parallel Group, Placebo Controlled Trial
Public Title of Study	Impact of effect of Ayurvedic treatment on novel Corona virus disease
Scientific Title of Study	Impact of Indian traditional Ayurvedic treatment regime for nCoV-2 (COVID-19)
Trial Acronym	

Secondary IDs if Any

Secondary ID	Identifier
NIL	NIL

Details of Principal Investigator or overall Trial Coordinator (multi-center study)

Name	Dr Ganpat Devpura
Designation	Professor Medicine
Affiliation	National Institute of Medical Sciences
Address	Professor Department of Medicine National Institute of Medical Sciences and Research, Jaipur India 303121 NH 11 C Jaipur Delhi Highway Nims University Campus Jaipur Rajasthan India Jaipur RAJASTHAN 303121 India
Phone	9829069669
Fax	
Email	gdevpura@yahoo.co.in

Details of Contact Person Scientific Query

Name	Dr Abhishek Sharma
Designation	Assistant Professor Medicine
Affiliation	National Institute of Medical Sciences
Address	Professor Department of Medicine National Institute of Medical Sciences and Research, Jaipur India 303121 NH 11 C Jaipur Delhi Highway Nims University Campus Jaipur Rajasthan India Jaipur RAJASTHAN 302021 India
Phone	9828816135
Fax	
Email	dr.abhisheksharma1987@gmail.com

CLINICAL TRIALS REGISTRY - INDIA
ICMR - National Institute of Medical Statistics

PDF of Trial
CTRI Website URL - http://ctri.nic.in

Clinical Trial Details (PDF Generation Date :- Thu, 24 Sep 2020 07:14:13 GMT)

CTRI Number	CTRI/2020/09/027882 [Registered on: 17/09/2020] - **Trial Registered Prospectively**
Last Modified On	17/09/2020
Post Graduate Thesis	No
Type of Trial	Interventional
Type of Study	Drug
Study Design	Randomized, Parallel Group, Placebo Controlled Trial
Public Title of Study	A Clinical Trial to Evaluate the effect of an Ayurvedic Regimen administered in (COVID – 19) Patients
Scientific Title of Study	A Randomized, Double-blind, Placebo-controlled Study to Evaluate the effect of an Ayurvedic Regimen administered in nCoV-2 (COVID – 19) Patients

Secondary IDs if Any

Secondary ID	Identifier
NIL	NIL

Details of Principal Investigator or overall Trial Coordinator (multi-center study)

Details of Principal Investigator	
Name	Dr Shirobhi Sharma
Designation	Assistant Professor,Department of Medicine
Affiliation	Subharti Medical College and Hospital
Address	Subharti Medical College and Hospital, Subhartipuram, NH 58, Meerut bypass (Delhi Haridwar Road) Meerut UTTAR PRADESH 250005 India
Phone	9456206192
Fax	
Email	shirobhisharma@yahoo.in

Details Contact Person (Scientific Query)

Details Contact Person (Scientific Query)	
Name	Dr Shirobhi Sharma
Designation	Assistant Professor,Department of Medicine
Affiliation	Subharti Medical College and Hospital
Address	Subharti Medical College and Hospital, Subhartipuram, NH 58, Meerut bypass (Delhi Haridwar Road) Meerut UTTAR PRADESH 250005 India
Phone	9456206192
Fax	
Email	shirobhisharma@yahoo.in

Details Contact Person (Public Query)

Details Contact Person (Public Query)	
Name	Dr Gaurav Kapil
Designation	Assistant Professor,Department of Pharmacology
Affiliation	Subharti Medical College and Hospital
Address	Subharti Medical College and Hospital, Subhartipuram, NH 58, Meerut bypass (Delhi Haridwar Road) Meerut UTTAR PRADESH 250005 India

Appendix – 6.2

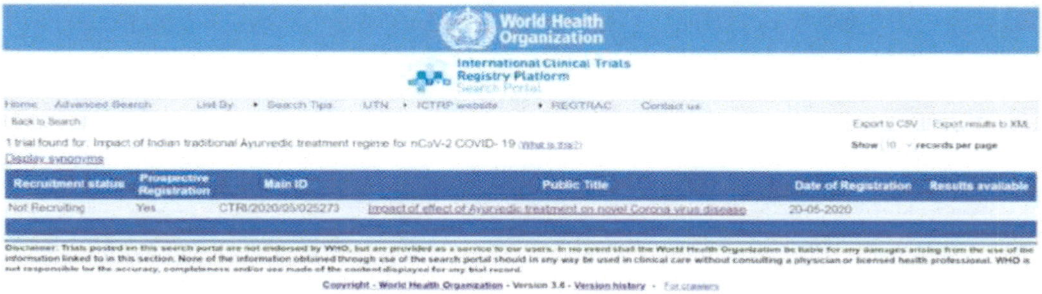
World Health Organization

International Clinical Trials Registry Platform
Search Portal

Home Advanced Search List By • Search Tips UTN • ICTRP website • REGTRAC Contact us

Back to Search

Export to CSV Export results to XML

1 trial found for: Impact of Indian traditional Ayurvedic treatment regime for nCoV-2 COVID- 19 (What is this?)

Display synonyms

Show 10 records per page

Recruitment status	Prospective Registration	Main ID	Public Title	Date of Registration	Results available
Not Recruiting	Yes	CTRI/2020/05/025273	Impact of effect of Ayurvedic treatment on novel Corona virus disease	20-05-2020	

Disclaimer: Trials posted on this search portal are not endorsed by WHO, but are provided as a service to our users. In no event shall the World Health Organization be liable for any damages arising from the use of the information linked to in this section. None of the information obtained through use of the search portal should in any way be used in clinical care without consulting a physician or licensed health professional. WHO is not responsible for the accuracy, completeness and/or use made of the content displayed for any trial record.

Copyright - World Health Organization - Version 3.6 - Version history - For crawlers

Snapshot from World Health Organization-International Clinical Trial Registry Platform exhibiting global accreditation of our Randomized Clinical Trial conducted for Ayurvedic medicines against COVID-19 positive patients

Bibliography

Abd El Motteleb D.M., Selim S.A., Mohamed A.M.. Differential effects of eugenol against hepatic inflammation and overall damage induced by ischemia/re-perfusion injury., *J. Immunotoxicol.*. **2014;** 11(3): 238-245.
[http://dx.doi.org/10.3109/1547691X.2013.832444] [PMID: 24099633]

Abu-Arafeh A., Andrews P.J.D.. Conducting feasibility studies in clinical trials are an investment to ensure a good study., *Resuscitation.* **2016;** 104: A1-A2.
[http://dx.doi.org/10.1016/j.resuscitation.2016.04.015] [PMID: 27155545]

Adedeji A.O., Severson W., Jonsson C., Singh K., Weiss S.R., Sarafianos S.G.. Novel inhibitors of severe acute respiratory syndrome coronavirus entry that act by three distinct mechanisms., *J. Virol.*. **2013;** 87(14): 8017-8028.
[http://dx.doi.org/10.1128/JVI.00998-13] [PMID: 23678171]

Adusumalli S., Madan Ranjit P., Sankaranarayan Harish M.. Antiasthmatic activity of aqueous extract of Pistacia Integerrima galls., *Int. J. Pharm. Pharm. Sci.*. **2013;** 5 Suppl. 2: 116-121.

Agarwal R., Diwanay S., Patki P., Patwardhan B.. Studies on immunomodulatory activity of Withania somnifera (Ashwagandha) extracts in experimental immune inflammation., *J. Ethnopharmacol.*. **1999;** 67(1): 27-35.
[http://dx.doi.org/10.1016/S0378-8741(99)00065-3] [PMID: 10616957]

Ahui M.L.B., Champy P., Ramadan A., Pham Van L., Araujo L., Brou André K., Diem S., Damotte D., Kati-Coulibaly S., Offoumou M.A., Dy M., Thieblemont N., Herbelin A.. Ginger prevents Th2-mediated immune responses in a mouse model of airway inflammation., *Int. Immunopharmacol.*. **2008;** 8(12): 1626-1632.
[http://dx.doi.org/10.1016/j.intimp.2008.07.009] [PMID: 18692598]

Ali Q., Wu Y., Hussain T.. Chronic AT2 receptor activation increases renal ACE2 activity, attenuates AT1 receptor function and blood pressure in obese Zucker rats., *Kidney Int.*. **2013;** 84(5): 931-939.
[http://dx.doi.org/10.1038/ki.2013.193] [PMID: 23823602]

Anand K., Ziebuhr J., Wadhwani P., Mesters J.R., Hilgenfeld R.. Coronavirus main proteinase (3CLpro) structure: basis for design of anti-SARS drugs., *Science.* **2003;** 300(5626): 1763-1767.
[http://dx.doi.org/10.1126/science.1085658] [PMID: 12746549]

API. 2016. Tulsi - Ayurvedic Pharmacopeia of India.; pp. 170.-172.

Avdesh A., Chen M., Martin-Iverson M.T., Mondal A., Ong D., Rainey-Smith S., Taddei K., Lardelli M., Groth D.M., Verdile G., Martins R.N.. Regular care and maintenance of a zebrafish (Danio rerio) laboratory: an introduction., *J. Vis. Exp.*. **2012;** (69): e4196.
[http://dx.doi.org/10.3791/4196] [PMID: 23183629]

Ayurvedic medicine: In depth (2019) National Center for Complementary and Integrative, U.S. Department of Health & Human Services, National Institutes of Health.. 2019.

Bae G.S., Kim M.S., Jeong J., Lee H.Y., Park K.C., Koo B.S., Kim B.J., Kim T.H., Lee S.H., Hwang S.Y., Shin Y.K., Song H.J., Park S.J.. Piperine ameliorates the severity of cerulein-induced acute pancreatitis by inhibiting the activation of mitogen activated protein kinases., *Biochem. Biophys. Res. Commun.*. **2011;** 410(3): 382-388.
[http://dx.doi.org/10.1016/j.bbrc.2011.05.136] [PMID: 21663734]

Acharya Balkrishna

Bale S., Venkatesh P., Sunkoju M., Godugu C.. An adaptogen: Withaferin a ameliorates *in vitro* and *in vivo* pulmonary fibrosis by modulating the interplay of fibrotic, matricelluar proteins, and cytokines., *Front. Pharmacol.*. **2018;** 9(MAR): 248.
[http://dx.doi.org/10.3389/fphar.2018.00248] [PMID: 29623041]

Balkrishna A., Solleti S.K., Verma S., Varshney A.. Application of Humanized Zebrafish Model in the Suppression of SARS-CoV-2 Spike Protein Induced Pathology by Tri-Herbal Medicine Coronil *via* Cytokine Modulation., *Molecules.* **2020;** 25(21): 5091.
[http://dx.doi.org/10.3390/molecules25215091] [PMID: 33147850] a

Balkrishna A., Solleti S.K., Singh H., Tomer M., Sharma N., Varshney A.. Calcio-herbal formulation, Divya-Swasari-Ras, alleviates chronic inflammation and suppresses airway remodelling in mouse model of allergic asthma by modulating pro-inflammatory cytokine response., *Biomedicine and Pharmacotherapy. Elsevier.* **2020;** 126(February): 110063.
[http://dx.doi.org/10.1016/j.biopha.2020.110063] [PMID: 32145582] a

Balkrishna A., Solleti S.K., Singh H., Tomer M., Sharma N., Varshney A.. Calcio-herbal formulation, Divya-Swasari-Ras, alleviates chronic inflammation and suppresses airway remodelling in mouse model of allergic asthma by modulating pro-inflammatory cytokine response., *Biomed. Pharmacother.*. **2020;** 126: 110063.
[http://dx.doi.org/10.1016/j.biopha.2020.110063] [PMID: 32145582] b

Balkrishna A., Verma S., Solleti S.K., Khandrika L., Varshney A.. Calcio-Herbal Medicine Divya-Swasari-Vati Ameliorates SARS-CoV-2 Spike Protein-Induced Pathological Features and Inflammation in Humanized Zebrafish Model by Moderating IL-6 and TNF-α Cytokines., *J. Inflamm. Res.*. **2020;** 13: 1219-1243.
[http://dx.doi.org/10.2147/JIR.S286199] [PMID: 33414643]

Balkrishna A., Haldar S., Singh H., Roy P., Varshney A.. Coronil, a Tri-Herbal Formulation, Attenuates Spike-Protein-Mediated SARS-CoV-2 Viral Entry into Human Alveolar Epithelial Cells and Pro-Inflammatory Cytokines Production by Inhibiting Spike Protein-ACE-2 Interaction., *J. Inflamm. Res.*. **2021;** 14: 869-884.
[http://dx.doi.org/10.2147/JIR.S298242] [PMID: 33758527]

Balkrishna A., Pokhrel S., Singh H., Joshi M., Mulay V.P., Haldar S., Varshney A.. Withanone from *Withania somnifera* Attenuates SARS-CoV-2 RBD and Host ACE2 Interactions to Rescue Spike Protein Induced Pathologies in Humanized Zebrafish Model., *Drug Des. Devel. Ther.*. **2021;** 15: 1111-1133.
[http://dx.doi.org/10.2147/DDDT.S292805] [PMID: 33737804]

Balkrishna A., Mittal R., Arya V.. Computational Evidences of Phytochemical Mediated Disruption of PLpro Driven Replication of SARS-CoV-2: A Therapeutic Approach Against COVID-19., *Current Pharmaceutical Biotechnology.*. **2020**

Balkrishna A., Pokhrel S., Varshney A.. Tinocordiside from Tinospora cordifolia (Giloy) May Curb SARS-CoV-2 Contagion by Disrupting the Electrostatic Interactions between Host ACE2 and Viral S-Protein Receptor Binding Domain., *Comb. Chem. High Throughput Screen.*. **2020;** 23
[http://dx.doi.org/10.2174/1386207323666201110152615] [PMID: 33172372]

Balkrishna A., Pokhrel S., Varshney A.. Phyto-compounds from a rather poisonous plant, Strychnos nux-vomica, show high potency against SARS-CoV-2 RNA-dependent RNA polymerase., *Curr. Mol. Med.*..
[http://dx.doi.org/10.2174/1566524021666210218113409] [PMID: 33602083] In Press

Barboza J.N., da Silva Maia Bezerra Filho C., Silva R.O., Medeiros J.V.R., de Sousa D.P.. An overview on the anti-inflammatory potential and antioxidant profile of eugenol., *Oxid. Med. Cell. Longev..* **2018;** 2018: 3957262.
[http://dx.doi.org/10.1155/2018/3957262] [PMID: 30425782]

Batlle D., et al. Acute Kidney Injury in COVID-19: Emerging Evidence of a Distinct Pathophysiology., *Journal of the American Society of Nephrology : JASN.* **2020**: 1380-1383.
[http://dx.doi.org/10.1681/ASN.2020040419]

Benedetti C., Waldman M., Zaza G., Riella L.V., Cravedi P.. COVID-19 and the Kidneys: An Update., *Front. Med. (Lausanne).* **2020;** 7: 423.
[http://dx.doi.org/10.3389/fmed.2020.00423] [PMID: 32793615]

Bhalla G., Kaur S., Kaur J., Kaur R., Raina P.. 'Antileishmanial and immunomodulatory potential of Ocimum sanctum Linn. and Cocos nucifera Linn. in murine visceral leishmaniasis', *Journal of Parasitic Diseases., J. Parasit. Dis..* **2017;** 41(1): 76-85.
[http://dx.doi.org/10.1007/s12639-016-0753-x] [PMID: 28316391]

Bosch B.J., Bartelink W., Rottier P.J.M.. Cathepsin L functionally cleaves the severe acute respiratory syndrome coronavirus class I fusion protein upstream of rather than adjacent to the fusion peptide., *J. Virol..* **2008;** 82(17): 8887-8890.
[http://dx.doi.org/10.1128/JVI.00415-08] [PMID: 18562523]

Brocker C., Thompson D., Matsumoto A., Nebert D.W., Vasiliou V.. Evolutionary divergence and functions of the human interleukin (IL) gene family., *Hum. Genomics.* **2010;** 5(1): 30-55.
[http://dx.doi.org/10.1186/1479-7364-5-1-30] [PMID: 21106488]

Bui T.T., Piao C.H., Song C.H., Shin H.S., Shon D.H., Chai O.H.. Piper nigrum extract ameliorated allergic inflammation through inhibiting Th2/Th17 responses and mast cells activation., *Cell. Immunol..* **2017;** 322: 64-73.
[http://dx.doi.org/10.1016/j.cellimm.2017.10.005] [PMID: 29066080]

Bupp K., Roth M.J.. Alteration and analyses of viral entry with library-derived peptides., *Adv. Virus Res..* **2005;** 65(5): 147-172.
[http://dx.doi.org/10.1016/S0065-3527(05)65005-1] [PMID: 16387196]

de Carvalho J.F., Draper N.R., Smith H.. , . Journal of the American Statistical Association. 1981. Applied Regression Analysis (2nd ed)..

Cava C., Bertoli G., Castiglioni I.. *In Silico* Discovery of Candidate Drugs against Covid-19., *Viruses 2020.* **2020;** 12: 404.
[http://dx.doi.org/10.3390/v12040404]

Chang J.S., Wang K.C., Yeh C.F., Shieh D.E., Chiang L.C.. Fresh ginger (Zingiber officinale) has anti-viral activity against human respiratory syncytial virus in human respiratory tract cell lines., *Journal of Ethnopharmacology. Elsevier.* **2013;** 145(1): 146-151.
[http://dx.doi.org/10.1016/j.jep.2012.10.043] [PMID: 23123794]

Chatterjee A., Dutta C.P.. Alkaloids of Piper longum Linn. I. Structure and synthesis of piperlongumine and piperlonguminine., *Tetrahedron.* **1967;** 23(4): 1769-1781.
[http://dx.doi.org/10.1016/S0040-4020(01)82575-8] [PMID: 6047519]

Chen J., Qi T., Liu L., Ling Y., Qian Z., Li T., Li F., Xu Q., Zhang Y., Xu S., Song Z., Zeng Y., Shen Y., Shi Y., Zhu T., Lu H.. Clinical progression of patients with COVID-19 in Shanghai, China., *J. Infect..* **2020;** 80(5): e1-e6.
[http://dx.doi.org/10.1016/j.jinf.2020.03.004] [PMID: 32171869]

Chericoni S., Prieto J.M., Iacopini P., Cioni P., Morelli I.. *In vitro* activity of the essential oil of Cinnamomum zeylanicum and eugenol in peroxynitrite-induced oxidative processes., *J. Agric. Food Chem.*. **2005;** 53(12): 4762-4765.
[http://dx.doi.org/10.1021/jf050183e] [PMID: 15941312]

Chidambaram A.G., Josephson M.. Clinical research study designs: The essentials., *Pediatr. Investig.*. **2019;** 3(4): 245-252.
[http://dx.doi.org/10.1002/ped4.12166] [PMID: 32851330]

Choudhury S.S., Bashyam L., Manthapuram N., Bitla P., Kollipara P., Tetali S.D.. Ocimum sanctum leaf extracts attenuate human monocytic (THP-1) cell activation., *Journal of Ethnopharmacology. Elsevier.* **2014;** 154(1): 148-155.
[http://dx.doi.org/10.1016/j.jep.2014.03.049] [PMID: 24732112]

Chu H., Chan C.M., Zhang X., Wang Y., Yuan S., Zhou J., Au-Yeung R.K., Sze K.H., Yang D., Shuai H., Hou Y., Li C., Zhao X., Poon V.K., Leung S.P., Yeung M.L., Yan J., Lu G., Jin D.Y., Gao G.F., Chan J.F., Yuen K.Y.. Middle East respiratory syndrome coronavirus and bat coronavirus HKU9 both can utilize GRP78 for attachment onto host cells., *J. Biol. Chem.*. **2018;** 293(30): 11709-11726.
[http://dx.doi.org/10.1074/jbc.RA118.001897] [PMID: 29887526]

Cinatl J., Morgenstern B., Bauer G., Chandra P., Rabenau H., Doerr H.W.. Glycyrrhizin, an active component of liquorice roots, and replication of SARS-associated coronavirus., *Lancet.* **2003;** 361(9374): 2045-2046.
[http://dx.doi.org/10.1016/S0140-6736(03)13615-X] [PMID: 12814717]

Cohen M.M.. Tulsi - Ocimum sanctum: A herb for all reasons., *J. Ayurveda Integr. Med.*. **2014;** 5(4): 251-259.
[http://dx.doi.org/10.4103/0975-9476.146554] [PMID: 25624701]

Conference I., et al. Specifications: test procedures and acceptance criteria for new drug substances and new drug products: chemical substances Q6A., *Ich harmonised tripartite guideline specifications.*. **1999**

Conference I., et al. Validation of analytical procedures: text and methodology Q2(R1)., *Ich harmonised tripartite guideline.*. **1994***VALIDATION OF ANALYTICAL PROCEDURES: TEXT AND METHODOLOGY Q2(R1).*.

Conti P., et al. Induction of pro-inflammatory cytokines (IL-1 and IL-6) and lung inflammation by COVID-19: anti-inflammatory strategies., *J. Biol. Regul. Homeost. Agents.* **2020;** 34(2): 327-331.
[http://dx.doi.org/10.23812/CONTI-E] [PMID: 32171193]

Coperchini F., Chiovato L., Croce L., Magri F., Rotondi M.. The cytokine storm in COVID-19: An overview of the involvement of the chemokine/chemokine-receptor system., *Cytokine Growth Factor Rev.*. **2020;** 53: 25-32.
[http://dx.doi.org/10.1016/j.cytogfr.2020.05.003] [PMID: 32446778]

Correa L.B., Pádua T.A., Seito L.N., Costa T.E., Silva M.A., Candéa A.L., Rosas E.C., Henriques M.G.. Anti-inflammatory Effect of Methyl Gallate on Experimental Arthritis: Inhibition of Neutrophil Recruitment, Production of Inflammatory Mediators, and Activation of Macrophages., *J. Nat. Prod.*. **2016;** 79(6): 1554-1566.
[http://dx.doi.org/10.1021/acs.jnatprod.5b01115] [PMID: 27227459]

Cyranoski D.. China is promoting coronavirus treatments based on unproven traditional medicines., *Nature.*. **2020**
[http://dx.doi.org/10.1038/d41586-020-01284-x] [PMID: 32376938]

Dau B., Holodniy M.. Novel targets for antiretroviral therapy: clinical progress to date., *Drugs.* **2009;** 69(1): 31-50.
[http://dx.doi.org/10.2165/00003495-200969010-00003] [PMID: 19192935]

Devpura G., Tomar B.S., Nathiya D., Sharma A., Bhandari D., Haldar S., Balkrishna A., Varshney A.. Randomized placebo-controlled pilot clinical trial on the efficacy of ayurvedic treatment regime on COVID-19 positive patients., *Phytomedicine.* **2021;** 84: 153494.
[http://dx.doi.org/10.1016/j.phymed.2021.153494] [PMID: 33596494]

Dosch S.F., Mahajan S.D., Collins A.R.. SARS coronavirus spike protein-induced innate immune response occurs *via* activation of the NF-kappaB pathway in human monocyte macrophages *in vitro.*, *Virus Res..* **2009;** 142(1-2): 19-27.
[http://dx.doi.org/10.1016/j.virusres.2009.01.005] [PMID: 19185596]

Douglas J.L., Panis M.L., Ho E., Lin K.Y., Krawczyk S.H., Grant D.M., Cai R., Swaminathan S., Cihlar T.. Inhibition of respiratory syncytial virus fusion by the small molecule VP-14637 *via* specific interactions with F protein., *J. Virol..* **2003;** 77(9): 5054-5064.
[http://dx.doi.org/10.1128/JVI.77.9.5054-5064.2003] [PMID: 12692208]

Dowell A.C., Hamilton S., McLeod D.K.. Job satisfaction, psychological morbidity and job stress among New Zealand general practitioners., *N. Z. Med. J..* **2000;** 113(1113): 269-272.
[PMID: 10935564]

Dubey N., et al. Toxicological and pharmacological assessment of Godanti bhasma., *Asian J. Chem..* **2012;** 24(10): 4653-4656.

Ernst E.. Major Herbs of Ayurveda., *Focus Altern. Complement. Ther..* **2010;** 8(1): 98.
[http://dx.doi.org/10.1111/j.2042-7166.2003.tb05765.x]

Ferrario C.M., Jessup J., Chappell M.C., Averill D.B., Brosnihan K.B., Tallant E.A., Diz D.I., Gallagher P.E.. Effect of angiotensin-converting enzyme inhibition and angiotensin II receptor blockers on cardiac angiotensin-converting enzyme 2., *Circulation.* **2005;** 111(20): 2605-2610.
[http://dx.doi.org/10.1161/CIRCULATIONAHA.104.510461] [PMID: 15897343]

Gautam M., Saha S., Bani S., Kaul A., Mishra S., Patil D., Satti N.K., Suri K.A., Gairola S., Suresh K., Jadhav S., Qazi G.N., Patwardhan B.. Immunomodulatory activity of Asparagus racemosus on systemic Th1/Th2 immunity: implications for immunoadjuvant potential., *J. Ethnopharmacol..* **2009;** 121(2): 241-247.
[http://dx.doi.org/10.1016/j.jep.2008.10.028] [PMID: 19038322]

Saha S., Ghosh S.. Tinospora cordifolia: One plant, many roles., *Anc. Sci. Life.* **2012;** 31(4): 151-159.
[http://dx.doi.org/10.4103/0257-7941.107344] [PMID: 23661861]

Girija P. L. T., Sivan N.. Ayurvedic treatment of COVID-19/SARS-CoV-2: A case report., *Journal of Ayurveda and Integrative Medicine..* Institute of Transdisciplinary Health Science and Technology and World Ayurveda Foundation.. **2020**
[http://dx.doi.org/10.1016/j.jaim.2020.06.001]

Gorbalenya A.E., et al. Coronaviridae Study Group of the International Committee on Taxonomy of VirusesThe species Severe acute respiratory syndrome-related coronavirus: classifying 2019-nCoV and naming it SARS-CoV-2., *Nat. Microbiol..* **2020;** 5(4): 536-544.
[http://dx.doi.org/10.1038/s41564-020-0695-z] [PMID: 32123347]

Gralinski L.E., Menachery V.D.. Return of the Coronavirus: 2019-nCoV., *Viruses.* **2020;** 12(2): 1-8.
[http://dx.doi.org/10.3390/v12020135] [PMID: 31991541]

Guo J., Huang Z., Lin L., Lv J.. Coronavirus Disease 2019 (COVID-19) and Cardiovascular Disease: A Viewpoint on the Potential Influence of Angiotensin-Converting Enzyme Inhibitors/Angiotensin Receptor Blockers on Onset and Severity of Severe Acute Respiratory Syndrome Coronavirus 2 Infection., *J. Am. Heart Assoc.*. **2020;** 9(7): e016219.
[http://dx.doi.org/10.1161/JAHA.120.016219] [PMID: 32233755]

Gupta P.K., Chakraborty P., Kumar S., Singh P.K., Rajan M.G., Sainis K.B., Kulkarni S.. G1-4A, a Polysaccharide from Tinospora cordifolia Inhibits the Survival of Mycobacterium tuberculosis by Modulating Host Immune Responses in TLR4 Dependent Manner., *PLoS One.* **2016;** 11(5): e0154725.
[http://dx.doi.org/10.1371/journal.pone.0154725] [PMID: 27148868]

Gupta S., Walia A., Malan R.. Phytochemistry and Pharmacology of Cedrus Deodera: an Overview., *Int. J. Pharm. Sci. Res.*. **2011;** 2(8): 2010-2020.
[http://dx.doi.org/10.13040/IJPSR.0975-8232.2(8).2010-20]

Haga S., Yamamoto N., Nakai-Murakami C., Osawa Y., Tokunaga K., Sata T., Yamamoto N., Sasazuki T., Ishizaka Y.. Modulation of TNF-α-converting enzyme by the spike protein of SARS-CoV and ACE2 induces TNF-α production and facilitates viral entry., *Proc. Natl. Acad. Sci. USA.* **2008;** 105(22): 7809-7814.
[http://dx.doi.org/10.1073/pnas.0711241105] [PMID: 18490652]

Hagenlocher Y., Bergheim I., Zacheja S., Schäffer M., Bischoff S.C., Lorentz A.. Cinnamon extract inhibits degranulation and de novo synthesis of inflammatory mediators in mast cells., *Allergy.* **2013;** 68(4): 490-497.
[http://dx.doi.org/10.1111/all.12122] [PMID: 23409834]

Haick A.K., Rzepka J.P., Brandon E., Balemba O.B., Miura T.A.. Neutrophils are needed for an effective immune response against pulmonary rat coronavirus infection, but also contribute to pathology., *J. Gen. Virol.*. **2014;** 95(Pt 3): 578-590.
[http://dx.doi.org/10.1099/vir.0.061986-0] [PMID: 24323639]

Hamming I., Timens W., Bulthuis M.L., Lely A.T., Navis G., van Goor H.. Tissue distribution of ACE2 protein, the functional receptor for SARS coronavirus. A first step in understanding SARS pathogenesis., *J. Pathol.*. **2004;** 203(2): 631-637.
[http://dx.doi.org/10.1002/path.1570] [PMID: 15141377]

Harada S.. The broad anti-viral agent glycyrrhizin directly modulates the fluidity of plasma membrane and HIV-1 envelope., *Biochem. J.*. **2005;** 392(Pt 1): 191-199.
[http://dx.doi.org/10.1042/BJ20051069] [PMID: 16053446]

Hassan Khattab H.A.R., et al. Licorice (Glycyrrhizza glabra) extract prevents production of th2 cytokines and free radicals induced by ova albumin in mice., *Int. J. Pharmacol.*. **2018;** 14(8): 1072-1079.
[http://dx.doi.org/10.3923/ijp.2018.1072.1079]

Hernandez-Baltazar D., Zavala-Flores L.M., Villanueva-Olivo A.. The 6-hydroxydopamine model and parkinsonian pathophysiology: Novel findings in an older model., *Neurologia.* **2017;** 32(8): 533-539.
[http://dx.doi.org/10.1016/j.nrl.2015.06.011] [PMID: 26304655]

Hershenberg R., Drabick D.A.G., Vivian D.. An opportunity to bridge the gap between clinical research and clinical practice: implications for clinical training., *Psychotherapy (Chic.).* **2012;** 49(2): 123-134.
[http://dx.doi.org/10.1037/a0027648] [PMID: 22642520]

Heurich A., Hofmann-Winkler H., Gierer S., Liepold T., Jahn O., Pöhlmann S.. TMPRSS2 and ADAM17 cleave ACE2 differentially and only proteolysis by TMPRSS2 augments entry driven by the severe acute respiratory syndrome coronavirus spike protein., *J. Virol.*. **2014;** 88(2): 1293-1307. [http://dx.doi.org/10.1128/JVI.02202-13] [PMID: 24227843]

Hoffmann M., Kleine-Weber H., Schroeder S., Krüger N., Herrler T., Erichsen S., Schiergens T.S., Herrler G., Wu N.H., Nitsche A., Müller M.A., Drosten C., Pöhlmann S.. SARS-CoV-2 Cell Entry Depends on ACE2 and TMPRSS2 and Is Blocked by a Clinically Proven Protease Inhibitor., *Cell.* **2020;** 181(2): 271-280.e8.
[http://dx.doi.org/10.1016/j.cell.2020.02.052] [PMID: 32142651]

Huang C., Wang Y., Li X., Ren L., Zhao J., Hu Y., Zhang L., Fan G., Xu J., Gu X., Cheng Z., Yu T., Xia J., Wei Y., Wu W., Xie X., Yin W., Li H., Liu M., Xiao Y., Gao H., Guo L., Xie J., Wang G., Jiang R., Gao Z., Jin Q., Wang J., Cao B.. Clinical features of patients infected with 2019 novel coronavirus in Wuhan, China., *Lancet.* **2020;** 395(10223): 497-506.
[http://dx.doi.org/10.1016/S0140-6736(20)30183-5] [PMID: 31986264]

Huang H., Morgan C.M., Asolkar R.N., Koivunen M.E., Marrone P.G.. Phytotoxicity of sarmentine isolated from long pepper (Piper longum) fruit., *J. Agric. Food Chem.*. **2010;** 58(18): 9994-10000.
[http://dx.doi.org/10.1021/jf102087c] [PMID: 20839888]

Hui D.S., I Azhar E., Madani T.A., Ntoumi F., Kock R., Dar O., Ippolito G., Mchugh T.D., Memish Z.A., Drosten C., Zumla A., Petersen E.. The continuing 2019-nCoV epidemic threat of novel coronaviruses to global health - The latest 2019 novel coronavirus outbreak in Wuhan, China., *Int. J. Infect. Dis.*. **2020;** 91: 264-266.
[http://dx.doi.org/10.1016/j.ijid.2020.01.009] [PMID: 31953166]

Hunter C.A., Jones S.A.. IL-6 as a keystone cytokine in health and disease., *Nat. Immunol.*. **2015;** 16(5): 448-457.
[http://dx.doi.org/10.1038/ni.3153] [PMID: 25898198]

Huynh J., Li S., Yount B., Smith A., Sturges L., Olsen J.C., Nagel J., Johnson J.B., Agnihothram S., Gates J.E., Frieman M.B., Baric R.S., Donaldson E.F.. Evidence supporting a zoonotic origin of human coronavirus strain NL63., *J. Virol.*. **2012;** 86(23): 12816-12825.
[http://dx.doi.org/10.1128/JVI.00906-12] [PMID: 22993147]

Illesca P., Valenzuela R., Espinosa A., Echeverría F., Soto-Alarcon S., Ortiz M., Videla L.A.. Hydroxytyrosol supplementation ameliorates the metabolic disturbances in white adipose tissue from mice fed a high-fat diet through recovery of transcription factors Nrf2, SREBP-1c, PPAR-γ and NF-κB., *Biomed. Pharmacother.*. **2019;** 109: 2472-2481.
[http://dx.doi.org/10.1016/j.biopha.2018.11.120] [PMID: 30551508]

India A.P.. , . 2016. Giloy - Ayurvedic Pharmacopeia of India; pp. 53.-56.

Jakovljevic M., Bjedov S., Jaksic N., Jakovljevic I.. Covid-19 pandemia and public and global mental health from the perspective of global health security., *Psychiatr. Danub.*. **2020;** 32(1): 6-14.
[http://dx.doi.org/10.24869/psyd.2020.6] [PMID: 32303023]

Jantan I., Haque M.A., Ilangkovan M., Arshad L.. An insight into the modulatory effects and mechanisms of action of phyllanthus species and their bioactive metabolites on the immune system., *Front. Pharmacol.*. **2019;** 10(JULY): 878.
[http://dx.doi.org/10.3389/fphar.2019.00878] [PMID: 31440162]

Jayaprakasha G.K., Jagan Mohan Rao L., Sakariah K.K.. Volatile constituents from Cinnamomum zeylanicum fruit stalks and their antioxidant activities., *J. Agric. Food Chem.*. **2003;** 51(15): 4344-4348.
[http://dx.doi.org/10.1021/jf034169i] [PMID: 12848508]

Jin Z., Du X., Xu Y., Deng Y., Liu M., Zhao Y., Zhang B., Li X., Zhang L., Peng C., Duan Y., Yu J., Wang L., Yang K., Liu F., Jiang R., Yang X., You T., Liu X., Yang X., Bai F., Liu H., Liu X., Guddat L.W., Xu W., Xiao G., Qin C., Shi Z., Jiang H., Rao Z., Yang H.. Structure of M^{pro} from SARS-CoV-2 and discovery of its inhibitors., *Nature*. **2020;** 582(7811): 289-293. [http://dx.doi.org/10.1038/s41586-020-2223-y] [PMID: 32272481]

Kandhare A.D., Bodhankar S.L., Singh V., Mohan V., Thakurdesai P.A.. 'Anti-asthmatic effects of type-A procyanidine polyphenols from cinnamon bark in ovalbumin-induced airway hyperresponsiveness in laboratory animals', *Biomedicine and Aging Pathology.*, *Biomed. Aging Pathol.*. **2013;** 3(1): 23-30. [http://dx.doi.org/10.1016/j.biomag.2013.01.003]

Kanwar A.S., Bhutani K.K.. Effects of Chlorophytum arundinaceum, Asparagus adscendens and Asparagus racemosus on pro-inflammatory cytokine and corticosterone levels produced by stress., *Phytother. Res.*. **2010;** 24(10): 1562-1566. [http://dx.doi.org/10.1002/ptr.3218] [PMID: 20564504]

Kaur G., Singh N., Samuel S.S., Bora H.K., Sharma S., Pachauri S.D., Dwivedi A.K., Siddiqui H.H., Hanif K.. Withania somnifera shows a protective effect in monocrotaline-induced pulmonary hypertension., *Pharm. Biol.*. **2015;** 53(1): 147-157. [http://dx.doi.org/10.3109/13880209.2014.912240] [PMID: 25237891]

Kim M.E., Na J.Y., Lee J.S.. Anti-inflammatory effects of trans-cinnamaldehyde on lipopolysaccharide-stimulated macrophage activation *via* MAPKs pathway regulation., *Inc.* **2018;** 40(3): 219-224. [http://dx.doi.org/10.1080/08923973.2018.1424902] [PMID: 29355056]

Kim S-H., Lee Y-C.. Piperine inhibits eosinophil infiltration and airway hyperresponsiveness by suppressing T cell activity and Th2 cytokine production in the ovalbumin-induced asthma model., *J. Pharm. Pharmacol.*. **2009;** 61(3): 353-359. [http://dx.doi.org/10.1211/jpp.61.03.0010] [PMID: 19222908]

Koe T.. It' s official : China adds three TCM formula to COVID-19 standard therapy, **2020**

Korber B., Fischer W.M., Gnanakaran S., Yoon H., Theiler J., Abfalterer W., Hengartner N., Giorgi E.E., Bhattacharya T., Foley B., Hastie K.M., Parker M.D., Partridge D.G., Evans C.M., Freeman T.M., de Silva T.I., McDanal C., Perez L.G., Tang H., Moon-Walker A., Whelan S.P., LaBranche C.C., Saphire E.O., Montefiori D.C., Angyal A., Brown R.L., Carrilero L., Green L.R., Groves D.C., Johnson K.J., Keeley A.J., Lindsey B.B., Parsons P.J., Raza M., Rowland-Jones S., Smith N., Tucker R.M., Wang D., Wyles M.D., Sheffield COVID-19 Genomics GroupTracking Changes in SARS-CoV-2 Spike: Evidence that D614G Increases Infectivity of the COVID-19 Virus., *Cell.* **2020;** 182(4): 812-827.e19. [http://dx.doi.org/10.1016/j.cell.2020.06.043] [PMID: 32697968]

Kruse R.L.. Therapeutic strategies in an outbreak scenario to treat the novel coronavirus originating in Wuhan, China., *F1000 Res.*. **2020;** 9: 72. [http://dx.doi.org/10.12688/f1000research.22211.2] [PMID: 32117569]

Ksiazek T.G., Erdman D., Goldsmith C.S., Zaki S.R., Peret T., Emery S., Tong S., Urbani C., Comer J.A., Lim W., Rollin P.E., Dowell S.F., Ling A.E., Humphrey C.D., Shieh W.J., Guarner J., Paddock C.D., Rota P., Fields B., DeRisi J., Yang J.Y., Cox N., Hughes J.M., LeDuc J.W., Bellini W.J., Anderson L.J., SARS Working GroupA novel coronavirus associated with severe acute respiratory syndrome., *N. Engl. J. Med.*. **2003;** 348(20): 1953-1966. [http://dx.doi.org/10.1056/NEJMoa030781] [PMID: 12690092]

Kulkarni S.K., Dhir A.. Withania somnifera: an Indian ginseng., *Prog. Neuropsychopharmacol. Biol. Psychiatry.* **2008;** 32(5): 1093-1105. [http://dx.doi.org/10.1016/j.pnpbp.2007.09.011] [PMID: 17959291]

Kumar V., Dhanjal J. K., Kaul S. C., et al. Withanone and caffeic acid phenethyl ester are predicted to interact with main protease (Mpro) of SARS-CoV-2 and inhibit its activity., *Journal of Biomolecular Structure and Dynamics.*. Taylor & Francis. **2020**
[http://dx.doi.org/10.1080/07391102.2020.1772108]

Kumar V., Dhanjal J.K., Bhargava P., Kaul A., Wang J., Zhang H., Kaul S.C., Wadhwa R., Sundar D.. Withanone and Withaferin-A are predicted to interact with transmembrane protease serine 2 (TMPRSS2) and block entry of SARS-CoV-2 into cells., *J. Biomol. Struct. Dyn.*. **2022;** 40(1): 1-13.
[http://dx.doi.org/10.1080/07391102.2020.1775704] [PMID: 32469279]

Lachin J.M., Matts J.P., Wei L.J.. Randomization in clinical trials: conclusions and recommendations., *Control. Clin. Trials.* **1988;** 9(4): 365-374.
[http://dx.doi.org/10.1016/0197-2456(88)90049-9] [PMID: 3203526]

Lan J., Ge J., Yu J., Shan S., Zhou H., Fan S., Zhang Q., Shi X., Wang Q., Zhang L., Wang X.. Structure of the SARS-CoV-2 spike receptor-binding domain bound to the ACE2 receptor., *Nature.* **2020;** 581(7807): 215-220.
[http://dx.doi.org/10.1038/s41586-020-2180-5] [PMID: 32225176]

Lee I.S., Cho D.H., Kim K.S., Kim K.H., Park J., Kim Y., Jung J.H., Kim K., Jung H.J., Jang H.J.. Anti-inflammatory effects of embelin in A549 cells and human asthmatic airway epithelial tissues., *Immunopharmacol. Immunotoxicol.*. **2018;** 40(1): 83-90.
[http://dx.doi.org/10.1080/08923973.2017.1414836] [PMID: 29299941]

Lee S.A., Lee S.H., Kim J.Y., Lee W.S.. Effects of glycyrrhizin on lipopolysaccharide-induced acute lung injury in a mouse model., *J. Thorac. Dis.*. **2019;** 11(4): 1287-1302.
[http://dx.doi.org/10.21037/jtd.2019.04.14] [PMID: 31179071]

Lee S.A.. How much "Thinking" about COVID-19 is clinically dysfunctional?, *Brain Behav. Immun.*. **2020;** 87: 97-98.
[http://dx.doi.org/10.1016/j.bbi.2020.04.067] [PMID: 32353520]

Lee W., Yoo H., Kim J.A., Lee S., Jee J.G., Lee M.Y., Lee Y.M., Bae J.S.. Barrier protective effects of piperlonguminine in LPS-induced inflammation *in vitro* and *in vivo*., *Food Chem. Toxicol.*. **2013;** 58: 149-157.
[http://dx.doi.org/10.1016/j.fct.2013.04.027] [PMID: 23619565]

Altman D.G., Schulz K.F., Moher D., Egger M., Davidoff F., Elbourne D., Gøtzsche P.C., Lang T., CONSORT GROUP (Consolidated Standards of Reporting Trials)The revised CONSORT statement for reporting randomized trials: explanation and elaboration., *Ann. Intern. Med.*. **2001;** 134(8): 663-694.
[http://dx.doi.org/10.7326/0003-4819-134-8-200104170-00012] [PMID: 11304107]

Li F., Li W., Farzan M., Harrison S.C.. Structure of SARS coronavirus spike receptor-binding domain complexed with receptor., *Science.* **2005;** 309(5742): 1864-1868.
[http://dx.doi.org/10.1126/science.1116480] [PMID: 16166518]

Li K., Wu J., Wu F., Guo D., Chen L., Fang Z., Li C.. The Clinical and Chest CT Features Associated With Severe and Critical COVID-19 Pneumonia., *Invest. Radiol.*. **2020;** 55(6): 327-331.
[http://dx.doi.org/10.1097/RLI.0000000000000672] [PMID: 32118615]

Li X.C., Zhang J., Zhuo J.L.. , . Pharmacological Research. 125. Elsevier Ltd; 2017. The vasoprotective axes of the renin-angiotensin system: Physiological relevance and therapeutic implications in cardiovascular, hypertensive and kidney diseases.; pp. 21.-38.

Lim G.Y.. , . TCM and COVID-19 : China conducting trials to test efficacy and safety of traditional herbal interventions. 2020. pp. 4.-6.

Ling Ren J., Zhang A. H, Wang X.J. Traditional Chinese medicine for COVID-19 treatment., *Pharmacological Research.* **2020**: 104743.
[http://dx.doi.org/10.1016/j.phrs.2020.104743]

Lu H.. Drug treatment options for the 2019-new coronavirus (2019-nCoV)., *Biosci. Trends.* **2020;** 14(1): 69-71.
[http://dx.doi.org/10.5582/bst.2020.01020] [PMID: 31996494]

Lu S., et al. , . Signal Transduction and Targeted Therapy. Springer US; 2020. Comparison of nonhuman primates identified the suitable model for COVID-19..

Ma C., Zou L., Xia Y., Tu Y., Xue D., Yang Y., Liu D., Liu Y., Wu H., Dan H., You P.. Extracts of Coleus forskohlii relieves cough and asthma symptoms *via* modulating inflammation and the extracellular matrix., *J. Cell. Biochem.*. **2019;** 120(6): 9648-9655.
[http://dx.doi.org/10.1002/jcb.28243] [PMID: 30520122]

Mahajan N., Rawal S., Verma M., Poddar M., Alok S.. 'A phytopharmacological overview on Ocimum species with special emphasis on Ocimum sanctum', *Biomedicine and Preventive Nutrition., Elsevier Masson SAS.* **2013;** 3(2): 185-192.
[http://dx.doi.org/10.1016/j.bionut.2012.08.002]

Majdalawieh A.F., Carr R.I.. *In vitro* investigation of the potential immunomodulatory and anti-cancer activities of black pepper (Piper nigrum) and cardamom (Elettaria cardamomum)., *J. Med. Food.* **2010;** 13(2): 371-381.
[http://dx.doi.org/10.1089/jmf.2009.1131] [PMID: 20210607]

Mantovani A., Cassatella M.A., Costantini C., Jaillon S.. Neutrophils in the activation and regulation of innate and adaptive immunity., *Nat. Rev. Immunol.*. **2011;** 11(8): 519-531.
[http://dx.doi.org/10.1038/nri3024] [PMID: 21785456]

Mathur R., Swaminathan S.. National Ethical Guidelines for Biomedical and Health Research Involving Human Participants, 2017: A commentary., *Indian J. Med. Ethics.* **2018;** 3(3): 201-204.
[http://dx.doi.org/10.20529/IJME.2018.065] [PMID: 30211674]

Matsuyama S., Nagata N., Shirato K., Kawase M., Takeda M., Taguchi F.. Efficient activation of the severe acute respiratory syndrome coronavirus spike protein by the transmembrane protease TMPRSS2., *J. Virol.*. **2010;** 84(24): 12658-12664.
[http://dx.doi.org/10.1128/JVI.01542-10] [PMID: 20926566]

Meghwani H., Prabhakar P., Mohammed S.A., Dua P., Seth S., Hote M.P., Banerjee S.K., Arava S., Ray R., Maulik S.K.. Beneficial Effect of *Ocimum sanctum* (Linn) against Monocrotaline-Induced Pulmonary Hypertension in Rats., *Medicines (Basel).* **2018;** 5(2): 34.
[http://dx.doi.org/10.3390/medicines5020034] [PMID: 29673152]

Mehla K., Balwani S., Agrawal A., Ghosh B.. Ethyl gallate attenuates acute lung injury through Nrf2 signaling., *Elsevier Masson SAS.* **2013;** 95(12): 2404-2414.
[http://dx.doi.org/10.1016/j.biochi.2013.08.030] [PMID: 24018486]

Michaelis M., Geiler J., Naczk P., Sithisarn P., Ogbomo H., Altenbrandt B., Leutz A., Doerr H.W., Cinatl J. Jr. Glycyrrhizin inhibits highly pathogenic H5N1 influenza A virus-induced pro-inflammatory cytokine and chemokine expression in human macrophages., *Med. Microbiol. Immunol. (Berl.).* **2010;** 199(4): 291-297.
[http://dx.doi.org/10.1007/s00430-010-0155-0] [PMID: 20386921]

Michaelis M., Geiler J., Naczk P., Sithisarn P., Leutz A., Doerr H.W., Cinatl J. Jr. Glycyrrhizin exerts antioxidative effects in H5N1 influenza A virus-infected cells and inhibits virus replication and pro-inflammatory gene expression., *PLoS One.* **2011;** 6(5): e19705.
[http://dx.doi.org/10.1371/journal.pone.0019705] [PMID: 21611183]

Mihajlovic-Madzarevic V.. , . Clinical Trials Audit Preparation. 2010. Appendix B: Guidance for Industry-E6 Good Clinical Practice: Consolidated Guidance..

Millet J.K., Whittaker G.R.. Host cell proteases: Critical determinants of coronavirus tropism and pathogenesis., *Elsevier B..* **2015;** 202: 120-134.
[http://dx.doi.org/10.1016/j.virusres.2014.11.021] [PMID: 25445340]

Ministry AYUSH. Interdisciplinary AYUSH Research & Development Task Force Guidelines for AYUSH Clinical Studies in COVID-19., **2020**

Mishra A., Gond S.K., Kumar A., Sharma V.K., Verma S.K., Kharwar R.N., Sieber T.N.. Season and tissue type affect fungal endophyte communities of the Indian medicinal plant Tinospora cordifolia more strongly than geographic location., *Microb. Ecol..* **2012;** 64(2): 388-398.
[http://dx.doi.org/10.1007/s00248-012-0029-7] [PMID: 22430503]

Mishra A., et al. In-house preparation and characterization of an Ayurvedic bhasma: Praval bhasma., *Journal of integrative medicine.* Journal of Integrative Medicine Editorial Office.. Elsevier; Singapore: **2014;** 12(1): 52-58.*In-house preparation and characterization of an Ayurvedic bhasma: Praval bhasma..*
[http://dx.doi.org/10.1016/S2095-4964(14)60005-4]

Mishra L.C., Singh B.B., Dagenais S.. Scientific basis for the therapeutic use of Withania somnifera (ashwagandha): a review., *Altern. Med. Rev..* **2000;** 5(4): 334-346.
[PMID: 10956379]

Moon C.. Fighting COVID-19 exhausts T cells., *Nat. Rev. Immunol..* **2020;** 20(5): 277.
[http://dx.doi.org/10.1038/s41577-020-0304-7] [PMID: 32249845]

Mucsi I., Gyulai Z., Béládi I.. Combined effects of flavonoids and acyclovir against herpesviruses in cell cultures., *Acta Microbiol. Hung..* **1992;** 39(2): 137-147.
[PMID: 1339152]

Nagata N., Iwata N., Hasegawa H., Fukushi S., Harashima A., Sato Y., Saijo M., Taguchi F., Morikawa S., Sata T.. Mouse-passaged severe acute respiratory syndrome-associated coronavirus leads to lethal pulmonary edema and diffuse alveolar damage in adult but not young mice., *Am. J. Pathol..* **2008;** 172(6): 1625-1637.
[http://dx.doi.org/10.2353/ajpath.2008.071060] [PMID: 18467696]

Nicolis E., Lampronti I., Dechecchi M.C., Borgatti M., Tamanini A., Bezzerri V., Bianchi N., Mazzon M., Mancini I., Giri M.G., Rizzotti P., Gambari R., Cabrini G.. Modulation of expression of IL-8 gene in bronchial epithelial cells by 5-methoxypsoralen., *Elsevier B..* **2009;** 9(12): 1411-1422.
[http://dx.doi.org/10.1016/j.intimp.2009.08.013] [PMID: 19720161]

Nishimoto Y., Hisatsune A., Katsuki H., Miyata T., Yokomizo K., Isohama Y.. Glycyrrhizin attenuates mucus production by inhibition of MUC5AC mRNA expression *in vivo* and *in vitro*., *J. Pharmacol. Sci..* **2010;** 113(1): 76-83.
[http://dx.doi.org/10.1254/jphs.09344FP] [PMID: 20453436]

Nolkemper S., Reichling J., Stintzing F.C., Carle R., Schnitzler P.. Antiviral effect of aqueous extracts from species of the Lamiaceae family against Herpes simplex virus type 1 and type 2 *in vitro*., *Planta Med..* **2006;** 72(15): 1378-1382.
[http://dx.doi.org/10.1055/s-2006-951719] [PMID: 17091431]

Ou J., et al. **2020**Emergence of RBD mutations in circulating SARS-CoV-2 strains enhancing the structural stability and human ACE2 receptor affinity of the spike protein, *bioRxiv.* : 1-30.
[http://dx.doi.org/10.1101/2020.03.15.991844]

Ou X., et al. , . Nature communications. 11. Springer; US: 2020. Characterization of spike glycoprotein of SARS-CoV-2 on virus entry and its immune cross-reactivity with SARS-CoV.; p. 1620

Padhi A.K., Tripathi T.. , . Can SARS-CoV-2 Accumulate Mutations in the S-Protein to Increase Pathogenicity?. ACS Pharmacology and Translational Science; 2020. pp. 17.-20.

Pal D., Sahu C.K., Haldar A.. Bhasma : The ancient Indian nanomedicine., *J. Adv. Pharm. Technol. Res..* **2014;** 5(1): 4-12.
[http://dx.doi.org/10.4103/2231-4040.126980] [PMID: 24696811]

Pan C., Dong Z.. Antiasthmatic Effects of Eugenol in a Mouse Model of Allergic Asthma by Regulation of Vitamin D3 Upregulated Protein 1/NF-κB Pathway., *Inflammation.* **2015;** 38(4): 1385-1393.
[http://dx.doi.org/10.1007/s10753-015-0110-8] [PMID: 25588851]

Panchabhai T.S., Kulkarni U.P., Rege N.N.. Validation of therapeutic claims of Tinospora cordifolia: a review., *Phytother. Res..* **2008;** 22(4): 425-441.
[http://dx.doi.org/10.1002/ptr.2347] [PMID: 18167043]

Parliament T. H. E. E.. Traditional herbal medicinal products, directive 2001/83/ec on the community code relating to medicinal products for human use., **2004;** 6: 85-90.

Pattanayak P., Behera P., Das D., Panda S.K.. Ocimum sanctum Linn. A reservoir plant for therapeutic applications: An overview., *Pharmacogn. Rev..* **2010;** 4(7): 95-105.
[http://dx.doi.org/10.4103/0973-7847.65323] [PMID: 22228948]

Pharmacopoeia I.. , . WHO EXPERT COMMITTEE ON SPECIFICATIONS FOR PHARMACEUTICAL PREPARATIONS', WHO Techincal Report Series.. Thirty-nin; 2005.

Prabakaran P., Gan J., Feng Y., Zhu Z., Choudhry V., Xiao X., Ji X., Dimitrov D.S.. Structure of severe acute respiratory syndrome coronavirus receptor-binding domain complexed with neutralizing antibody., *J. Biol. Chem..* **2006;** 281(23): 15829-15836.
[http://dx.doi.org/10.1074/jbc.M600697200] [PMID: 16597622]

Priyashree S., Jha S., Pattanayak S.P.. A review on Cressa cretica Linn.: A halophytic plant., *Pharmacogn. Rev..* **2010;** 4(8): 161-166.
[http://dx.doi.org/10.4103/0973-7847.70910] [PMID: 22228956]

Pynam H., Dharmesh S.M.. Antioxidant and anti-inflammatory properties of marmelosin from Bael (Aegle marmelos L.); Inhibition of TNF-α mediated inflammatory/tumor markers., *Biomed. Pharmacother..* **2018;** 106(January): 98-108.
[http://dx.doi.org/10.1016/j.biopha.2018.06.053] [PMID: 29957472]

Qin C., Zhou L., Hu Z., Zhang S., Yang S., Tao Y., Xie C., Ma K., Shang K., Wang W., Tian D.S.. Dysregulation of Immune Response in Patients With Coronavirus 2019 (COVID-19) in Wuhan, China., *Clin. Infect. Dis..* **2020;** 71(15): 762-768.
[http://dx.doi.org/10.1093/cid/ciaa248] [PMID: 32161940]

Rajadhyaksha V.. Conducting feasibilities in clinical trials: an investment to ensure a good study., *Perspect. Clin. Res..* **2010;** 1(3): 106-109.
[PMID: 21814631]

Rajaram A., Vanaja G.R., Vyakaranam P., Rachamallu A., Reddy G.V., Anilkumar K., Arunasree K.M., Dhyani A., Prasad N.K., Sharma S., Chandra Joshi M., Kimothi G.P., Brindavanam N.B., Reddanna P.. Anti-inflammatory profile of Aegle marmelos (L) Correa (Bilva) with special reference to young roots grown in different parts of India., *J. Ayurveda Integr. Med.*. **2018;** 9(2): 90-98.
[http://dx.doi.org/10.1016/j.jaim.2017.03.006] [PMID: 29239790]

Ram A., Mabalirajan U., Das M., Bhattacharya I., Dinda A.K., Gangal S.V., Ghosh B.. Glycyrrhizin alleviates experimental allergic asthma in mice., *Int. Immunopharmacol.*. **2006;** 6(9): 1468-1477.
[http://dx.doi.org/10.1016/j.intimp.2006.04.020] [PMID: 16846841]

Ram A., Balachandar S., Vijayananth P., Singh V.P.. Medicinal plants useful for treating chronic obstructive pulmonary disease (COPD): current status and future perspectives., *Elsevier B.*. **2011;** 82(2): 141-151.
[http://dx.doi.org/10.1016/j.fitote.2010.09.005] [PMID: 20851752]

Rana S., Shahzad M., Shabbir A.. Pistacia integerrima ameliorates airway inflammation by attenuation of TNF-α, IL-4, and IL-5 expression levels, and pulmonary edema by elevation of AQP1 and AQP5 expression levels in mouse model of ovalbumin-induced allergic asthma., *Phytomedicine.* **2016;** 23(8): 838-845.
[http://dx.doi.org/10.1016/j.phymed.2016.04.006] [PMID: 27288919]

Rastogi S., Pandey D.N., Singh R.H.. COVID-19 pandemic: A pragmatic plan for ayurveda intervention., *J. Ayurveda Integr. Med...* **2020**
[http://dx.doi.org/10.1016/j.jaim.2020.04.002] [PMID: 32382220]

Rauf A., Saleem M., Uddin G., Siddiqui B.S., Khan H., Raza M., Hamid S.Z., Khan A., Maione F., Mascolo N., De Feo V.. Phosphodiesterase-1 inhibitory activity of two flavonoids isolated from pistacia integerrima J. L. Stewart galls., *Evid. Based Complement. Alternat. Med.*. **2015;** 2015: 506564.
[http://dx.doi.org/10.1155/2015/506564] [PMID: 25945110]

Razinkov V., Gazumyan A., Nikitenko A., Ellestad G., Krishnamurthy G.. RFI-641 inhibits entry of respiratory syncytial virus *via* interactions with fusion protein., *Chem. Biol.*. **2001;** 8(7): 645-659.
[http://dx.doi.org/10.1016/S1074-5521(01)00042-4] [PMID: 11451666]

Reichling J., Schnitzler P., Suschke U., Saller R.. Essential oils of aromatic plants with antibacterial, antifungal, antiviral, and cytotoxic properties--an overview., *Forsch. Komplement. Med.*. **2009;** 16(2): 79-90.
[http://dx.doi.org/10.1159/000207196] [PMID: 19420953]

Sahoo I., More S.S., Jadhav V., Dalai S., Sahoo M.. Clinical Appraisal on Therapeutic Efficacy of Tankana & Sphatika Bhasma With Madhu Pratisarana In Tundikeri., *J. Drug Deliv. Ther.*. **2019;** 9(6): 130-134.
[http://dx.doi.org/10.22270/jddt.v9i6.3707]

Salata C., Calistri A., Parolin C., Palù G.. Coronaviruses: a paradigm of new emerging zoonotic diseases., *Pathog. Dis.*. **2019;** 77(9): 1-5.
[http://dx.doi.org/10.1093/femspd/ftaa006] [PMID: 32065221]

Schlede E., Genschow E., Spielmann H., Stropp G., Kayser D.. Oral acute toxic class method: a successful alternative to the oral LD50 test., *Regul. Toxicol. Pharmacol.*. **2005;** 42(1): 15-23.
[http://dx.doi.org/10.1016/j.yrtph.2004.12.006] [PMID: 15896439]

Schulz K.F., Grimes D.A.. Blinding in randomised trials: hiding who got what., *Lancet.* **2002;** 359(9307): 696-700.
[http://dx.doi.org/10.1016/S0140-6736(02)07816-9] [PMID: 11879884]

Serafini G., Parmigiani B., Amerio A., Aguglia A., Sher L., Amore M.. The psychological impact of COVID-19 on the mental health in the general population., *QJM.* **2020;** 113(8): hcaa201.
[http://dx.doi.org/10.1093/qjmed/hcaa201] [PMID: 32569360]

Sharma P., Dwivedee B.P., Bisht D., Dash A.K., Kumar D.. The chemical constituents and diverse pharmacological importance of *Tinospora cordifolia.*, *Heliyon.* **2019;** 5(9): e02437.
[http://dx.doi.org/10.1016/j.heliyon.2019.e02437] [PMID: 31701036]

Shirole R.L., Shirole N.L., Saraf M.N.. Embelia ribes ameliorates lipopolysaccharide-induced acute respiratory distress syndrome., *Journal of Ethnopharmacology. Elsevier.* **2015;** 168: 356-363.
[http://dx.doi.org/10.1016/j.jep.2015.03.009] [PMID: 25818695]

Shree P., et al. Targeting COVID-19 (SARS-CoV-2) main protease through active phytochemicals of ayurvedic medicinal plants–Withania somnifera (Ashwagandha), Tinospora cordifolia (Giloy) and Ocimum sanctum (Tulsi)–a molecular docking study., *J. Biomol. Struct. Dyn..* **2020;** 19(August)
[http://dx.doi.org/10.1080/07391102.2020.1810778] [PMID: 32851919]

Ayurvedic Treatment of Chronic Obstructive Pulmonary Disease World Famous Sexologist Ayurvedic medicines for COPD., **2015**: 1-8.

Singh H.B., Srivastava M., Singh A.B., Srivastava A.K.. Cinnamon bark oil, a potent fungitoxicant against fungi causing respiratory tract mycoses., *Allergy.* **1995;** 50(12): 995-999.
[http://dx.doi.org/10.1111/j.1398-9995.1995.tb02515.x] [PMID: 8834832]

Singh S., Agrawal S.S.. 'Anti-Asthmatic and Anti-Inflammatory Activity of Ocimum sanctum', *Int. J. Pharmacognosy*, 29(4), pp. 306–310. doi: Singh, S., & Agrawal, S. S. (1991). Anti-Asthmatic and Anti-Inflammatory Activity of Ocimum sanctum., *International Journal of Pharmacognosy.* **1991;** 29(4): 306-310.
[http://dx.doi.org/10.3109/13880209109082904]

Sinha K., et al. Tinospora cordifolia (Guduchi), a reservoir plant for therapeutic applications: A Review., *Indian J. Tradit. Knowl..* **2004;** 3(3): 257-270.[IJTK].

Stadler K., Masignani V., Eickmann M., Becker S., Abrignani S., Klenk H.D., Rappuoli R.. SARS--beginning to understand a new virus., *Nat. Rev. Microbiol..* **2003;** 1(3): 209-218.
[http://dx.doi.org/10.1038/nrmicro775] [PMID: 15035025]

Sudeep H.V., Gouthamchandra K., Shyamprasad K.. Molecular docking analysis of Withaferin A from Withania somnifera with the Glucose regulated protein 78 (GRP78) receptor and the SARS-CoV-2 main protease., *Bioinformation.* **2020;** 16(5): 411-417.
[http://dx.doi.org/10.6026/97320630016411] [PMID: 32831523]

Sujith K., Darwin C.R., Suba V.. Antioxidant Activity of Ethanolic Root Extract of Anacyclus Pyrethrum., *International Research Journal of Pharmacy.* **2011;** 2(12): 222-226.

Sunita P., Jha S., Pattanayak S.. *In-vivo* Antitussive Activity of Cressa cretica Linn. using Cough Model in Rodents., *Pharmacognosy Res..* **2009;** 1(3): 157-161.

Suresh K.. An overview of randomization techniques: An unbiased assessment of outcome in clinical research., *J. Hum. Reprod. Sci..* **2011;** 4(1): 8-11.
[http://dx.doi.org/10.4103/0974-1208.82352] [PMID: 21772732]

Tao L., et al. Metabolic Control of Viral Infection through PPAR-α Regulation of STING Signaling, *bioRxiv.* **2019**: 731208.
[http://dx.doi.org/10.1101/731208]

Tay M.Z., Poh C.M., Rénia L., MacAry P.A., Ng L.F.P.. The trinity of COVID-19: immunity, inflammation and intervention., *Nat. Rev. Immunol.*. **2020;** 20(6): 363-374. [http://dx.doi.org/10.1038/s41577-020-0311-8] [PMID: 32346093]

Thaker S.J., Gogtay N.J., Thatte U.M.. Pharmacoepidemiology: The essentials., *Clin. Epidemiol. Glob. Health.* **2015;** 3(2): 52-57. [http://dx.doi.org/10.1016/j.cegh.2014.04.003]

The World Bank (2020) COVID-19 to Plunge Global Economy into Worst Recession since World War II, The World Bank..

Tian X., Li C., Huang A., Xia S., Lu S., Shi Z., Lu L., Jiang S., Yang Z., Wu Y., Ying T.. Potent binding of 2019 novel coronavirus spike protein by a SARS coronavirus-specific human monoclonal antibody., *Emerg. Microbes Infect.*. **2020;** 9(1): 382-385. [http://dx.doi.org/10.1080/22221751.2020.1729069] [PMID: 32065055]

Tiwari M., Dwivedi U.N., Kakkar P.. Tinospora cordifolia extract modulates COX-2, iNOS, ICAM-1, pro-inflammatory cytokines and redox status in murine model of asthma., *J. Ethnopharmacol.*. **2014;** 153(2): 326-337. [http://dx.doi.org/10.1016/j.jep.2014.01.031] [PMID: 24556222]

Tripathi S., Maier K.G., Bruch D., Kittur D.S.. Effect of 6-gingerol on pro-inflammatory cytokine production and costimulatory molecule expression in murine peritoneal macrophages., *J. Surg. Res.*. **2007;** 138(2): 209-213. [http://dx.doi.org/10.1016/j.jss.2006.07.051] [PMID: 17291534]

Tsui P.T., Kwok M.L., Yuen H., Lai S.T.. Severe acute respiratory syndrome: clinical outcome and prognostic correlates., *Emerg. Infect. Dis.*. **2003;** 9(9): 1064-1069. [http://dx.doi.org/10.3201/eid0909.030362] [PMID: 14519241]

United States Phamacopeia - USPChemical Tests/<467>RESIDUAL SOLVENTS., *USP.* **2007;** 30: 1-10.

United States Phamacopeia - USPElemental impurities- Limits. 2016.

United States Phamacopeia - USP38'<561 > ARTICLES OF BOTANICAL ORIGIN'., *Articles of Botanical Origin.* (20): 1-54.no date

Vadnere G.P., Pathan A.R., Singhai A.K.. Characterization of indigenous traditional medicine - Muktashukti Bhasma., *Indian J. Tradit. Knowl.*. **2013;** 12(3): 483-488.

Varga Z., Flammer A.J., Steiger P., Haberecker M., Andermatt R., Zinkernagel A.S., Mehra M.R., Schuepbach R.A., Ruschitzka F., Moch H.. Endothelial cell infection and endotheliitis in COVID-19., *Lancet.* **2020;** 395(10234): 1417-1418. [http://dx.doi.org/10.1016/S0140-6736(20)30937-5] [PMID: 32325026]

Vinay S., et al. Pharmacognostical and Phytochemical Study of Piper Longum L. and., *Journal of Pharmaceutical and Scientific Innovation.* **2012;** 1(1): 62-66.

Vinaya, et al. Bronchodilator activity of Ocimum sanctum Linn. (tulsi) in mild and moderate asthmatic patients in comparison with salbutamol: a single-blind cross-over study., *Int. J. Basic Clin. Pharmacol.*. **2017;** 6(3): 511. [http://dx.doi.org/10.18203/2319-2003.ijbcp20170543]

Vivek-Ananth R. P., et al. *In silico* identification of potential natural product inhibitors of human proteases key to SARS-CoV-2 infection R.P., : 1-51.**2020**

Vyas P., Chandola H.M., Ghanchi F., Ranthem S.. Clinical evaluation of Rasayana compound as an adjuvant in the management of tuberculosis with anti-Koch's treatment., *Ayu.* **2012;** 33(1): 38-43. [http://dx.doi.org/10.4103/0974-8520.100307] [PMID: 23049182]

Vyas V.K., Bhandari P., Patidar R.. A comprehensive review on Withania somnifera dunal., *J. Nat. Rem...* **2011**
[http://dx.doi.org/10.18311/jnr/2011/43]

Wagner J., et al. Absolute lymphocyte count is a prognostic marker in Covid□19: A retrospective cohort review., *International Journal of Laboratory Hematology..* **2020**
[http://dx.doi.org/10.1111/ijlh.13288]

Walls A.C., Xiong X., Park Y.J., Tortorici M.A., Snijder J., Quispe J., Cameroni E., Gopal R., Dai M., Lanzavecchia A., Zambon M., Rey F.A., Corti D., Veesler D.. Unexpected Receptor Functional Mimicry Elucidates Activation of Coronavirus Fusion., *Cell.* **2019;** 176(5): 1026-1039.e15. [http://dx.doi.org/10.1016/j.cell.2018.12.028] [PMID: 30712865]

Wan Y., Shang J., Graham R., Baric R.S., Li F.. Receptor Recognition by the Novel Coronavirus from Wuhan: an Analysis Based on Decade-Long Structural Studies of SARS Coronavirus., *J. Virol..* **2020;** 94(7): e00127-20.
[http://dx.doi.org/10.1128/JVI.00127-20] [PMID: 31996437]

WHO (2020) WHO Director-General's opening remarks at the media briefing on COVID-19, World Health Organization.. 2020.

Wolkerstorfer A., Kurz H., Bachhofner N., Szolar O.H.. Glycyrrhizin inhibits influenza A virus uptake into the cell., *Antiviral Res..* **2009;** 83(2): 171-178.
[http://dx.doi.org/10.1016/j.antiviral.2009.04.012] [PMID: 19416738]

Wright B. (2017). , . A Comprehensive and Practical Guide to Clinical Trials. Setting Up of Site, Site Assessment Visits, and Selection..

Wu C.A., Wu J.J., Tsai M.J., Chen R.Y.. Immunomodulatory effects of a traditional Chinese medicine, Chi-Shie-Shuang-Bu-An-Shen-Tang, on BALB/c mice., *J. Ethnopharmacol..* **2007;** 113(2): 300-305. [http://dx.doi.org/10.1016/j.jep.2007.06.021] [PMID: 17681444]

Xie G., Chen N., Soromou L.W., Liu F., Xiong Y., Wu Q., Li H., Feng H., Liu G.. p-Cymene protects mice against lipopolysaccharide-induced acute lung injury by inhibiting inflammatory cell activation., *Molecules.* **2012;** 17(7): 8159-8173.
[http://dx.doi.org/10.3390/molecules17078159] [PMID: 22772811]

K Yadav A., Agrawal J., Pal A., Gupta M.M.. Novel anti-inflammatory phytoconstituents from Desmodium gangeticum., *Nat. Prod. Res..* **2013;** 27(18): 1639-1645.
[http://dx.doi.org/10.1080/14786419.2012.761620] [PMID: 23336435]

Yadav D.K., Mudgal V., Agrawal J., Maurya A.K., Bawankule D.U., Chanotiya C.S., Khan F., Thul S.T.. Molecular docking and ADME studies of natural compounds of Agarwood oil for topical anti-inflammatory activity., *Curr. Computeraided Drug Des..* **2013;** 9(3): 360-370.
[http://dx.doi.org/10.2174/1573409911309030012] [PMID: 23566359]

Yang H.M., et al. , . International Immunopharmacology. Elsevier; 2018. Pogostone attenuates TNF-- -induced injury in A549 cells *via* inhibiting NF-κB and activating Nrf2 pathways.; pp. 15.-22.

Yang L., et al. , . COVID-19: immunopathogenesis and Immunotherapeutics.. Signal Transduction and Targeted Therapy; 2020. p. 128

Yu M.S., Lee J., Lee J.M., Kim Y., Chin Y.W., Jee J.G., Keum Y.S., Jeong Y.J.. Identification of myricetin and scutellarein as novel chemical inhibitors of the SARS coronavirus helicase, nsP13., *Bioorg. Med. Chem. Lett.*. **2012;** 22(12): 4049-4054.
[http://dx.doi.org/10.1016/j.bmcl.2012.04.081] [PMID: 22578462]

Yu P., et al. A familial cluster of infection associated with the 2019 novel coronavirus indicating potential person-to-person transmission during the incubation period., *Prog. Polym. Sci.*.. **2015**
[http://dx.doi.org/10.1016/j.progpolymsci.2015.10.006]

Zaki A.M., van Boheemen S., Bestebroer T.M., Osterhaus A.D., Fouchier R.A.. Isolation of a novel coronavirus from a man with pneumonia in Saudi Arabia., *N. Engl. J. Med.*. **2012;** 367(19): 1814-1820.
[http://dx.doi.org/10.1056/NEJMoa1211721] [PMID: 23075143]

Zeng Z.Q., Chen D.H., Tan W.P., Qiu S.Y., Xu D., Liang H.X., Chen M.X., Li X., Lin Z.S., Liu W.K., Zhou R.. Epidemiology and clinical characteristics of human coronaviruses OC43, 229E, NL63, and HKU1: a study of hospitalized children with acute respiratory tract infection in Guangzhou, China., *Eur. J. Clin. Microbiol. Infect. Dis.*. **2018;** 37(2): 363-369.
[http://dx.doi.org/10.1007/s10096-017-3144-z] [PMID: 29214503]

Zhang P., Zhang E., Xiao M., Chen C., Xu W.. Study of anti-inflammatory activities of α--glucosylated eugenol., *Arch. Pharm. Res.*. **2013;** 36(1): 109-115.
[http://dx.doi.org/10.1007/s12272-013-0003-z] [PMID: 23325490]

Zhao L., Wang X., Chang Q., Xu J., Huang Y., Guo Q., Zhang S., Wang W., Chen X., Wang J.. Neferine, a bisbenzylisoquinline alkaloid attenuates bleomycin-induced pulmonary fibrosis., *Elsevier B.*. **2010;** 627(1-3): 304-312.
[http://dx.doi.org/10.1016/j.ejphar.2009.11.007] [PMID: 19909737]

Zhao Q., Meng M., Kumar R., Wu Y., Huang J., Deng Y., Weng Z., Yang L.. Lymphopenia is associated with severe coronavirus disease 2019 (COVID-19) infections: A systemic review and meta-analysis., *Int. J. Infect. Dis.*. **2020;** 96: 131-135.
[http://dx.doi.org/10.1016/j.ijid.2020.04.086] [PMID: 32376308]

Zheng L., Zelen M.. Randomized clinical trials., *Wiley Interdiscip. Rev. Comput. Stat.*. **2010;** 2(1): 49-53.
[http://dx.doi.org/10.1002/wics.63]

Zhu N., Zhang D., Wang W., Li X., Yang B., Song J., Zhao X., Huang B., Shi W., Lu R., Niu P., Zhan F., Ma X., Wang D., Xu W., Wu G., Gao G.F., Tan W., China Novel Coronavirus Investigating and Research TeamA novel coronavirus from patients with pneumonia in China, 2019., *N. Engl. J. Med.*. **2020;** 382(8): 727-733.
[http://dx.doi.org/10.1056/NEJMoa2001017] [PMID: 31978945]

Zu Z.Y., Jiang M.D., Xu P.P., Chen W., Ni Q.Q., Lu G.M., Zhang L.J.. Coronavirus Disease 2019 (COVID-19): A Perspective from China., *Radiology*. **2020;** 296(2): E15-E25.
[http://dx.doi.org/10.1148/radiol.2020200490] [PMID: 32083985]

SUBJECT INDEX

A

B

C

D

E

F

G

H

K

L

M

N

O

P

Q

R

S

T

U

V

W

Z

Made in the USA
Las Vegas, NV
14 August 2025

40175d9a-2ea1-4280-a7b3-af09eb949096R01